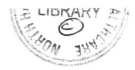
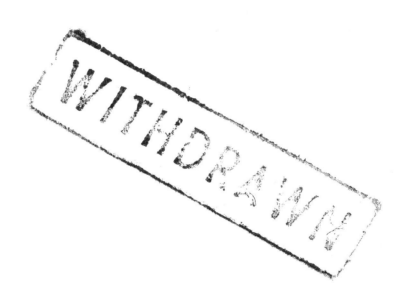

Acquired Damage to the Developing Brain: Timing and Causation

Edited by

Waney Squier MBChB MRCP FRCPath

Consultant Neuropathologist and Honorary Clinical Lecturer,
Department of Neuropathology, The Radcliffe Infirmary, Oxford, UK

A member of the Hodder Headline Group
LONDON • NEW YORK • NEW DELHI

First published in Great Britain in 2002 by
Arnold, a member of the Hodder Headline Group,
338 Euston Road, London NW1 3BH

http://www.arnoldpublishers.com

Distributed in the USA by
Oxford University Press Inc.,
198 Madison Avenue, New York, NY10016
Oxford is a registered trademark of Oxford University Press

Whilst the advice and information in this book are believed to be true and
accurate at the date of going to press, neither the authors nor the publisher
can accept any legal responsibility or liability for any errors or omissions
that may be made. In particular (but without limiting the generality of the
preceding disclaimer) every effort has been made to check drug dosages;
however, it is still possible that errors have been missed. Furthermore,
dosage schedules are constantly being revised and new side-effects
recognized. For these reasons the reader is strongly urged to consult the
drug companies' printed instructions before administering any of the drugs
recommended in this book.

British Library Cataloguing in Publication Data
A catalogue record for this book is available from the British Library

Library of Congress Cataloging-in-Publication Data
A catalog record for this book is available from the Library of Congress

ISBN 0 340 75930 5

1 2 3 4 5 6 7 8 9 10

Commissioning Editor: Georgina Bentliff
Production Editor: Wendy Rooke
Production Controller: Bryan Eccleshall
Project Manager: Tim Wale

Typeset in 10/12pt Palatino by Integra Software Services Pvt Ltd, Pondicherry, India
www.integra-india.com
Printed and bound in Italy by Giunti

What do you think about this book? Or any other Arnold title?
Please send your comments to feedback.arnold@hodder.co.uk

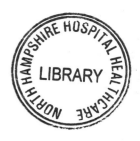

To Anna and Bindi

Contents

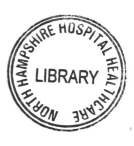

Contributors

Philip Anslow FRCR
Consultant Neuroradiologist
The Radcliffe Infirmary
Oxford
UK

Laura Bennet PhD
Senior Lecturer
Department of Paediatrics
The Liggins Institute
The University of Auckland
Auckland
New Zealand

Paul Chamberlain MD
University Lecturer/Honorary
Consultant
Nuffield Department of Obstetrics
and Gynecology
The Radcliffe Infirmary
Oxford
UK

David Evans BM MA MRCP FRCPCH
Consultant Neonatologist and Honorary
Senior Clinical Lecturer
Department of Neonatal Medicine
Southmead Hospital
Bristol
UK

Geraldine Gaffney MD MRCOG
Senior Lecturer/Consultant in Obstetrics
and Gynaecology
University College Hospital
Galway
Eire

Peter D Gluckman MBChB, MMedSc, DSc, FRSNZ,
FRACP
Professor of Perinatal and
Paediatric Biology
The Liggins Institute
The University of Auckland
Auckland
New Zealand

Alistair J Gunn MBChB PhD FRACP
Senior Lecturer
Department of Paediatrics
The Liggins Institute
The University of Auckland
Auckland
New Zealand

Ann Johnson MD FRCP
Reader in Perinatal Epidemiology
National Perinatal Epidemiology
Unit
Institute of Health Sciences
Oxford
UK

Malcolm Levene MD FRCP FRCPCH
Professor of Paediatrics and
Child Health
University of Leeds
The General Infirmary at Leeds
Leeds
UK

Gillian T McCarthy FRCP FRCPCH
Honorary Consultant Neuropaediatrician
Chailey Heritage Clinical Services
East Sussex
UK

Michael A Patton MA MSc FRCP FRCPCH
Professor of Medical Genetics
St George's Hospital Medical School
London
UK

Michael J Powers QC
4 Paper Buildings
Temple
London
UK

Mary A Rutherford MD MRCP
Honorary Senior Lecturer in Paediatrics
Robert Steiner MR Unit
Imperial College School of Medicine
London
UK

Waney Squier MBChB MRCP FRCPath
Consultant Neuropathologist and
Honorary Clinical Lecturer
Department of Neuropathology
The Radcliffe Infirmary
Oxford
UK

Robert C Vannucci MD
Professor of Pediatrics
The Pennsylvania State
University
College of Medicine
Hershey
Pennsylvania
USA

Acknowledgements

I would like to thank Samantha Cragg for willing and expert secretarial and editorial assistance, Helene Beard for her skill in producing many of the images, and Hilary Brown for constant and discrete facilitation of the project. Nick Dunton, Georgina Bentliff, and Tim Wale, among others from Arnold, initiated and guided the project. I owe thanks to my teacher Jeanne-Claudie Larroche and to my mother and my two daughters for their encouragement, tolerance, and support.

Introduction

The object of this communication is to show that the act of birth does occasionally imprint upon the nervous and muscular systems of the nascent infantile organism very serious and peculiar evils. When we investigate the evils in question, and their causative influences, we find that the same laws of pathology apply to diseases incidental to the act of birth as to those which originate before and after birth.
William Little, 1861

The object of this book is almost identical to that of William Little's paper published almost one and a half centuries ago.[1] Those 'very serious and peculiar evils' imprinted on the nervous and muscular systems are now usually called cerebral palsy and in the following chapters the 'causative influences' will be explored in detail, in particular those which can damage the developing brain before birth.

Little's outstanding contribution to the understanding of cerebral palsy has been widely interpreted and remembered as an association of cerebral palsy with birth injury, while many of the details of his observations and insights have been overlooked.

In the last decade it has become increasingly well recognized that the majority of children with cerebral palsy have no evidence of difficulties at birth and the causes of damage must be sought at other times, particularly in intrauterine life, as indeed Little himself had noted.

Not all developmental brain damage is cerebral palsy, this term implies a component of motor impairment. Other manifestations include impairment of cognition, language, hearing, and vision, as well as epilepsy. Although the term cerebral palsy is used in this book, we examine the entire spectrum of insults which can result in any or all of these forms of disability.

The scale of the problem is enormous. Some 2 per 1000 children have cerebral palsy, while many more have other forms of developmental brain damage; a recent study has shown that among very preterm infants followed up until their teenage years over 50 percent show abnormalities on MRI scan and they have an excess of neurological, cognitive and behavioral problems.[2]

This book seeks to address the nature of developmental brain damage and, in particular, how and when brain damage has occurred, and which investigations may be fruitful and valid. Cerebral palsy places enormous emotional, physical, and financial burdens on affected families and we owe them every possible investigation which may establish the cause of the damage.

Many cases of cerebral palsy will come to litigation; an increasing trend in recent decades. Families resort to litigation for a number of reasons; many simply want to find out the truth about what happened to damage their child. It is a sad reflection of the state of communication between doctors and patients if there is a need to resort to the legal process to obtain detailed information about the clinical management of a pregnancy and childbirth. Many such cases might be avoided if the medical profession were able to offer a full, open, and honest explanation of events.

In other cases litigation is seen as the only possible avenue for obtaining sufficient funds to provide for the lifetime needs of a severely disabled child. State provision for such children is clearly inadequate.

This book intends to inform all those involved in preparing cases of brain damage in infants. Much of the book is devoted to the clinical, pathological, and scientific evidence which can establish the nature and timing of damage to the developing brain.

The success of a case depends on adequate initial assessment of a claim to establish at an early stage that it is appropriate and has a reasonable chance of success thus avoiding lengthy and distressing delays. Once a claim is established as reasonable then all the relevant information, clinical investigations and statements must be assembled and medical experts instructed to assist in preparing the case. The medical experts play a crucial role in assisting the legal preparation of the case. They must have sufficient experience and knowledge of their subject and the relevant literature to be able to present their views robustly and defend them under cross-examination. An instructing solicitor has the responsibility of making medical experts aware of the legal process and the rules which apply to preparing and presenting a report.

The final chapter of this book deals in some depth with the legal and philosophical aspects of causation and its proof.

The book is written by an international team of experts from many disciplines who bring to the book clinical, scientific, and legal perspectives. While there may be some overlap between chapters, editing has been kept to a minimum so that the individual chapters stand alone and retain the style and character of the author.

It is hoped that the whole will provide a comprehensive, factual base to inform all of those who are involved in the care of children who have acquired brain damage early in their development. Only when we have a better understanding of the causes and timing of this kind of brain damage can we begin to implement measures for its prevention.

REFERENCES

1 Little WJ. On the influence of abnormal parturition, difficult labours, premature birth, and asphyxia neonatorum, on the mental and physical condition of the child, especially in relation to deformities. Transcribed from The Obsteric Society of London 1861–2; **3**: 293.

2 Stewart AL, Rifkin L, Amess PN *et al.* Brain structure and neurocognitive and behavioural function in adolescents who were born very preterm. Lancet 1999; **353**: 1653–7.

1 Cerebral palsy: the clinical problem

Gillian T McCarthy

The clinician faced with a neurologically damaged child must be willing to accept a complicated and time-consuming role. The developing child needs regular review. The perceptions, anxieties, expectations, fears, and predicament of the child and family must be acknowledged if a partnership is to be effective.[1] It is important to listen to the child and family, to observe and analyze the child's abilities and disabilities, to be open-minded and ready to review the evidence and consult colleagues from other specialties. Pediatric neurology and neurodisability are rapidly developing disciplines and there is much to learn.

The fetal and neonatal brain may be damaged in many different ways and at any time during development. The clinician has the task of diagnosis and management of neurological problems, which may appear similar whatever the underlying causes. Neurological examination and multi-disciplinary clinical assessment will give clues to possible etiology and outcome and will be augmented by investigations, including neuro-imaging and biochemistry. Clinical management and assessment are required throughout childhood to encourage optimum development.

1.1 DEFINITION OF TERMS

Term: 37 to <42 completed weeks of gestation.
Post-term: >42 completed weeks of gestation.
Preterm: <37 completed weeks of gestation.
Neonatal period: <28 days from birth.
Perinatal period: from 28 weeks gestation to <7 days of life.
Low birthweight (LBW): <2500 g.
Very low birthweight (VLBW): <1500 g.
Extremely low birthweight (ELBW): <1000 g.

1.2 CEREBRAL PALSY

1.2.1 Definition

Cerebral palsy is a non-progressive, but not necessarily unchanging, disorder of movement and posture caused by damage to the developing brain at or around birth. Cerebral palsy is not a single condition – cerebral palsies would be a more accurate description, since a wide spectrum of disorders is covered. Other neurological conditions may masquerade as cerebral palsy. It is important to take a careful history including family history. The timing of appearance of neurological signs and symptoms can give a clue to the diagnosis.

Careful sequential observations and examination of the infant and child are also vital in order to arrive at the correct diagnosis. The brain is rarely simply damaged in the motor control areas, many other possible associated neurological disorders may develop, particularly affecting cognitive ability, vision, and hearing. Causes of damage to the developing brain are described in Chapter 3, 6, and 8.

The gestational age at which damage occurs has an effect upon the clinical picture. The preterm infant may sustain damage which may only become clinically apparent with time and we know that some preterm infants may suffer hemorrhage or hydrocephalus which may not cause long-term neurological signs. Studies have looked particularly at the development of speech and sensory and motor function.[2] There is increasing evidence of plasticity of neural function in the very young infant.[3]

1.2.2 Neurological development

Normal development depends upon an intact nervous system interacting with an environment that provides appropriate stimulation, nutrition, care, and attention. The complex interaction of the sensory systems with the maturing motor system ensures normal postural development with increasing motor ability. Children with cerebral palsy lack the reciprocal inhibition necessary for smooth, co-ordinated movement. The spastic stretch reflex in children with cerebral palsy differs from that seen in adults or children with acquired brain injury. It has been suggested that there is lack of control from supra spinal centers, although it is not possible to exclude impairment of spinal mechanisms.[4] The demonstration of a supraspinal element to reciprocal inhibition is of particular relevance, since it shows the potential influence of cognitive and emotional factors in treatment. Automatic anticipatory postural responses also use reciprocal inhibition to prevent antagonist co-contraction. The extent of the pathway damage will dictate the ability of the child to respond to physical therapy. However, motivation and cognitive ability will also play a part in the outcome.

Mechanisms involved in acquisition of normal motor skills include progressive increase in conduction velocity within the descending motor pathways, progressive myelination of nerve fibers and increasing synaptic connections in the cortex and spinal cord.

Children also develop their motor skills by laying down memory patterns via visual and sensory systems as they build up their anticipatory postural control. These systems may be damaged in children with cerebral palsy.[5]

1.2.3 Management of cerebral palsy

1.2.3.1 *Posture management, mobility, and orthopedic management*

All types of cerebral palsy have in common abnormal postural development. The patterns of abnormality depend on the anatomical areas of damage. Good clinical management of posture, movement, and deformity will affect the final outcome improving mobility, function, and quality of life.

1.2.3.1.1 Posture

Assessment of postural maturity can be made using the levels of lying, sitting, and standing ability described by Pountney *et al.*[6] These levels give an opportunity to assess ability and asymmetry in supine, prone, and sitting.

Correct positioning prevents the development of deformity caused by spasticity acting across joints. Muscle shortening may cause pain, dislocation and weakness of the opposing lengthened muscle. Fixed positions may be caused by persistent automatisms such as the abnormal asymmetric tonic neck reflex (ATNR), which results in head turn, flattening of the skull, extension of the arm and leg on one side and flexion on the other – the 'fencing position'. Over time this results in the development of a windswept deformity and scoliosis (Fig. 1.1)

Persistence of the primitive grasp reflex, symmetric tonic extension, extensor thrust, persistent sucking or rooting reflexes may all interfere with normal balance and movement.

Researchers have shown that muscles require periods of stretch of at least 6 hours a day to main-

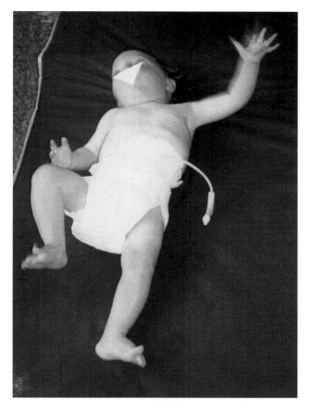

Figure 1.1 Young child showing a combination of asymmetric tonic neck reflex (ATNR) and startle reflex. Note the gastrostomy tube.

tain or increase length.[7,8] Equipment providing biomechanically appropriate support in a variety of positions can provide these periods of stretch whilst allowing a child to participate in daily life.[9]

The pelvis is the key to good management of the trunk and legs. Since many children remain at a primitive level of lying posture (i.e. at lying ability levels 1 or 2), the pelvis remains tilted posteriorly when placed in a sitting position, the lumbar spine remains kyphotic and the whole trunk will follow. When seating the child a sacral pad and ramped cushion allow better positioning of the pelvis. If there is also asymmetry of the hips caused by an ATNR, a knee block with or without abduction pads will maintain the hips in a good position when sitting.

A correct sitting position can facilitate movement and function and aid learning in children with cerebral palsy. Fixation in a good posture not only aids hand function and visual fixation but also attention.[10]

Intermittent stretching, active exercise, passive movements, regular changes of position, repetitions of actions with the environment have been shown to be the most effective methods of improving motor skills and practical activity whilst preventing progression of deformity (Fig. 1.2, p. 6).

1.2.3.1.2 Motor function and mobility

Management of motor function and mobility requires a multidisciplinary approach led by an experienced physiotherapist providing active therapy, advice to parents and carers and regular multidisciplinary assessments and discussions. In the early years attention to posture, movement, and walking may be a priority but it is important to have goal-directed activities with the child as an active participant.

In general, the natural history of cerebral palsy follows certain patterns. The study of Crothers and Paine still holds important lessons today.[11] All children with hemiplegia will walk, as will 80 percent of children with extrapyramidal or mixed types of cerebral palsy. Seventy percent of children who have hemiplegia will walk by the age of 2 years and 90 percent by age 4, while only half of children with bilateral cerebral palsy will walk by 4 years. Most children sitting unsupported by age 2 will be community ambulators whilst the proportion falls to 50 percent if sitting is not achieved until 2–3 years.[12]

In Scrutton's study of 346 children with bilateral cerebral palsy, by age 5 years, 39 percent could walk 10 steps alone (with splints if needed); 60 percent could get to sitting on the floor and sit without propping; 28 percent of hips had a problem requiring surgery or other intervention.[13]

1.2.3.1.3 Therapy, medication, and rhizotomy

Baclofen is an antispastic medication, which can be used to aid therapy for some children. It blocks the excitatory effects of the sensory input from limb muscles. When given by mouth it works for about 8 hours and the dose needs to be regulated for the individual child. Side effects may occur.

Continuous intrathecal baclofen infusion (CIBI) therapy has been used since June 1996 for the treatment of spasticity in children with cerebral palsy. It is administered by a metered programmable pump implanted under the skin of the abdomen via a catheter placed in the spinal subarachnoid space. The dosage is approximately 1/100th of the oral dose. Problems include excessive reduction of muscle tone, loss of bladder control, nausea, and tiredness. Pump malfunction and infection occur in 5 percent of cases.[14]

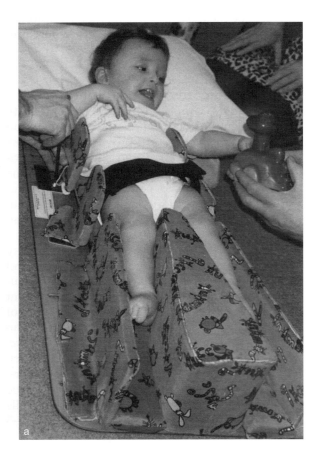
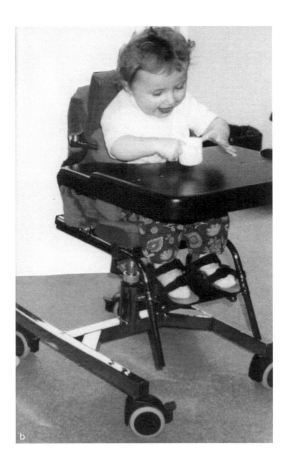
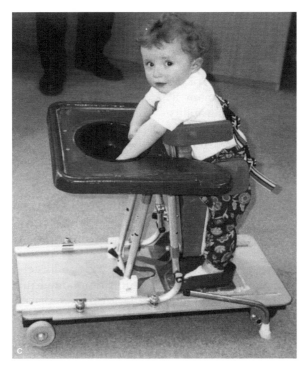

Figure 1.2 Posture management. (a) Lying; (b) sitting; (c) standing.

Selective dorsal rhizotomy to reduce spasticity has become re-popularized in North America in the past 20 years. The rationale of treatment is reduction of spasticity by selective division of posterior nerve rootlets at the second to the fifth lumbar spinal levels (L2 to L5). The rootlets are selected by electrical stimulation and divided neurosurgically. Suitable candidates are children with spastic diplegia who are able to walk. Good results are dependent on careful selection and children should be treated in centers equipped for accurate evaluation.

There is some evidence that the benefit of the operation could be due to the intensive physiotherapy strengthening program prior to surgery[15] although results differ.[16] Comparison of CIBI and selective dorsal rhizotomy (SDR) showed no significant difference in results, but CIBI was significantly more expensive and also had more side effects and complications than the SDR.[17]

1.2.3.1.4   Orthopedic management

Orthopedic intervention is often required in children with cerebral palsy. Gait analysis is an important, though expensive, tool using videotape, linear measurements, kinematics, dynamic electromyography (EMG), kinetics, and energy assessment for presurgical assessment of patients.

Early and active *management of the hips* is essential in prevention of dislocation and the need for bony surgery. Non-ambulant children with bilateral cerebral palsy are most at risk of developing problems. Soft tissue surgery to release shortened or contracted muscles may prevent progressive subluxation and the subsequent need for major bony surgery. However, division of spastic muscle may result in the loss of normal muscle fibers with increasing fibrosis and contractures. The use of botulinum toxin injections to allow stretching of muscles is another intervention that is helpful in orthopedic management.

Almost one-third of hips of children with bilateral cerebral palsy have a problem by the age of 5 years.[13] Significant modeling of the acetabulum occurs in the first 3 or 4 years, which explains why soft tissue surgery is more effective if carried out in the early years. Changes may occur throughout childhood, so regular monitoring is necessary.

The importance of symmetrical positioning has already been mentioned. Referral to a surgeon experienced in management of children with cerebral palsy is also essential.

Approximately 40 percent of children with cerebral palsy have a structural *spinal deformity* of 10 percent or more. Many of these curves are severe, especially in non-ambulant quadriplegic and the more severe diplegic patients. The debate as to whether spinal surgery should be carried out on this group of patients is discussed well in recent papers.[18,19] If there is no intervention progression will continue, with associated loss of sitting balance, pressure problems and often associated eating problems. Eventually premature death may occur from respiratory failure or pneumonia.

Spinal fusion is major surgery often done in two stages (Fig. 1.3, p.8), with associated risks and postoperative complications. Essential prerequisites before surgery are:

1   The curve should be within the surgical range and showing progression and problems with sitting
2   The child should be over 10 years of age
3   The child should be aware of his/her surroundings and others
4   There should be adequate range of movement of the hips to allow seating afterwards
5   Nutritional status must be adequate
6   All other medical problems must be stable and not considered to present undue risk for surgery
7   The surgeon should be experienced in treating this type of problem.

1.2.3.2   Feeding and nutrition

Oral difficulties are common in cerebral palsy and are often the presenting symptom. Bulbar signs include poor movements of the tongue and lips, with a tongue thrust, poor coordination of suck and swallow and incoordination of esophageal stripping, therefore affecting the pre-oral, oral, pharyngeal, and swallowing phases of feeding.

Gastroesophageal reflux and hiatus hernia are commonly associated with athetoid and other forms of cerebral palsy. Moderate to severe gastroesophageal reflux is reported in between 11 and 75 percent of infants and children with cerebral palsy.

Complications of gastroesophageal reflux include poor nutrition and growth retardation; esophagitis and bleeding; recurrent respiratory symptoms – laryngospasm, reflex bronchospasm and reflex central apnea.[20] Constipation is also a common problem caused by poor fluid and dietary intake and difficulty coordinating expulsion of feces.

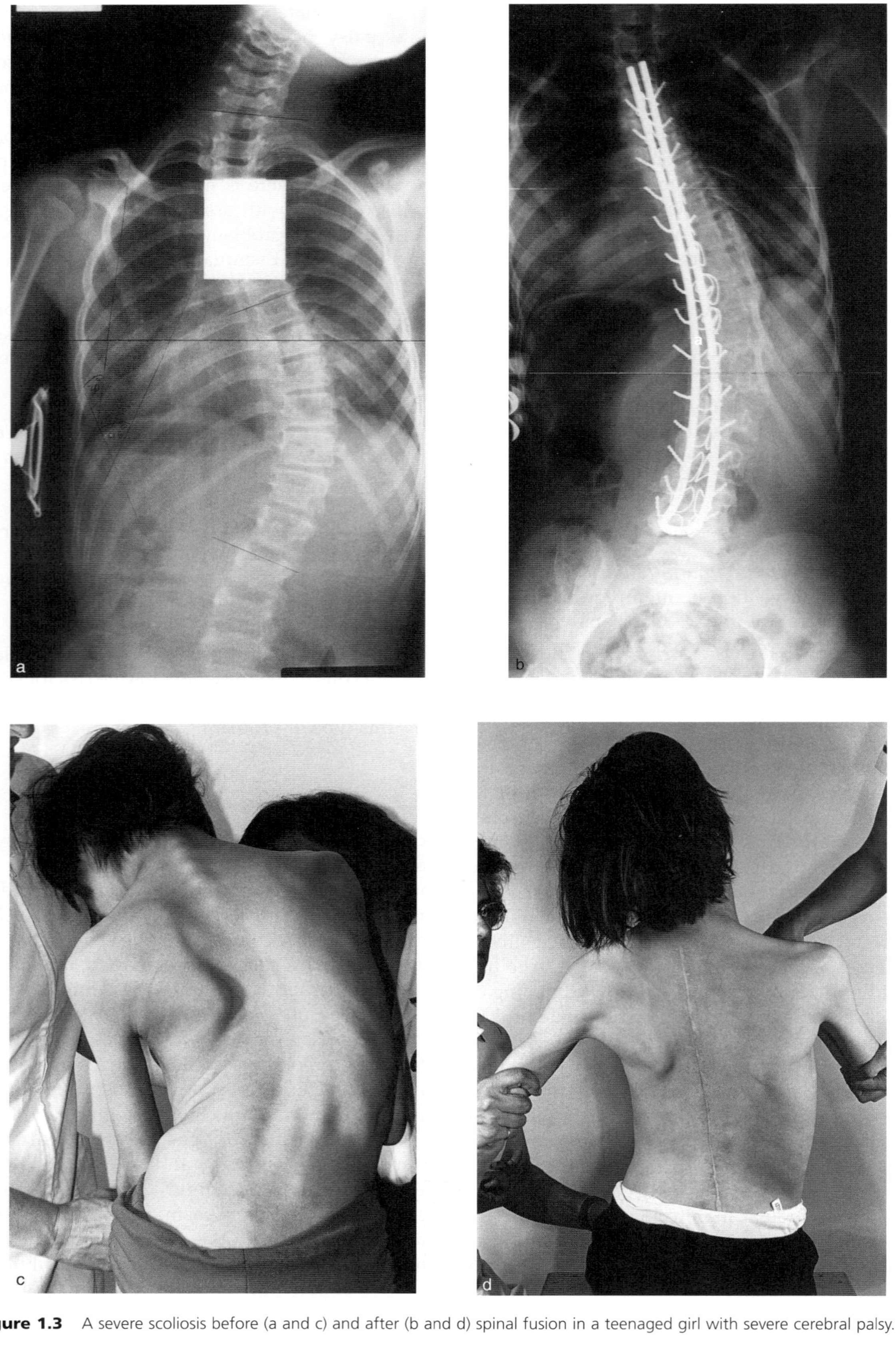

Figure 1.3   A severe scoliosis before (a and c) and after (b and d) spinal fusion in a teenaged girl with severe cerebral palsy.

Nutrition may be insufficient due to oral and swallowing problems. Children with severe cerebral palsy tend to be small and light for their age and poor nutrition is compounded by lack of normal movement leading to reduction of linear growth of bones and muscles; and hormonal imbalance with delay in the onset of puberty.

Surgical repair of hiatus hernias is often necessary in children with severe reflux problems. At the same time a gastrostomy may be fashioned, which allows ease of feeding and administration of medications and reduces the stress on the family and carers.

1.2.3.3   *Speech and language problems and communication*

Impairment of oral function often accompanies dyskinetic cerebral palsy and quadriplegia when limited speech and poor articulation are complicated by cognitive impairment. Oral competence should be assessed at an early stage by an experienced speech and language therapist. Considerable information about the child's potential for speech can be obtained by using the Pediatric Oral Skills Package.[21,22]

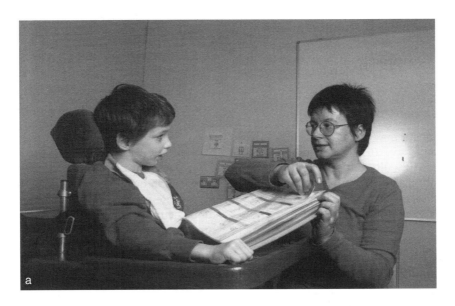

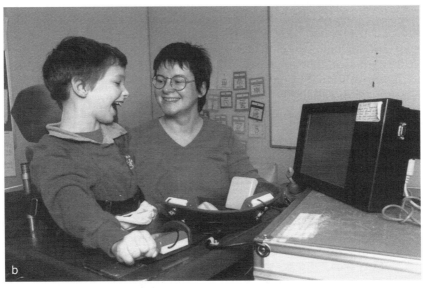

Figure 1.4   Communication aids and electronic assistive equipment. (a) Child using a REBUS Symbol Dictionary with a listener scanning access. (b) Switch access to Chailey Communication System software on the Cameleon II computer (a voice output communication aid).

Communication is a basic human need. Assessment of communication includes non-verbal and social skills as well as verbal comprehension, expressive language, and articulation.

Augmentative communication is required for severely speech-impaired people. Early intervention is required to establish a good basis of language comprehension. Constant language stimulation is essential. Simple methods of interaction include eye pointing, reaching, pointing, vocalization, gesture, sign language, pictures, symbols and the written word (Fig. 1.4, p.9).

A wide range of electronic communication aids and other electronic assistive equipment is available. Mobility and communication are developmentally interrelated skills and the acquisition of driving skills by multiply handicapped young people who are unable to speak frequently brings benefits in many areas, including the desire to communicate.[23]

1.2.3.4   Bladder control

Children with spasticity may be late acquiring bladder control and may have urgency of micturition, giggle incontinence, difficulty initiating micturition, and urinary retention. Urodynamic studies may show evidence of a neuropathic bladder with detrusor hyperreflexia, deficient vesico-urethral sensation or detrusor-sphincter dyssynergia.[24] Anticholinergic medication may reduce the detrusor activity or in the case of retention problems baclofen may reduce perineal muscle tone.

1.2.3.5   Vision

Perinatal brain damage is the second most important cause of visual impairment in childhood in Europe and North America. The majority of blind children now have additional impairments, mostly neurodevelopmental disorders.[25]

Visual problems are common in children with all types of cerebral palsy, due to damage to optic nerves and pathways or to the visual cortex. In addition retinopathy of prematurity (ROP) occurs in very preterm infants, causing variable morbidity from retinal damage and myopia of varying degree. Careful ophthalmological follow-up is therefore mandatory. ROP accounted for 12 percent of childhood blindness in a study in 1977, a more important cause was visual pathway disease which accounted for 42 percent of cases.[26]

Children with brain damage often have difficulty in directing their vision, detecting, and aiming their gaze. They may have difficulty separating figure from ground, piecemeal vision, difficulties with tracking and tracing and inaccurate reaching or placing.[27]

Active visual scanning is required for normal visual perception. Damage to one occipito-frontal fasciculus in periventricular leukomalacia accounts for the frequency of defects of voluntary eye movements enabling following and looking in children with quadriplegia and diplegia.

It is possible to assess vision in the newborn infant using neurophysiological techniques. The visual evoked potentials (VEPs) offer a window on visual function and more generally on cerebral or neurological function.[28–30]

The visual stimulus can be elicited by light flashes or by pattern stimuli (reversing, onset/offset, clicks, bars or pinwheels). The pattern stimuli are more sensitive measures of visual function and are the only way to give an estimate of visual acuity neurophysiologically. The state of arousal of the infant needs to be constant to make valid comparisons of latency or amplitude changes.

VEPs in older children require a reasonable level of attention and the ability to fix gaze.[31]

Visual field defects may occur if the optic radiations are damaged. Children with hemiplegia caused by middle cerebral artery infarction have homonymous hemianopia. Hemianopic children will usually turn their heads towards the non-seeing field and then rotate their eyes back to the object of interest.[32]

1.2.3.6   Hearing

The prevalence of hearing loss in cerebral palsy is falling. Prevalence in the 1940s and 1950s was 25 percent, falling to 12.5 percent by 1970.[33] After 1970, 5 percent of children with athetoid cerebral palsy had sensorineural deafness, with 1.6–3 percent in other types of cerebral palsy.[34,35]

Most at risk are preterm babies who have anoxic seizures and jaundice and those with prenatal infections of rubella and cytomegalovirus.[36,37] Children with abnormal oropharyngeal function may be at greater risk of middle ear problems.

The age at diagnosis of deafness tends to be later than in the non-handicapped population as there is a 65 percent risk of an added defect – mental, visual, or epilepsy. This makes accurate behavioral testing very difficult. Also parents and professionals may be concentrating on what is seen as the primary disability.

With neonatal screening and careful follow-up, deafness should be identified and treated at an early stage, although in the presence of severe postural disability and cognitive difficulties it will never be an easy task. In view of the complexities of testing children with cerebral palsy it is suggested that their hearing should be tested by a specialist team.[38]

1.2.3.7 Cognitive problems

Formal psychometric assessment is difficult or impossible to carry out in children with severe levels of motor and speech impairment. In general the more severe the damage to the brain the greater the overall effects on cognitive development. The problems are compounded by damage to the visual systems, language areas, and hearing and motor impairment. Epilepsy also increases the risk of cognitive impairment.

Although approximately two-thirds of children with hemiplegia are of normal intelligence, the mean IQ of the group is shifted downwards, to a mean of around 81, but the shift is most marked for those with the greatest neurological involvement.[39] There is no significant difference between the children with right or left hemiplegia and a normal distribution of verbal and performance discrepancies. The mean IQ of children with early-acquired hemiplegia is significantly lower than that of children with congenital hemiplegia.

The verbal IQ is probably the best indicator of overall intelligence, partly because the performance items require normal manipulative ability. Also the developing brain's response to damage seems to be to preserve language at the expense of visuo-spatial skills.[40] The presence of seizures has an adverse effect on IQ and learning abilities.[41]

1.2.3.8 Emotional and behavioral problems

Children with severe forms of cerebral palsy are limited by their disability from developing normal detachment from parents and carers. This may result in extreme dependence and difficulty in separating from parents. Sleep problems are common and may be compounded by lack of physical ability to move in bed or to maintain a comfortable position.

Parents may not be able to see the disabled child as a growing, developing person needing to be treated emotionally at an age-appropriate level. The child may be dependent upon parents for communication. Early intervention by a sensitive multidisciplinary team will enable families to understand and cope with their many problems more successfully.

Children with spastic forms of cerebral palsy are often hypersensitive to new situations, sounds and visual stimuli. Children with hydrocephalus often suffer from hyperacusis, becoming extremely distressed by sharp or unusual sounds. Flashing lights or sharp sounds may trigger epileptic seizures, causing distress to child and carers.

Athetosis and ataxia may be associated with extreme shyness. Children with these conditions may find integration into mainstream school very difficult. Their often precarious motor performance may be impaired by their anxiety, especially if they are teased or bullied.

Goodman and Graham in a large study of around 900 children with hemiplegia, showed that approximately 50 percent of them had psychiatric disorders. The children had problems with behavior, emotions, or relationships, which interfered markedly with their everyday lives, causing them substantial distress, or resulting in considerable disruption for others.[42] Common problems were anxiety, irritability, and hyperactivity/inattention. Inappropriate school placement, unrecognized special needs or victimization may contribute to difficulties. Emotional and behavioral problems respond well to the normal psychiatric interventions such as medication or family therapy.

1.2.3.9 Peer relationships

Although children with hemiplegia tend to be placed in mainstream schools they have problems getting on with other children. There is increasing evidence for constitutional impairments in social understanding, which contribute to their emotional and social immaturity.[43]

1.2.3.10 Epilepsy

Epilepsy occurs commonly in children with cerebral palsy; its overall incidence is reported to be between 15 and 60 percent.[44] It is more common in spastic quadriplegia and hemiplegia than in diplegia or dyskinetic cerebral palsy. Children who develop seizures in the first year of life are more likely to have associated cognitive impairment.

Seizures may occur in the neonatal period and persist into the first year of life, particularly in children who have suffered severe anoxic-ischemic brain injury.

1.2.3.10.1 Infantile spasms

Infantile spasms (IS) are a rare severe form of generalized epilepsy occurring in infancy and associated with previous brain pathology in a proportion of cases. Up to 60 percent present in the first 6 months of life and 90 percent in the first year of life.[45] The attacks are usually in the form of flexion, or salaam spasms, which occur in runs, often on waking or falling asleep. Further loss of developmental skills occurs with the onset of the spasms. The electroencephalogram (EEG) pattern is diagnostic with hypsarrythmia, that is irregular, diffuse, high voltage slow waves interspersed with sharp waves and spikes.

Causes of IS include anoxic-ischemic encephalopathy, intrauterine infections, tuberous sclerosis, cerebral malformations or dysgenesis. Conditions such as Aicardi syndrome in girls may present with IS. Treatment of IS may be difficult. The first-line treatment is with corticosteroids. Second-line treatment is with sodium valproate and benzodiazepines such as clobazam or nitrazepam.

Infantile spasms tend to a grave prognosis with mortality of 20 percent reported in several series.[46,47] In survivors, mental retardation of severe degree occurs in up to 50 percent and sensory defects are common. Cerebral palsy is present in up to a half of affected children.

Other types of epilepsy follow IS in 50–60 percent of affected children. Partial seizures and Lennox Gastaut syndrome are the most common sequelae.[48,49]

1.2.3.10.2 Other seizure types associated with cerebral palsy

- *Generalized seizures* – often with focal onset.
- *Focal myoclonus* – occurs in cortical dysplasia syndromes.
- *Gelastic seizures* – seizures associated with forced laughter which is loud and mirthless and unprovoked; occur rarely. Sometimes associated with a hamartoma of the third ventricle, they can be associated with difficult behavior and precocious puberty.[50]
- *Partial continuous epilepsy* – a rare form of epilepsy associated with a hemiplegia and progressive cortical atrophy.
- *Simple partial seizures* – tend to occur in children with a variety of cerebral lesions including cortical dysplasias, brain malformations, and porencephalies. Onset of severe epilepsy tends to occur before the age of 3 years in 53 percent of cases and 84 percent have severe types of seizure, often complex partial type. Seizures induced by movement or startle are always of lesional origin.[51,52]

1.2.3.10.3 Prognosis

Several authors have reported the course of lesional partial epilepsy with reported remission rates of between 30.6 and 63.5 percent after a 2-year follow-up.[53]

Children with significant epilepsy accompanying cerebral palsy are likely to have severely impaired cognitive development. The double insult may be aggravated by the effects of medication unless this is carefully monitored. Even after a period of frequent seizures, control may be restored over time and medication successfully discontinued after a seizure-free period of 2 years.

1.2.3.11 The burden of care: emotional and financial factors

The burden of care placed on the families of children with cerebral palsy may be unbearable for some, whilst accepted by others. The strengths and weaknesses of families will be exposed by the stress. Marriage breakdown, whilst not markedly greater than in the population as a whole, is more likely to occur at the time of diagnosis or illness or need for surgery. Assessment and treatment become bound in as measures of the emergent child and the functioning of the family, and consequently these are issues of great sensitivity.[1]

Parents will have expectations of their child, the child that they have is not the one that they imagined they would have. The loss and grief are initially profound and unlike a death it is impossible to mourn, the child's presence precludes a proper grief. The continuity of the handicapped child gives a sense of guilt to the grief, an explanation for the chronic sorrow. Each contact with professionals may rekindle the reminiscence of the original pain felt at the first discovery of differentness.

As children become aware of their limitations they too will experience pain and loss. The importance of empathizing with children and giving them the space and possibility of expression is vital to their development and maturity. Children's right to self-expression and personal autonomy, although limited by their disability, may still be encouraged by a sympathetic and understanding environment. Social integration is still a long way from being solved in the UK, although there are encouraging signs of movement.

Adolescence is a particularly difficult time for young people constrained by disability and psychiatric disorders such as depression; suicide and suicidal behaviors are more common at this time. The task of maximizing experience and opportunity for growth is one of education, in its wider sense, with the best enabling of the handicapped young person from earliest childhood. The quality of life will be a direct function of the sort of personality that has been formed.

The financial costs of caring for a disabled child are also great. In a study in Liverpool, UK, it was estimated that the cost of hospital and family practitioner care from birth to the age of 8–9 years was on average about 6 times greater than for a normal child and 9 times greater if the child was of low birthweight.[54]

The costs to the family are also considerable in terms of the loss of potential earnings of the mother who may be unable to pursue her career. The general costs of day-to-day care are also increased even when statutory allowances are available.

1.3   SPASTIC CEREBRAL PALSIES

1.3.1   Spastic quadriplegia

Four-limb and trunk involvement may be called spastic quadriplegia or tetraplegia, or bilateral hemiplegia. Asymmetrical involvement is common.

Children with spastic quadriplegia typically have more severe problems with cognitive function and more associated complications. Increased muscle tone may become apparent early in the first year and the arms and legs are equally affected. This group of children may merge into the more severe spastic diplegic group in whom hand function may be impaired but is less severely affected than lower limb function. Visual problems, squints, and seizures are common.

It is clear that a proportion of affected infants have lost a twin *in utero*. In monochorionic twin pregnancies death of one twin late in gestation is recognized as being an important risk factor for the surviving twin to have cerebral palsy. It has been suggested that a significant number of singletons with spastic cerebral palsy may be the result of the death of a co-twin in the second half of gestation.[55] If both twins are live at birth there is a 1 in 56 probability that one has cerebral palsy and 1 in 430 that both have it. If one twin is stillborn there is a 1 in 10 probability that the other has cerebral palsy.[56] (The mechanism of the brain damage is different if the twin has died intrapartum.)

1.3.1.1   Clinical presentation

Initial muscle tone may be low with poor head control and paucity of movement and feeding problems. Visual attention may be poor and squints may be present from an early stage.

Pupillary reflexes may be sluggish and there may be a convergent squint. However, visual following responses at brainstem level may be deceptively good in the young baby.

Some infants may be very irritable and startle excessively to sound. The sleep pattern may be poor and early postural difficulties cause the infant to be difficult to place in supine. Primitive reflexes may be prominent and pathological reflexes may be present. Seizures will occur in some babies.

The evolution of signs in the first year depends on the severity of damage but good management can reduce symptoms. The head circumference, initially within normal limits, fails to grow or does so at a reduced rate.

Hearing responses are difficult to assess and auditory brainstem evoked responses (BSER) may be intact without normal relay of hearing in the cortex. Attention and arousal heavily influence the late cortical components of the responses.[57]

1.3.1.2   Evolution of quadriplegia

Children with quadriplegia may have severely compromised postural development. Typical deformities arise from persistent reflex postures associated with

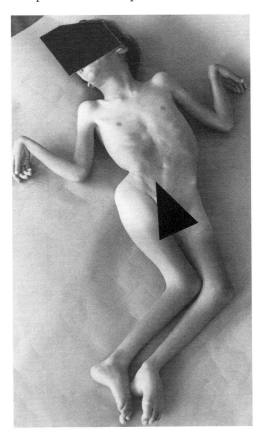

Figure 1.5   Severe deformities in a boy with spastic quadriplegia.

altered muscle tone and contractures of muscles. An example is the asymmetric tonic neck reflex (ATNR) (See Fig. 1.1). Correct positioning is important for this group of children using a variety of positions throughout the day.

Marked arm and hand involvement limits the ability to reach and grasp. Supination of the wrist is usually limited and the thumb may be flexed and abducted across the palm. Independent finger movements are usually impaired and a persistent grasp reflex may inhibit any useful hand function.

Oral function, feeding, and speech are affected and growth and nutrition are poor. Cognitive function is impaired and epilepsy is more common. In the more severe cases of quadriplegia puberty is delayed. Orthopedic deformities such as scoliosis, hip dislocation, deformities of the hands and feet, are common and progress in puberty (Fig. 1.5, p. 13)

1.3.2   Spastic diplegia

1.3.2.1   Clinical presentation

In diplegia the legs are primarily affected. Hand function often improves markedly during development but it is rare for the arms to be completely normal. There is an evolving motor picture depending on the severity of the neurological damage. Associated disorders are common in diplegia including squints, visual problems, perceptual difficulties, problems of eye–hand coordination, dysarthria, and cognitive disorders. This pattern of cerebral palsy

was first recognized as a condition occurring in children following premature or abnormal birth by Little in 1862[58] and Freud in 1897.[59]

1.3.2.2   Evolution of diplegia

After birth there may be signs of cerebral irritation with feeding difficulties, irritability, and jitteriness, or conversely drowsiness and hypotonia. Seizures occur in some children. Following this there may be an apparent silent period when development appears to be normal, although careful observation of the lying posture in prone and supine will show delay in maturation.

During the hypotonic phase neurological examination will reveal poor head control, persistence of neonatal reflexes and reduction of spontaneous movement of the legs. The development of sitting balance may be very delayed; indeed some children with severe diplegia never attain normal sitting balance on the floor.

Early gross motor signs are associated with poor pelvic control, late sitting, a tendency to persistent lumbar kyphosis and late trunk righting reactions. In prone the baby may never crawl properly but pull along in 'commando' fashion.

A dystonic phase may follow, with increasing stiffness and fixed postures. The muscle tone feels rigid and mass movements and poor balance indicate the lack of postural control. The deep tendon reflexes are increased, especially in the legs.

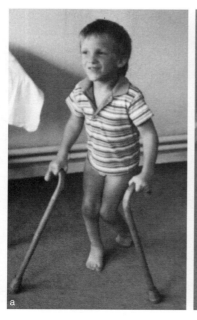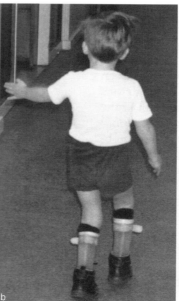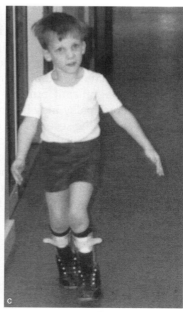

Figure 1.6   A boy aged 6 years standing with support before orthopedic surgery (a), and walking independently in splints after surgery (b and c).

Persistence of the ATNR and 'scissoring' of the legs are often present. These may interfere with spontaneous movement and cause asymmetry and limit function. As in other types of cerebral palsy the pelvis is the key to successful management of trunk posture and ambulation. Prevention of subluxation of the hips and maintenance of symmetry help to prevent dislocation of the hips and later deformity of the spine. It has been shown that the hips are at greater risk of developing subluxation leading on to dislocation if the child is not weight bearing.[60]

Following the dystonic phase the rigid-spastic phase occurs, with increased extensor tone and increasing spasticity and very brisk reflexes with ankle clonus. When standing the child may adopt either an equinus position with knees flexed and hips tightly adducted, or a crouch position with flexion at hips, knees, and ankles.

The development of standing and walking depends upon pelvic stability. Children with weak hip abductors may be very slow in walking independently since they are unable to control the pelvis in order to transfer weight and step. Strong hip adductors may be used as stabilizers of the pelvis but cause increasing hip subluxation and a sinking posture. Trunk balance may be achieved by leaning forward and balancing on the toes. The typical posture of the spastic diplegic gait is leaning forward and teetering along on the toes, being unable to stand still (Fig. 1.6, p.14).

Gait analysis to define the biomechanical factors that may impede walking is useful to target orthopedic intervention effectively.[61]

1.4 HEMIPLEGIA

The term hemiplegia is used when spasticity or dyskinesia affects only one side of the body. The onset can be before or after birth and both

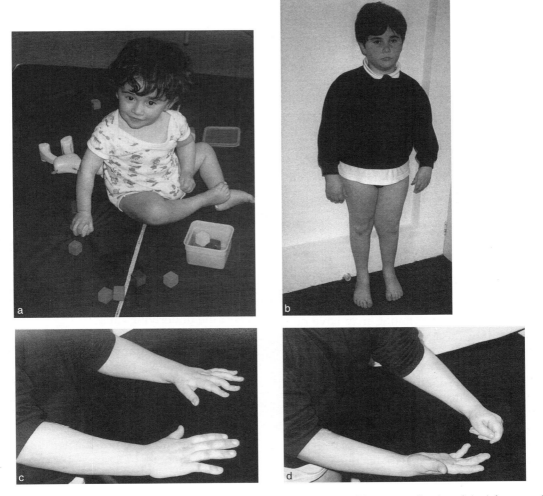

Figure 1.7 Boy with a left hemiplegia at the ages of 10 months (a) and 13 years (b). Note smaller size of the left arm and leg and inability to supinate the left arm.

preterm and term babies can be affected. Hemiplegia has been studied extensively as it produces such a good paradigm of neurological disorder within the same person.[2] It is not surprising that hemiplegia can be associated with a wide spectrum of difficulties as the neurological lesion producing the visible motor disorder may be very small or very extensive and the under lying brain may be malformed or normally formed. The advent of magnetic resonance imaging has allowed us to look more closely at the underlying pathology.

1.4.1　Clinical presentation

Congenital hemiplegia commonly presents around the age of 6 months when parents or professionals note the poor use of one hand or persistence of fisting (Fig. 1.7, p. 15).

The alteration in muscle tone and activity of the affected side can vary markedly and careful neurological and physiotherapy assessments are required. A strong grasp response and inability to open the hand may impair hand function, as may sensory loss, particularly poor proprioception causing sensory inattention.

The main motor impairment may be spastic, dyskinetic, or a mixture of both. The presence of a unilateral cerebral infarct does not inevitably cause long-term motor deficit; over 50 percent of infants with neonatal cerebral infarction are entirely normal at age 12–18 months.[62]

A visual field defect caused by interruption of the visual pathway may occur after middle cerebral artery infarction.[30]

1.4.2　Evolution of hemiplegia

The development of hand function should be encouraged in babies and young children by regular physiotherapy, including group work to encourage two-handed activities. The position of the wrists affects hand function but splinting may have only partial success. If by the age of 2 years hand function is very limited despite adequate therapy, it is likely to remain poor. In cases of dyskinesia there may be major difficulties in damping down unwanted movements in the affected limb, and children may devise their own methods of control, for example by clamping the arm under the desk.

The hemiplegic leg usually grows less well than the normal side and this exacerbates the tendency for toe walking. A shoe raise may help to keep the pelvis level during growth and a heel raise later. Elongation of the tendo calcaneus may be necessary. In some children scoliosis develops and the spine may need to be braced. Surgical fusion may be necessary later.

1.5　DYSKINETIC CEREBRAL PALSY

1.5.1　Definitions

All abnormal movements arising from disturbance of the extrapyramidal system may be grouped under the term dyskinesia.

- *Athetosis* describes large-amplitude, writhing, involuntary movements, exacerbated by intentional movements or emotion. These movements are present when awake and can involve any movement or part of the body, depending on the severity of the damage.
- *Chorea* describes smaller amplitude, jerky, quasi-purposive involuntary movements that may be present at rest, often involving the face and head, mouth and tongue, as well as the limbs. They may occur with athetoid movements.
- *Hemiballismus* describes violent, often large-amplitude movements of one half of the body, which can occur when any movement of the body is attempted. It is due to a lesion of the opposite subthalamic nucleus.
- *Dystonia* is a disorder of tone causing a fixed posture of a segment of the body or limbs and is caused by excessive muscle tone in antagonist muscle groups. It may occur in a limb at rest or when voluntarily maintained in a certain position.

For practical purposes, chorea, athetosis, and dystonia may be regarded as parts of a spectrum of movement disorder, which merge into one another. However, it is worthwhile spending time analyzing the type of involuntary movements, which may reflect the underlying cause.

Dyskinetic cerebral palsy may be caused by asphyxial brain damage. However, there is increasing evidence of other underlying causes. A recurrence risk for siblings of patients with dyskinetic cerebral palsy and a normal birth history could be as high as 10 percent.[63,64] The metabolic forms of dopa-sensitive dystonia, described later, have only recently been delineated. It is clear that some of these potentially treatable cases are being missed.[65]

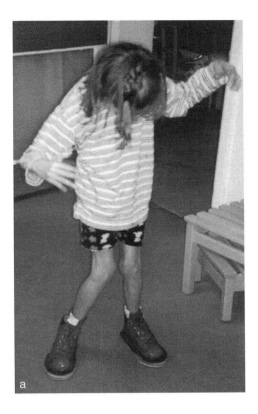

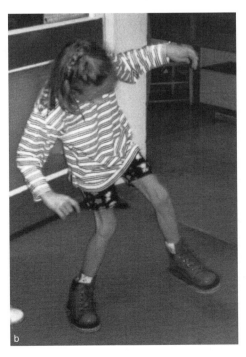

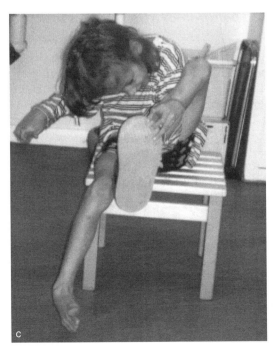

Figure 1.8 A girl aged 9 with dyskinetic cerebral palsy showing determination to balance and succeed in spite of her movement problems.

1.5.2   Athetoid cerebral palsy

1.5.2.1   Clinical presentation

Typically children who have suffered asphyxia have a relatively 'silent period' before the appearance of problems. Most infants have feeding problems and constipation, which may not be recognized as significant. Low muscle tone, associated poor head control and dysconjugate eye movements may be present.

Children with evolving athetoid cerebral palsy may show very poor postural reactions in the first year but their level of alertness and developing situational understanding will give clues to their underlying cognitive ability. Athetoid movements usually appear in the second year.

Associated damage, which increases concern for eventual outcome, includes the early onset of seizures and the presence of severe feeding difficulties.

Strong primitive reflexes (or automatisms – the asymmetric tonic neck reflex (ATNR), symmetric neck response (SNR), involuntary grasp reflex and extensor response of the legs) may intrude upon the normal movement repertoire. Asymmetry causes difficulty in sitting and standing and later problems associated with pelvic control and position that may lead to orthopedic complications.

1.5.2.2   Evolution of athetoid cerebral palsy

The child with a movement disorder has to learn to balance within the framework of his own proprioceptive ability. There has to be sufficient neurological potential for the child to gain control.

It can be difficult to predict future mobility in the first year of life, as there is often marked hypotonia. As tone increases, the severity of the involuntary movements may affect balance. Motivation is important and children should be encouraged, for example by group work (Fig. 1.8, p.17).

However, if there is severe damage the child may never be able to attain critical balance. Good postural management is then vital for functional independence.

Control of oral muscles may be seriously impaired. Feeding skills give a good idea of eventual oral and speaking skills. Group work can be vital to success. Augmentative communication may be necessary using symbols, words, and communication aids. The use of switches to access computers and other activities such as driving a powered wheelchair allows a measure of independence despite limited physical ability.

Many children with dyskinesia have problems of eye movements that may have arisen from lack of fixation of the head or from imbalance of eye muscle control.

Gastro-esophageal reflux and hiatus hernias are commonly associated with athetoid and other forms of cerebral palsy.

1.5.3   Metabolic diseases causing dystonia

1.5.3.1   Hyperbilirubinemia

Rarely seen in developed countries now, this complication of high level of bilirubin in the blood in the newborn period is typically associated with athetosis and high-frequency hearing loss. The infant is severely ill with cerebral irritation, decerebrate posture, 'sun-setting' eye signs, seizures and a high-pitched cry. Death may occur unless the level of bilirubin is reduced by exchange transfusion.

1.5.3.2   Dopa-responsive dystonia

Segawa first described dopa-responsive dystonia in the early 1970s.[66] Children may present with signs suggesting spastic diplegia. Signs of progression with extrapyramidal features or dystonia with diurnal fluctuation suggest possible dopa-responsive dystonia. Clinical response to levodopa therapy can then be demonstrated. A family history should be sought in these cases. We now know there is a wider phenotype, which includes apparent athetoid cerebral palsy, which may resemble idiopathic Parkinson's disease.[67]

Point mutations of the GTP cyclohydrolase gene have been mapped.[68] Clinical heterogeneity may exist within the same family. Dystonia is the important clinical feature even in the case of apparent athetoid cerebral palsy.[69]

1.5.3.3   Lesch-Nyhan syndrome

This is another condition that may be misdiagnosed as cerebral palsy. There is usually no perinatal cause but there may be a family history. It is a very rare, X-linked, metabolic disorder of purine metabolism caused by a deficiency of the enzyme hypoxanthine guanine phosphoribosyl transferase (HPRT).

A dystonic motor disorder develops, associated with self-injurious behavior that usually develops around the second year. This purine abnormality is associated with development of raised plasma uric acid leading to uric aciduria that can be treated with allopurinol. An early sign of the disease may be 'sand' in the diaper, caused by deposition of uric acid crystals from the urine.[70]

1.6 ATAXIC CEREBRAL PALSY

1.6.1 Incidence and causes of ataxia

The incidence of non-progressive congenital ataxia (NPCA) is reported as 0.13 per 1000 children.[71] It is therefore a relatively rare form of cerebral palsy accounting for less than 10 percent of cases.

The etiology of NPCA differs from other types of cerebral palsy; causes include hydrocephalus with aqueduct stenosis, congenital posterior fossa tumors, cysts or malformations such as Dandy Walker syndrome, cerebellar agenesis, hypoplasia or dysgenesis. These abnormalities are associated with clinically identifiable syndromes and have been reviewed in detail.[72,73]

Progressive neurological diseases of early onset may be misdiagnosed as cerebral palsy; these include metachromatic leukodystrophy, Batten's disease, ataxia telangiectasia, and Friedreich's ataxia.

Joubert's syndrome[74] is an inherited condition associated with abnormal respiration, episodic hyperpnea in the neonatal period, unusual jerky eye movements and later cerebellar ataxia and mental handicap.

Lesions of the parietal lobe controlling posture may also result in ataxia.[75]

1.6.2 Clinical presentation

Congenital ataxia presents with marked hypotonia and delay in postural development. Truncal ataxia with titubation of the head may become evident as sitting balance develops. Squints are more common in cerebral palsy and nystagmus in other causes of ataxia. Cognitive impairment and dysarthria are also common.

Information on long-term outcome of children with NPCA is scarce. In a recent report, cognitive impairment occurred in two thirds of subjects, epilepsy was a feature in one third, spasticity and focal dystonias were uncommon.[76]

1.6.3 Evolution of ataxic diplegia

In ataxic diplegia early hypotonia is replaced towards the end of the first year by spasticity in the legs with increased reflexes. The gait is wide based; contractures are less common than in pure spastic diplegia. There is a tendency to hyperextension of the knees and valgus position of the feet. Independent walking may be attained later than expected due to the impaired balance and muscle weakness.

1.7 HYDROCEPHALUS WITH CEREBRAL PALSY

1.7.1 Hydrocephalus in preterm infants

Thirteen percent of preterm infants with intraventricular hemorrhage develop progressive hydrocephalus with 6 percent requiring shunting.[77] Intraventricular hemorrhage may cause both malabsorption and obstruction of cerebrospinal fluid pathways. Clinical signs are of increasing head circumference, full anterior fontanel, sun-setting eye signs, lethargy or irritability, feeding difficulties, and vomiting.

The effects of intraventricular hemorrhage and hydrocephalus on long-term neurobehavioral outcome in preterm very low birthweight (VLBW) infants has been studied in comparison to normal VLBW infants.[78] Infants who require shunts for progressive hydrocephalus had significant difficulties with attentional and academic skills compared with infants with arrested hydrocephalus. Virtually all the infants with arrested hydrocephalus had abnormalities on their MRI scans.[79]

1.7.2 Hydrocephalus in term infants

Hydrocephalus may develop in term infants following hemorrhage, infarction, tumor, or infection. It can be a complication in twin delivery.

In destructive lesions varying degrees of motor disturbance may accompany the hydrocephalus from hemiplegia to severe symmetric or asymmetric diplegia or quadriplegia.

Associated problems are common, especially visual damage, including optic atrophy and visual pathway damage. Cognitive visual problems are common in children with shunted hydrocephalus and should be sought by active history taking.[80]

Other clinical signs are as in the preterm infant, increasing occipito-frontal circumference (OFC), tense anterior fontanel, feeding difficulties, poor suck and swallow or vomiting.

Visual evoked potentials (VEPs) may be delayed, with some improvement post shunting.[81]

1.8 PROBLEMS IN LOW BIRTHWEIGHT CHILDREN

There has been progressive improvement in the care of preterm and VLBW infants in the past 40 years accompanied by an increasing understanding of the risks and awareness of long-term outcome.

Longitudinal studies of survivors in the 1970s initially suggested that the prevalence of cerebral palsy remained constant, but over time the prevalence of children with clearly defined cerebral palsy has increased and there are more children with subtle perceptual-motor difficulties, visual and hearing problems.

More very immature babies of less than 26 weeks gestation are surviving and there are reports from around the world of increasingly preterm survivors.[82]

1.8.1 Motor and functional outcomes

The incidence of cerebral palsy in the preterm, VLBW and extremely low birthweight (ELBW) relates gestational age, birthweight, and place of birth.

A study from Hammersmith Hospital, London, of children born between 1984 and 1986 of less than 35 weeks gestation with no congenital abnormalities showed an incidence of cerebral palsy of 14.2 percent of survivors.[83] No child with a normal ultrasound scan developed cerebral palsy, whereas nearly all with major lesions did. Minor lesions, however, were not generally predictive of later outcome. This study group was derived from a tertiary referral center so there is bound to be a skewing effect compared with a population-based study. The infants with the lowest birthweight and gestational age were most affected at 6 years of age in their neurological and perceptual-motor development.

A study population comprising all liveborn infants born in Scotland in 1984 with birthweights less than 1500 g gives helpful information.[84] Four hundred and five survived the neonatal period and 371 (62 percent of the study population) survived to the age of 8 years. Fifteen percent of those with birthweights less than 1000 g (ELBW) and 6 percent of those weighing less than 1500 g (VLBW) attended special schools. Index children attending mainstream schools performed significantly less well in tests of neuromotor function than their comparison groups. Their mean IQs were 90.4 for ELBW and 93.7 for VLBW, while the comparison groups' IQs were 102.5 and 101.2. They were also less able in reading and number skills.

Fifty-two percent of ELBW children and 37 percent of the VLBW children required learning support compared with 16 percent in both comparison groups.[84]

In another, longitudinal study, the educational, motor, and behavioral performance of a hospital-based cohort of 51 VLBW children (in this study birthweight 1250 g or less) at the age of 6 years was reported.[85] The VLBW children performed less well in basic mathematics, spelling, reading, and motor skills. Forty-three percent of the VLBW group were having difficulty with one or more school subjects, compared with 11 percent of controls and 15 percent with two or more areas compared with 5 percent of controls.

Teachers identified emotional disorders and overactivity more often in the VLBW group.[85] Motor testing at 6 years of age was the best predictor of school problems at 8 years.[86]

By the age of 13 years 36 percent of VLBW children had significant motor impairment compared with 5 percent of controls. Visual impairments were present in 63 percent, compared with 36 percent of controls. Psychological problems were also more common in the index group.[87]

1.8.2 Vision in very low birthweight children without cerebral palsy

As has already been mentioned, retinopathy of prematurity is one of the major causes of blindness or severe visual handicap in a large group of VLBW and ELBW survivors and contributes to their cognitive difficulties.

In a follow-up study of visual impairment in VLBW children, reduced visual function was present in 63.5 percent compared with 36 percent of controls. Poor contrast sensitivity and poor visual acuity were predictive of lower IQ. Low birthweight, intraventricular hemorrhage, intrauterine growth retardation and low 1-minute Apgar scores predicted reduced visual function.

Measures were made of stereopsis and contrast sensitivity, which identified impaired vision that was not detected by normal screening and were related to impaired neurodevelopmental outcome in both motor and cognitive areas.

There are two possible explanations for the association between visual and neurodevelopmental impairments: both areas of disability may have a common etiology or poor visual function may directly affect the development of motor and cognitive skills.[88]

When preterm children with intraventricular hemorrhage (IVH) were compared over the first 4 years of life with 73 healthy preterm children without IVH, it was shown that children with IVH were at greater risk for ocular abnormalities, for deficits in grating acuity, and for deficits in recognition (letter) at ages 3 and 4 years. Children with IVH were also at risk for visual field deficits during the first postnatal year. Visual deficits were not related to the grade of IVH or to the co-occurrence of periventricular leukomalacia (PVL), but were associated in some subjects with ocular abnormalities and cerebral palsy.[89,90]

1.8.3 Hearing problems in low birthweight survivors

Hospital-based studies have placed the rate of moderate to severe sensorineural hearing loss between 2 and 10 percent. Aminoglycoside antibiotics, exposure to high levels of bilirubin, and major intracranial hemorrhage may be etiological factors. Middle ear pathology associated with recurrent infections is also a cause of significant hearing loss.[91]

1.8.4 Differential effects of preterm birth and small for gestational age

The adverse effects of being small for gestational age (SGA) have been recognized and studied over a long period. Differential effects of early and late growth retardation may be due to the term, growth-retarded infant having experienced the adverse environment for longer than the preterm infant or to the stage of organ development at the time of exposure.

Neonatal mortality of VLBW infants has decreased from 564 per 1000 live births in 1971 to 211 per 1000 live births in 1991. Infants who were SGA and preterm would have died previously but are now surviving.

Hutton's study of infants weighing less than 2000 g at birth, gestational age at birth 32 weeks or less, born in 1980 and 1981 in the county of Merseyside were assessed at age 8 or 9 years. Results showed that there was a difference in the effects of being preterm or SGA. Cognitive ability and motor ability were negatively associated with the degree of fetal growth retardation. Motor ability was positively associated with gestational age. Reading rate and reading accuracy were socially determined.

It is important to recognize that this study was of infants under 32 weeks gestational age so that any growth retardation will have occurred predominantly in the first two trimesters and may differ both in etiology and consequences from growth retardation taking place later in pregnancy.[92]

1.8.5 Health-related quality of life in high-risk babies[93]

A challenge to the conventional approach of assessing outcome for survivors looks at quality of life from the child's and family's perspectives. This approach acknowledges the individual's contribution to outcome and the changing perspective of the developing child over time.

1.9 LIFE EXPECTANCY IN CEREBRAL PALSY

There have been a number of studies of life expectancy in cerebral palsy. It is clearly difficult to be precise about prognosis as changing practices in both medical care and community living will have long-term effects on quality and length of life.

Mortality statistics from death certificates are not reliable; infantile cerebral palsy and learning disabilities are rarely mentioned (International Classification of Diseases code 343) as part of the diagnosis. Cerebral palsy is grossly under-represented in the mortality statistics for England and Wales.[94]

A cohort of children with cerebral palsy from the south-east of England born between 1970 and 1979 showed a 90 percent survival rate in 1990.[95] Immobility and severe mental handicap were the two strongest predictors of mortality.

In a study from British Columbia of children born between 1952 and 1989, 9.8 percent of the females and 9.6 percent of the males had died by 1989. In this group profound mental retardation and severe spastic quadriplegia were major hazards for survival.[96]

In a study from London of people with learning disability, respiratory disease was documented as the major cause of death in 52 percent of the study population compared with 16 percent of the whole population. The risk of dying before the age of 50 was 58 times higher than in England and Wales generally.[94]

Early death was significantly associated with cerebral palsy, incontinence, problems with mobility, and residence in hospital.

Severe epilepsy shortens life expectancy, particularly in young children and those who have severe feeding difficulties and gastroesophageal reflux. Sudden deaths also occur in this group of children.

1.10   REFERENCES

1 Taylor DC. Mechanisms of coping with handicap. In: McCarthy GT ed. *Physical disability in childhood. An interdisciplinary approach to management.* London: Churchill Livingstone, 1992: 53–64.

2 Carr LJ, Stephens JA. The development of descending motor pathways in children with hemiplegic cerebral palsy: the effects of early brain damage. In: Connolly KJ, Forssberg H eds. *Neurophysiology and neuropsychology of motor development.* Clinics in Developmental Medicine 143/144. London: MacKeith Press, 1997: 177–200.

3 Vargha-Khadem F, O'Gorman AM, Watters GV. Aphasia and handedness in relation to hemispheric side, age at injury and severity of cerebral lesion during childhood. *Brain* 1985; **108**: 677–93.

4 Leonard CT, Moritani T, Hirschfield H, Forssberg H. Deficits in reciprocal inhibition of children with cerebral palsy as revealed by H reflex testing *Developmental Medicine and Child Neurology* 1990; **32**: 974–84.

5 Gordon AM, Forssberg H. Development of neural mechanisms underlying grasping in children. In: Conolly KJ, Forssberg H eds. *Neurophysiology and neuropsychology of motor development.* Clinics in Developmental Medicine 143/144. London: MacKeith Press, 1997: 214–31.

6 Pountney TE, Mulcahy CM, Green EM. Early development of postural control. *Physiotherapy* 1990; **76**(12): 799–802.

7 Tardieu C, Lespargot A, Tabary C. For how long must the soleus be stretched each day to prevent contracture? *Developmental Medicine and Child Neurology* 1988; **30**: 3–10.

8 Lespargot A, Renaudin E, Khouri N, Robert M. Extensibility of hip adductors in children with cerebral palsy. *Developmental Medicine and Child Neurology* 1994; **36**: 980.

9 Mulcahy CM, Pountney TE, Nelham RL, Green EM, Billington GD. Adaptive seating for motor handicap: problems, a solution, assessment and prescription. *British Journal of Occupational Therapy* 1988; **51**(10): 347–52 and *Physiotherapy* 1988; **74**(10): 531–6.

10 Green EM. Does correct positioning affect the performance of a physically handicapped child? MD thesis, University of Dundee, 1990.

11 Crothers B, Paine R. *The natural history of cerebral palsy.* Classics in Developmental Medicine No 2. MacKeith Press, London: 1988.

12 Lin JP. Dorsal rhizotomy and physical therapy. Editorial. *Developmental Medicine and Child Neurology* 1998; **40**: 219–19.

13 Scrutton D. A study of hips in children with bilateral cerebral palsy *APCP Journal* 1999; **90**: 10–13

14 Gerszten PC, Albright AL, Johnstone GF. Intrathecal baclofen and subsequent orthopedic surgery in patients with spastic cerebral palsy. *Journal of Neurosurgery USA* 1998; **88**: 1009–13.

15 McLaughlin JF, Bjornson KF, Astley SJ *et al.* Selective dorsal rhizotomy: efficacy and safety in an investigator-masked clinical trial. *Developmental Medicine and Child Neurology* 1998; **40**: 220–32.

16 Steinbok P, Reiner AM, Armstrong RW, Cochrane DD. A randomised clinical trial to compare selective posterior rhizotomy plus physiotherapy with physiotherapy alone in children with spastic diplegic cerebral palsy. *Developmental Medicine and Child Neurology* 1997; **39**: 178–84.

17 Steinbok P, Daneshvar H, Evans D, Kestle JR. Cost analysis of continuous intrathecal baclofen versus selective posterior rhizotomy in the treatment of spastic quadriplegia associated with cerebral palsy. *Paediatric Neurosurgery* 1995; **22**(5): 255–64.

18 Banta JV, Lubicky JP. Resolution: a 15-year-old with spastic quadriplegia and a 60° scoliosis should have a posterior spinal fusion with instrumentation. The American Academy for Cerebral Palsy and Developmental Medicine 50th Anniversary Meeting Debate. *Developmental Medicine and Child Neurology* 1998; **40**: 278–83.

19 Cassidy C, Craig CI, Perry A, Karlin LI, Goldberg MJ. A reassessment of spinal stabilisation in severe cerebral palsy. *Journal of Pediatric Orthopedics* 1994; **14**: 731–9.

20 Lloyd DA, Pierro A. The therapeutic approach to the child with feeding difficulty: III Enteral feeding. In: Sullivan P, Rosenbloom L eds. *Feeding the disabled child.* Clinics in Developmental Medicine 140. London: MacKeith Press, 1997; 132–49.

21 Brindley C, Cave D, Crane S, Lees J, Moffat V. *Paediatric Oral Skills Package (POSP).* London: Whurr, 1996.

22 *Eating and drinking skills for children with motor disorders.* East Sussex, UK: Chailey Heritage Clinical Services, 1998.

23 Butler C. Effects of powered mobility on self-initiated behaviours of very young children with locomotor disability. *Developmental Medicine and Child Neurology* 1986; **28**: 325–32.

24 Drigo P, Seren F, Artibani W, Laverda AM, Battestella PA, Zacchello G. Neurogenic vesico-urethral dysfunction in children with cerebral palsy. *Journal of Neurological Science* 1988; **9**: 151–4.

25 Baird G, Moore AT. Epidemiology. In: *The management of visual impairment in childhood.* London: MacKeith Press, 1993: 1–8.

26 Bryars JH, Archer DB. Aetiological survey of visually handicapped children in Northern Ireland. *Transactions of the Ophthalmological Society of the United Kingdom* 1977; **97**: 26–9.

27 Foley J. Central visual disturbances. *Developmental Medicine and Child Neurology* 1987; **29**: 110–20.

28 Taylor MJ. Visual evoked potentials. In: Eyre JA ed. *The neurophysiological examination of the newborn*

infant. Clinics in Developmental Medicine 120. London: MacKeith Press, 1992: 93–111.

29 Taylor MJ, Menzies R, MacMillan LJ, Whyte HE. VEPs in normal full-term and premature neonates: longitudinal versus cross-sectional data. *Electroencephalography and Clinical Neurophysiology* 1987; **68**: 149–52.

30 Mercurio E, Atkinson J, Braddick O *et al.* Visual function and perinatal focal cerebral infarction. *Archives of Disease in Childhood* 1996; **75**: F76–81.

31 Hoyt CS. The clinical usefulness of the visual evoked responses. *Journal of Pediatric Ophthalmology and Strabismus* 1984; **21**: 231–4.

32 Good WV. Behaviors of visually impaired children. *Seminars in Ophthalmology* 1991; **6**: 158–60.

33 Fisch L. The aetiology of congenital deafness and audiometric patterns. *Journal of Laryngology* 1955; **69**: 7.

34 Robinson RO. The frequency of other handicaps in children with cerebral palsy. *Developmental Medicine and Child Neurology* 1973; **15**: 305.

35 Robson P. *ACHSHIP Reports.* London: *DHSS*, 1981.

36 Cremers CWRJ. Prevention of serious hearing impairment or deafness in the young child. *Journal of the Royal Society of Medicine* 1989; **82:** 484.

37 Preece PM, Peckham CS, Pearl KN. Congenital cytomegalovirus infection. *Archives of Disease in Childhood* 1984; **59**: 1120–6.

38 Baird G. Assessment of hearing and management of hearing problems. In: McCarthy GT ed. *Physical disability in childhood.* London: Churchill Livingstone, 1992: 89–94.

39 Goodman R, Yude C. IQ and its predictors in childhood hemiplegia. *Developmental Medicine and Child Neurology* 1996; **38**: 881–90.

40 Vargha-Khadem F, Isaacs E, Muter VA. A review of cognitive outcome after unilateral lesions sustained during childhood. *Journal of Child Neurology* 1994; **9**: 2S67–2S73.

41 Vargha-Kadem F, Isaacs EB, Van der Werf S, Robb S, Wilson J. Development of intelligence and memory in children with hemiplegic cerebral palsy. The deleterious consequences of early seizures. *Brain* 1992; **115**: 315–29.

42 Goodman R, Graham P. Psychiatric problems in children with hemiplegia; cross sectional epidemiological survey. *British Medical Journal* 1996; **312**: 1065–9.

43 Balleny H. Are the concepts of 'theory of mind' and 'executive function' useful in understanding social impairment in children with hemiplegic cerebral palsy? Clin Psy D thesis, University of East Anglia, Norwich, 1996.

44 Aicardi J. Epilepsy in brain injured children. *Developmental Medicine and Child Neurology* 1990; **32**: 191–202.

45 Chevrie JJ, Aicardi J. Le prognostic psychique des spasmes infantile traite par l'ACTH ou des corticoides. Analyse stastique de 78 cas suivis plus d'un an. *Journal of Neurological Science* 1971; **12**: 351–7.

46 Riikonen R, Donner M. Incidence and aetiology of infantile spasms from 1960 to 1976: a population study in Finland. *Developmental Medicine and Child Neurology* 1972; **21**: 333–43.

47 Jeavons P, Bower BD, Dimitrakoudi M. Long term prognosis of 150 cases of 'West Syndrome'. *Epilepsia* 1973; **14**: 153–64.

48 Ohtahara S, Yamatogi Y, Ohtsuka Y, Oka E, Ishida T. Prognosis of West Syndrome with special reference to Lennox Syndrome: a developmental study. In: Wade J, Penry JK eds. *Advances in epileptology. The Xth Epilepsy International Symposium.* New York: Raven Press, 1980: 149–54.

49 Aicardi J. Infantile spasms and related syndromes. In: Aicardi J ed. *Epilepsy in children*, 2nd edn. New York: Raven Press, 1994: 18–43.

50 Berkovic SF, Andermann F, Melanson D *et al.* Hypothalamic hamartomas and ictal laughter: evolution of a characteristic epileptic syndrome and diagnostic value of magnetic resonance. *Annals of Neurology* 1988; **23**: 429–39.

51 Pazzaglia P, D'Alessandro R, Lozito A, Lugaresi E. Classification of partial epilepsy according to the symptomology of the seizures. Practical value and prognostic implications. *Epilepsia* 1982; **23**: 343–50.

52 Henriksen O. Specific problems of children with epilepsy. *Epilepsia* **29**(suppl. 3): S6–S9.

53 Sorgijanov NG. Clinical evolution and prognosis of childhood epilepsies. *Epilepsia* 1982; **23**: 81–9.

54 Stevenson RC, Pharoah POD, Stevenson CJ, McCabe CJ, Cooke RWI. Cost of care for a geographically determined population of low birthweight infants to age 8–9 years. II. Children with disability. *Archives of Disease in Childhood* 1996; **74**: F118–21.

55 Pharoah POD, Cooke RWI. A hypothesis for the etiology of spastic cerebral palsy – the vanishing twin. *Developmental Medicine and Child Neurology* 1997; **39**: 292–6.

56 Pharoah POD, Cooke T. Cerebral palsy and multiple births. *Archives of Disease in Childhood* 1996; **75**(3): 174–7.

57 Kennedy CR. The assessment of hearing and brain stem function. In: Eyre JA ed. *The neurophysiological examination of the newborn infant.* Clinics in Developmental Medicine No 120. London: MacKeith Press, 1992: 79–92.

58 Little WJ. On the influence of abnormal parturition, labour, premature birth and asphyxia neonatorum on the mental and physical condition of the child, especially in relation to deformities. *Transactions of the Obstetrical Society of London* 1862; **111**: 293.

59 Freud S. *Die infantile Cerebrallahmung (Northnagel's specielle pathologie und therapie).* div 2, pt 2, vol 9 Vienna: Holder, 1897.

60 Scrutton D. The early management of the hip in cerebral palsy. *Developmental Medicine and Child Neurology* 1989; **31**: 108–16.

61 Gage JR. *Gait analysis in cerebral palsy.* Clinics in Developmental Medicine No. 121. London: MacKeith Press, 1991.

62 de Vries LS, Levene MI. Cerebral ischaemic lesions. In: Levene MI, Lilford RJ eds. *Fetal and neonatal neurology and neurosurgery*, 2nd edn. Edinburgh: Churchill Livingstone, 1995: 379–82.

63 Fletcher NA, Marsden CD. Dyskinetic cerebral palsy: a clinical and genetic study. *Developmental Medicine and Child Neurology* 1996; **38**: 873–80.

64 Bundey S, Griffiths M. Recurrence risks in families of children with symmetrical spasticity. *Developmental Medicine and Child Neurology* 1977; **19**: 179–91.

65 Boyd K, Patterson V. Dopa responsive dystonia: a treatable condition misdiagnosed as cerebral palsy. *British Medical Journal* 1989; **298**: 1019–20.

66 Segawa M, Hosaka A, Miyagawa F, Imai H. Hereditary progressive dystonia with marked diurnal fluctuation. *Advances in Neurology* 1976; **14**: 215–33.

67 Torbjoern G, Nygaard MD, Waran SP, Levine RA, Naini AB, Chutorian AM. Dopa-responsive dystonia simulating cerebral palsy. *Pediatric Neurology* 1994; **11**: 236–40.

68 Bandmann O, Nygaard TG, Surtees R, Marsden CD, Wood NW, Harding AE. Dopa-responsive dystonia in British patients: new mutations of the GTP-cyclo-hydrolase gene and evidence of heterogeneity. *Human Molecular Genetics* 1996; **5**: 403–6.

69 Robinson RO, McCarthy GT, Bandmann O, Dobbie M, Surtees R, Wood NW. GTP cyclohydrolase deficiency; intra-familial variation in clinical phenotype, including levodopa responsiveness. *Journal of Neurology, Neurosurgery and Psychiatry* 1999; **66**: 86–9.

70 Lesch M, Nyhan WL. A familial disorder of uric acid metabolism and central nervous system dysfunction. *American Journal of Medicine* 1964; **36**: 561–70.

71 Brett EM. Ataxia syndromes associated with agenesis of the cerebellar vermis. In: Brett EM ed. *Paediatric neurology*, 3rd edn. New York: Churchill Livingstone, 1997: 272–4.

72 Bordarier C, Aicardi J. Dandy-Walker syndrome and agenesis of the cerebellar vermis: diagnostic problems and genetic counselling. *Developmental Medicine and Child Neurology* 1990; **32**: 285–94.

73 Esscher E, Flodmark O, Hagberg G, Hagberg B. Non-progressive ataxia: origins, brain pathology and impairments in 78 Swedish children. *Developmental Medicine and Child Neurology* 1996; **38**: 285–96.

74 Boltshauser E, Isler W. Joubert syndrome: episodic hyperpnoea, abnormal eye movements, retardation and ataxia, associated with dysplasia of the cerebellar vermis. *Neuropediatrie* 1977; **8**: 57–66.

75 Gordon N. Ataxia of parietal lobe origin. *Developmental Medicine and Child Neurology* 1999; **41**: 353–5.

76 Steinlin M, Zangger B, Boltshauser E. Non-progressive congenital ataxia with or without cerebellar hypoplasia: a review of 34 subjects. *Developmental Medicine and Child Neurology* 1998; **40**: 148–54.

77 Dykes FD, Dunbar B, Lazarra A, Ahmann PA. Post-hemorrhagic hydrocephalus in high-risk preterm infants: natural history, management and long term outcome. *Journal of Pediatrics* 1989; **114**: 611–18.

78 Fletcher JM, Landry SH, Bohan TP *et al*. Effects of intraventricular hemorrhage and hydrocephalus on the long-term neurobehavioral development of preterm very-low-birthweight infants. *Developmental Medicine and Child Neurology* 1997; **39**: 596–606.

79 Hanlo PW, Gooskens RHJM, van Schooneveld M *et al*. The effect of intracranial pressure on myelination and the relationship with neurodevelopment in infantile hydrocephalus. *Developmental Medicine and Child Neurology* 1997; **39**: 286–91.

80 Houliston MJ, Taguri AH, Dutton GN, Hajivassiliou, C, Young DG. Evidence of cognitive visual problems in children with hydrocephalus: a structured clinical history-taking strategy. *Developmental Medicine and Child Neurology* 1999; **41**: 298–306.

81 Guthkelch AN, Hirsch RP, Vries JK. Visual evoked potentials in hydrocephalus: relationship to head size, shunting, and mental development. *Neurosurgery* 1984; **14**: 283–6.

82 Cooke RWI. Factors affecting survival and development in extremely tiny babies. *Seminars in Neonatology* 1996; **1**: 267–76.

83 Jongmans M, Mercuri E, de Vries LS *et al*. Minor neurological signs and perceptual-motor difficulties in prematurely born children. *Archives of Disease in Childhood* 1997; **76**: F9–14.

84 Hall A, McLeod A, Counsell C, Thomson L, Mutch L. School attainment, cognitive ability and motor function in a total Scottish very-low-birthweight population at eight years: a controlled study. *Developmental Medicine and Child Neurology* 1995; **37**: 1037–50.

85 Marlow N, Roberts BL, Cooke RWI. Motor skills in extremely low birth weight children at age six years. *Archives of Disease in Childhood* 1989; **64**: 839–47.

86 Marlow N, Roberts L, Cooke R. Outcome at 8 years for children with birth weights of 1250 g or less. *Archives of Disease in Childhood* 1993; **68**: 286–90.

87 Powls A, Botting N, Cooke RWI. Motor impairment in children 12 to 13 year olds with a birth weight of less than 1250 grams. *Archives of Disease in Childhood* 1995; **73**: F62–6.

88 Powls A, Botting N, Cooke RWI, Stephenson G, Marlow N. Visual impairment in very low birth-weight children. *Archives of Disease in Childhood* 1997; **76**: F82–7.

89 Eken P, De Vries LS, Van der Graaf Y, Meiners LC, Van Nieuwenhuizen O. Haemorrhagic-ischaemic lesions of the neonatal brain. Correlation between cerebral visual impairment, neurodevelopmental outcome and MRI in infancy. *Developmental Medicine and Child Neurology* 1995; **37**: 41–55.

90 Harvey E, Dobson V, Luna B, Scher M. Grating acuity and visual field development in children with intraventricular hemorrhage. *Developmental Medicine and Child Neurology* 1997; **39**: 305–12.

91 Hack M, Klein N, Taylor HG. School-age outcomes of children of extremely low birth weight and gestational age. *Seminars in Neonatology* 1996; **1**: 277–88.

92 Hutton JL, Pharoah POD, Cooke RWI, Stevenson RC. Differential effects of preterm birth and small gestational age on cognitive and motor development. *Archives of Disease in Childhood* 1997; **76**: F75–81.

93 Saigal S, Rosenbaum P. Health related quality of life considerations in the outcome of high-risk babies. *Seminars in Neonatology* 1996; **1**: 305–12.

94 Holling S, Attard MT, von Fraunhofer N, McGuigan S, Sedgewick P. Mortality in people with learning disability: risks, causes, and death certification findings in London. *Developmental Medicine and Child Neurology* 1998; **40**: 50–6.

95 Evans PM, Evans SJW, Alberman E. Cerebral palsy: why we must plan for survival. *Archives of Disease in Childhood* 1990; **65**: 1329–53.

96 Crichton JU, Mackinnon M, White CP. The life expectancy of persons with cerebral palsy. *Developmental Medicine and Child Neurology* 1995; **37**: 567–76.

2 Epidemiology of fetal and neonatal brain damage

Ann Johnson

In recent years, advances in neurobiology, neuropathology, and neuroimaging have furthered our understanding of fetal and neonatal brain damage. However, much of our current thinking on the causes of brain damage is based on the use and misuse of data arising from epidemiological studies.

Epidemiology is the basic science of clinical, preventive and community medicine. It has three main aims: (1) to describe the frequency and distribution of conditions in the population, (2) to identify risk factors for these conditions, and (3) to provide information which can be used to plan and evaluate services for the prevention and treatment of the conditions. In more general terms it has been described as a 'search for patterns'.

Epidemiology is a science which therefore demands (a) definitions of both the conditions being considered and the characteristics of the risk factors described; (b) denominators which apply to geographically defined populations in order to express rates or prevalence of conditions; (c) caution in interpreting research findings, in particular, distinguishing between risk factors (associations) and causal pathways.

In this chapter we will first try to define the term 'damage', identify the clinical conditions that may plausibly result from brain damage, and discuss the terminology used when investigating their etiology. Then, focusing particularly on cerebral palsy, we will review what is known about its prevalence (rate) and distribution, and consider some of the social and biological risk factors.

2.1 DEFINITIONS

2.1.1 Fetal and neonatal brain damage

The term 'damage' ('harm' which results in impairment of function) implies that the finely tuned process of normal development has been disturbed or interrupted in some way. Normal brain development is under the control of genetic, metabolic, nutritional, and hormonal factors and so it follows that abnormality or imbalance in any of these can potentially damage the growing maturing brain. Similarly, external agents such as infections, toxic substances, or acute or chronic hypoxia can cause damage.

The term 'injury' (to 'injure' is to cause harm) is often used to describe the effect of hypoxia-ischemia and usually carries the implication of avoidability. As we will see, contrary to earlier assumptions, brain damage is rarely caused by preventable hypoxic-ischemic injury around the time of birth. The terms 'brain damage' and 'brain injury' now need to encompass a much wider concept, to include a range of factors which can have their effect at any point from conception onwards, right through into childhood. Many of these factors appear unrelated to care and most remain unidentified.

2.1.2 Birth asphyxia

Although this topic will be dealt with fully elsewhere, it would be useful to address some of the problems surrounding the definition of 'birth asphyxia'. Blair[1] has identified the key issue as confusion about the sequence 'exposure – response – outcome'. She points out that the term 'birth asphyxia' is used to describe any part of this sequence and more importantly that the presence of an 'exposure' is inferred from the response or outcome even in the absence of evidence of a causal sequence. For example, fetal heart rate abnormality, acidosis, low Apgar score, and neonatal seizures may all be responses to a hypoxic-ischemic exposure, i.e. be markers of recent or concurrent hypoxic-ischemic injury at a cellular level. However, these clinically observable signs have a low specificity for such injury. They may, in fact, reflect much earlier hypoxic-ischemic damage, a 'normal physiological response' to hypoxic stress, or be due to a totally different cause. Recently, a consensus statement has been agreed in which the essential criteria for defining an acute intrapartum hypoxic event are included.[2] This was drawn up by a multidisciplinary group and endorsed by a large number of professional bodies. Although it is based on current epidemiological evidence, it is anticipated that as more precise ways of assessing fetal state, both antenatally and intrapartum, become available, the criteria will need to be refined and their sensitivity and specificity improved.[3]

2.2 CLINICAL EFFECTS OF BRAIN DAMAGE

The clinical effects of damage will be diverse, depending on the timing, the location, and the extent of the damage. Traditionally, clinical conditions which are thought to reflect abnormal brain development have been broadly classified into cerebral palsy, learning disabilities, specific learning disorders, sensory deficits, epilepsy, and behavioral abnormalities, including autism.

Although there is an argument for examining what is known about the epidemiology of all these clinical entities, in this chapter we will focus on cerebral palsy, and make some reference to learning disability and specific learning disorders.

2.3 EPIDEMIOLOGICAL TERMS

There are a few epidemiological terms which it might be helpful to consider at this stage. When describing the proportion of children in a population with a condition such as cerebral palsy, the term *prevalence rate* is used and a useful concept is *birth cohort prevalence rate*. This is the proportion of children with cerebral palsy in a 1-year cohort of livebirths. The cohort is best defined as livebirths to mothers resident in a particular geographic area rather than livebirths in a particular unit. This is because populations defined by unit of birth are prone to 'selection bias' and variations in rates over time or between units may be accounted for by differences in case-mix.

Cohorts defined by geographic boundaries are often listed on population registers. There are a number of such registers of children with cerebral palsy in the UK,[4–7] Sweden,[8] Denmark,[9] Western Australia,[10] California,[11] and elsewhere. Children are usually 'counted' as 'cases' on these registers at a particular age, often at 5 years. Earlier ascertainment of cases in the population may 'miss' children with mild disease that becomes clinically apparent at a later age, or conversely, clinical signs suggesting a diagnosis of cerebral palsy in the first 2 years after birth may disappear later in preschool years. These registers are an important source of information for those planning and providing services as well as providing a useful framework for research, both evaluative and etiological.[12]

The birth cohort prevalence rate may be expressed as *birthweight-specific prevalence rate*, that is, the proportion of children with cerebral palsy among births defined by birthweight group, such as <1000 g (extremely low birthweight (ELBW) babies), <1500 g (very low birthweight (VLBW) babies) and so on. This is a useful way of expressing the rate of cerebral palsy, as the risk of the condition increases with decreasing birthweight and the impacts of risk factors appear to differ in different birthweight groups.

Birthweight-specific prevalence rate is usually expressed as the number of cases per 1000 live-births in a cohort. However, among VLBW babies and particularly ELBW babies, *stillbirth and neonatal mortality rates* may have an impact on cerebral palsy rate. Over the years, neonatal intensive care techniques have been refined and the survival rates among these tiny babies have increased. This has been accompanied by an increase in VLBW cerebral palsy rates, presumably because of the survival of babies who are particularly vulnerable to antenatal or neonatal brain injury and who previously would have died. Expressing the rate as numbers of children with cerebral palsy per 1000 *survivors* takes changing mortality rates into account and is, after all, the information needed by parents and neonatologists.

One final point, if more VLBW babies survive, the number of children with cerebral palsy will increase even if the rate of cerebral palsy remains constant.[13] This has important implications for provision of health services well beyond the neonatal period and also for later educational and social services.

2.3.1   Risk factors

A risk factor is any factor that is associated with an increased frequency of a condition. For example, maternal chorioamnionitis is a risk factor for cerebral palsy in the baby. This does not mean that maternal chorioamnionitis is necessarily the cause of cerebral palsy, but is said to be an *association*. Low gestational age is also a risk factor for cerebral palsy. If maternal chorioamnionitis is more frequent in mothers who deliver preterm than mothers at or near term, then the increased risk of cerebral palsy in babies of mothers with maternal chorioamnionitis may be explained by the fact that they are more likely to be preterm. Gestational age would then be termed a *confounding factor*, that is, it confuses the apparent association of maternal chorioamnionitis and cerebral palsy.

The size of an association between a risk factor and cerebral palsy is expressed as a *relative risk*. The relative risk (RR) of maternal chorioamnionitis would be expressed as the rate of cerebral palsy among mothers with chorioamnionitis divided by the rate of cerebral palsy among mothers without chorioamnionitis. If the RR = 3, then mothers with

chorioamnionitis have three times the risk of having a baby with cerebral palsy compared with mothers without chorioamnionitis.

The association of risk factors and cerebral palsy is examined in observational studies, such as cohort and case–control studies. These are difficult to interpret for a number of reasons. Not only must known (and unknown) confounding factors be taken into account (as described above), but also possible sources of bias and the possibility of chance associations need to be considered.

Bias usually arises when the methods of selection of the populations with and without the condition differ in some way, or the information on the two populations is collected in a different way. For example, in a study of the association of 'intrapartum suboptimal care' and cerebral palsy, the observer collecting information from hospital notes needs to be 'blind' to whether the notes are those of a mother whose child does or does not have cerebral palsy. Otherwise there is a strong tendency to search more critically for evidence of suboptimal care among 'cases' than 'controls'. Finally, in studies particularly where there is an extensive search for risk factors, an association may occur by chance.

These are just a few of the problems which confront us when examining the epidemiological evidence related to the etiology of cerebral plasy. Extreme caution is needed when interpreting these findings and particularly when applying such evidence to individual children. Before an association can be considered to have a cause and effect relationship, a number of criteria must be met. The association is:

- usually strong, i.e. the relative risk is high;
- biologically plausible, i.e. there is a known mechanism or pathway whereby brain damage could have occurred;
- 'dose-dependent', i.e. the degree of association increases with increasing levels of exposure;
- found consistently in different studies using different methodologies.

In particular, the factor causing the brain damage needs to precede the onset of damage and be in the 'causal pathway'. It is in this area that so much confusion has arisen in cerebral palsy epidemiology studies. Defining 'causal pathways' for cerebral palsy, that is the sequences of events which end in cerebral palsy, has proved a useful way of conceptualizing the role of risk factors.[14] Taking our earlier example of the widely recognized association between maternal chorioamnionitis, preterm birth, and cerebral palsy, two of the many possible causal pathways might be:

1   Maternal infection $\longrightarrow$ preterm birth $\longrightarrow$

2   Maternal infection $\underset{\longleftarrow}{\overset{\longrightarrow}{}}$ fetal brain damage / preterm birth $\longrightarrow$ cerebral palsy

In pathway 1, preterm birth is in the causal pathway, whereas in pathway 2 it is an incidental event or 'epiphenomenon'. Clearly preventive strategies would differ in these two possibilities.

The most conclusive evidence of causality, however, is to be obtained from randomized controlled trials. If an intervention reduces the frequency of the risk factor and the frequency of cerebral palsy also falls then there is strong support for a causal link. This emphasizes the need for long-term follow-up in clinical trials of obstetric and neonatal interventions.[15]

We will now consider the frequency and distribution of three conditions that appear to reflect damage to the developing brain.

2.4   CEREBRAL PALSY

Cerebral palsy is an umbrella term used to describe 'a group of disorders in the development of posture or motor control, occurring as a result of a non-progressive lesion of the developing central nervous system'.[16] Although it is described as non-progressive, the clinical condition will change over time and overall life expectancy is reduced. The term encompasses people with similar health, educational, and social needs but the clinical features and the level of disability will vary depending on the extent and nature of the underlying brain damage. There are, therefore, considerable difficulties in deciding which children to include or exclude under this umbrella term.

2.4.1   Inclusions and exclusions

There are three main areas where there is uncertainty about which children to include or exclude. First, with the increasing use of neuro-imaging techniques, and genetic and metabolic studies, it has become clear that some children with cerebral palsy have underlying genetically determined disorders or maldevelopment of the brain. Secondly, children

with severe learning disability or a chronic debilitating condition may have profound hypotonia with associated loss of motor function. A third area of

infant vulnerable to neonatal cerebral hemorrhage and ischemia $\longrightarrow$ cerebral palsy

uncertainty is the boundary between 'clumsiness' with motor incoordination and cerebral palsy.

For the purposes of comparing data from different areas or monitoring changes in rate over time, inclusion and exclusion criteria need to be constant so that like is compared with like. Guidelines for inclusion and exclusion have been suggested which recommend that children who would previously have been included as a case of cerebral palsy should remain on a cerebral palsy register and the diagnostic label remain.[17] An alternative approach has been adopted in a consensus document developed by a European collaboration of cerebral palsy registers.[18] In this, it has been agreed that children with newly recognized brain malformations, neuronal migration defects, and chromosome translocations and deletions but who have the clinical features of cerebral palsy will be included under the umbrella term of cerebral palsy, but with these etiologic factors clearly indicated. On the other hand, it is recommended that hypotonic children with severe learning disability should be excluded from the umbrella term. These criteria have been incorporated into an algorithm and, using this, it has been possible to develop a European database of children with cerebral palsy. These criteria for inclusion and exclusion will need refining and updating as the underlying 'causes' of cerebral palsy are unravelled. Indeed the time may come when the overall term cerebral palsy will need to be dropped in favor of terms which more precisely describe the etiologic subgroups of this heterogeneous condition.

The third area of uncertainty, the inclusion or exclusion of children with very mild motor impairment, is more difficult. As different observers will draw the borderline between motor incoordination and cerebral palsy at different points, wide differences in prevalence rates between areas may be due to differing perceptions of mild cases. One way around the problem that occurs when comparing prevalence rates would be to 'count' only children who transgress a particular level of motor severity. This, of course, demands a consensus in grading the level of severity of motor disability and this leads us on to consider ways of describing and classifying children with cerebral palsy.

2.4.2 Standard description and subclassification of children with cerebral palsy

There are a number of possible ways of classifying children with cerebral palsy. These may be based on:

- pathophysiological or neuroanatomical characteristics;
- distribution of neurological impairment;
- level of severity of motor disability; or
- co-morbidity – association of sensory and intellectual deficit.

2.4.2.1 Classification by distribution of neurological impairment

There is considerable confusion in the terminology currently used to classify children by the extent and distribution of the motor impairment (in terms of altered muscle tone, reflex activity and added unwanted movements). For example, a child with four limb involvement may be described as having quadriplegia, tetraplegia, double-hemiplegia or even diplegia. A system whereby each limb is described in turn overcomes some of the terminology problems,[19] although inter- and intra-observer differences may still lead to inconsistencies in classification.

However, despite these difficulties, the traditional type of grouping of cerebral palsy children has been extensively used and three main clinical subtypes have been defined: four limb involvement – quadriplegia, lower limb – diplegia, and ipsilateral arm and leg – hemiplegia. In general there is increased muscle tone and the term 'spastic' is used to describe these subtypes. In addition, the terms dystonic, ataxic, and athetoid cerebral palsy are used to describe children with varying muscle tone and additional unwanted movements. Many children show features of more than one clinical subtype but the question is still often posed – are the clinical subtypes etiologically distinct?

There is some evidence of a relationship between birthweight or gestational age and clinical type of cerebral palsy. For example, for years it was claimed that diplegia (involvement of lower limbs) was the typical clinical manifestation of cerebral palsy in children born preterm, and overall was the commonest clinical subtype. On the well-established Swedish register, diplegia still accounts for 45 percent of all cerebral palsy cases, with most occurring among the preterm population.[8] On other registers, diplegia accounts for less than 20 percent of all cases although three-quarters of these children weigh less than 2500 g at birth[20] (Fig. 2.1). This clinical subtype is thought to reflect postnatal periventricular injury. A number of observers have reported that the proportion of cerebral palsy children with diplegia has decreased in recent years and there now appears to be an increasing proportion of children with severe quadriplegia (four limb involvement) among both preterm and full-term children.[6,8] This probably reflects the survival of severely affected babies with more extensive lesions who previously would have died. A third of all children on three UK registers now have four limb involvement, often with additional intellectual and sensory deficit[20] (Fig. 2.1).

In general, a higher proportion of full-term cerebral palsy children than preterm cerebral palsy children have hemiplegia and this clinical subtype accounts for a further third of all cases. Based on both the study of risk factors and neuro-imaging, it seems that hemiplegia in full-term cerebral palsy children is usually of prenatal origin, whereas preterm hemiplegia is related to early postnatal events.[21] It is of interest that right hemiplegia is more common than left-sided hemiplegia and it has been suggested that embolic episodes affect the left hemisphere more frequently than the right.

Dyskinetic, ataxic, and athetoid types of cerebral palsy are now rare. Dyskinetic clinical subtypes have been associated with 'birth asphyxia' in full-term babies with neuropathological evidence of injury to basal ganglia; athetoid types are very uncommon since bilirubin encephalopathy now rarely occurs; ataxic forms often have a genetic origin. In recent years there has been an increase in the number of children with atypical patterns of cerebral palsy, often presenting a complex clinical picture which cannot readily be classified.

2.4.2.2 Classification by severity of loss of motor function

There have been two approaches to this. In a standard form developed by Evans et al., the level of motor function is described using a simple four-point scale to define head, neck, and trunk control, upper limb function and lower limb function.[19] In a second approach, overall motor function at different ages is described, using a five-level system.[22] These types of classification are particularly useful

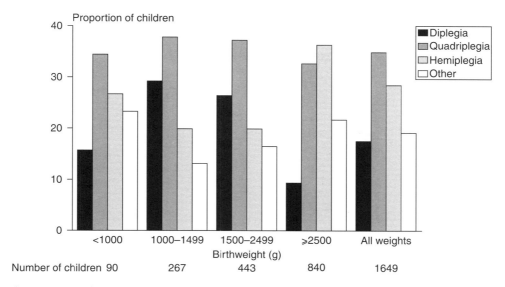

Figure 2.1 Clinical subtype of cerebral palsy by birthweight group. Combined Mersey, Scottish, and Oxford data, 1984–1989.[20]

in defining the needs of children with cerebral palsy, in evaluating the effects of treatments for cerebral palsy, in communicating with parents about the level of severity, in monitoring change over time and in examining differences in motor severity by birthweight group. In addition, they avoid the use of terms that carry value judgements, such as 'mild, moderate, and severe' disability.

Using the simple Evans classification system, a third of children with cerebral palsy are unable to walk even with aids and there is a tendency for non-walking to be more frequent among preterm cerebral palsy (Fig. 2.2). One in five children with

cerebral palsy have no useful hand use and there appears to be no difference in this proportion in the birthweight groups.

2.4.2.3 Classification by presence of additional sensory and/or intellectual deficits

A further aspect of functional loss is the coexistence of vision loss, hearing loss, intellectual deficit, and/or seizures. This co-morbidity will clearly alter the quality of life for children with

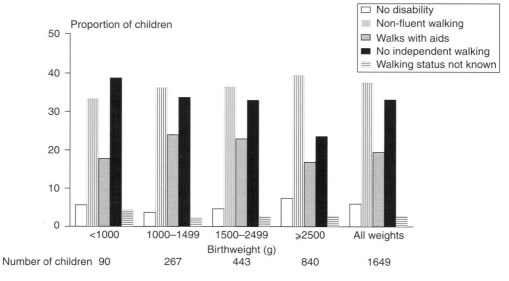

Figure 2.2 Level of walking by birthweight group. Mersey, Scottish, and Oxford data, 1984–1989.[20]

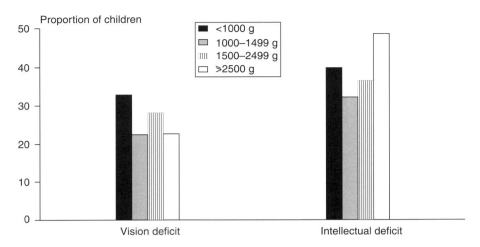

Figure 2.3   Vision deficit and learning disability among children with cerebal palsy by birthweight group. Mersey, Scottish, and Oxford data, 1984–1989.[20]

cerebral palsy. Although it may be difficult to assess both the level of vision and intellectual function in severely motor-impaired children, it appears that over a fifth of the children have severe vision loss, that is are blind or near blind, and moderate or severe intellectual impairment occurs in 40 percent of children with cerebral palsy.[20] A higher proportion of ELBW children with cerebral palsy have a vision defect compared with normal birthweight children with cerebral palsy, but intellectual deficit is more common in the larger babies (Fig. 2.3). In planning service provision this high rate of co-morbidity needs to be taken into account.

2.4.2.4   *Classification by impact of disability and quality of life measures*

An alternative approach is to measure the impact of disability on the child and the family. Using an instrument developed in the Northern Region (UK), a global measure of severity is obtained which reflects 'everyday reality'.[5] Similarly, instruments which measure quality of life are being developed, although many of these are unsuitable for use in children.[23] This approach to measuring 'severity' of disease is attractive and further reliable and valid instruments for use with children with cerebral palsy and their families are needed.

2.4.3   Life expectancy

There is a close relationship between severity of disability and life expectancy. In recent analyses, mobility, level of manual dexterity, and level of intellectual impairment have been used to predict life expectancy.[24,25] Children with milder levels of disability appear to have survival rates similar to those of children without cerebral palsy and yet may well need additional health and educational services. Those with severe disability do have a reduced life expectancy but will require a high level of support and care during their lifetime. Work in analyzing the care-load in terms of human and material resources has highlighted the immense commitment of families and the cost to society.[26]

2.4.4   Prevalence of cerebral palsy

Information on prevalence has almost entirely arisen from population registers of cerebral palsy. Despite the uncertainties of classification and inclusion/exclusion already highlighted, the prevalence rates for cerebral palsy reported from centers in the developed world have been very similar at about 2 per 1000 livebirths.[27] Table 2.1 summarizes the more recent estimates of prevalence in the 1980s and early 1990s.[28–36] The rates remain between 2 and 3 per 1000 livebirths with relatively little geographic variation. Further, there is no clear evidence of changes over time in the overall rate of cerebral palsy, despite falling perinatal mortality rates associated with changes in obstetric and neonatal care.

There are few data from less developed countries. In these areas it is likely that a tendency to higher rates of cerebral palsy due to traumatic, infective, and nutritional factors may be offset by higher mortality rates. Population-based prevalence studies are needed in these other parts of the world.

Table 2.1 Comparison of prevalence rates of cerebral palsy between centers

Geographical area	Birth years	Cerebral palsy prevalence rate per 1000 livebirths
Avon (UK)[28]	1984–88	2.0
Oxford (UK)[29]	1984–94	2.4
Cork (Eire)[30]	1968–90	2.1
Northern Ireland[31]	1987–89	2.8
Scotland[20]	1984–89	2.2
California[11]	1983–85	1.2[a]
Sweden[8]	1987–90	2.4
Mersey (UK)[6]	1982–89	2.5
Denmark[32]	1979–86	2.8
Northern (UK)[5]	1989–93	2.5[b]
W. Australia[33]	1980–94	2.6
Norway[34]	1971–89	2.4
Italy[35]	1989–92	2.5
Slovenia[36]	1987–90	3.0[b]

[a] Moderate or severe cerebral palsy only included and rate expressed as per 1000 neonatal survivors.

[b] Rate expressed as per 1000 neonatal survivors.

2.4.5 Risk factors for cerebral palsy

2.4.5.1 Low birthweight and cerebral palsy

Low birthweight is probably the best-defined risk factor for cerebral palsy. The risk of cerebral palsy increases as birthweight decreases; the rate for babies weighing under 1500 g at birth is nearly 80 times that of babies who weigh over 2500 g (Fig. 2.4). However, only one in five of the children with cerebral palsy in the community had a very low birthweight (<1500 g).

Babies weighing between 1500 g and 2499 g at birth have a rate of cerebral palsy 10 times higher than that of babies weighing more than 2500 g and contribute as many children with cerebral palsy to the community as the very low birthweight group. This group of larger low birthweight babies is probably etiologically heterogeneous, and includes a number of babies who are small for gestational age. As a group they merit further study to determine the extent to which prenatal and perinatal factors contribute to their brain injury.

2.4.5.2 Trends over time in rate of cerebral palsy among LBW babies

During the late 1970s and early 1980s, there was an increase in the number and rate of cerebral palsy among babies weighing less than 1500 g at birth[37] (Fig. 2.5). This was thought to reflect increased survival of very small babies who either had a prenatal brain injury or whose vulnerability to cerebral ischemia and hemorrhage after birth resulted in postnatal brain injury. In the late 1980s and early 1990s, the earlier steep rise in VLBW cerebral palsy rate seems to have leveled off, although one in 12 surviving babies weighing less than 1500 g at birth will have cerebral palsy (Table 2.2). It will be important to continue to monitor trends in cerebral palsy rates as the effects of new therapies such as surfactant, high-frequency ventilation and other new technologies become apparent.

These trends in birthweight-specific cerebral palsy over time have resulted in changes in the proportion

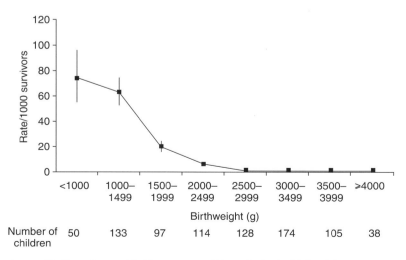

Figure 2.4 Cerebral palsy rate/1000 survivors, with 95 percent confidence limits, by birthweight group among children born 1984–1994 (excluding postneonatal cases).[29]

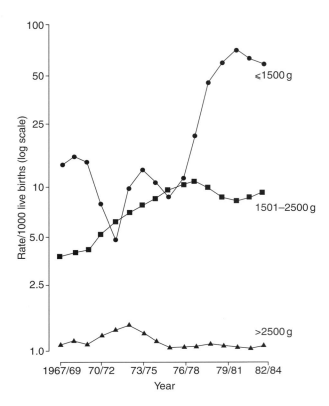

Figure 2.5 Birthweight-specific trends in cerebral palsy.[37] Reproduced from Pharoah *et al.* Birthweight specific trends in cerebral palsy. *Archives of Disease in Childhood* 1990; **65:** 602–6, with permission from BMJ Publishing Group.

of all children with cerebral palsy who weigh <1500 g at birth. In the 1970s, this proportion was less than 10 percent, but by the 1990s it was almost 25 percent (Fig. 2.6). The contribution of babies weighing less than 1000 g has also increased and there is evidence that the severity of disability is increasing over time in the VLBW cerebral palsy group.[5,6,8]

2.4.5.3 Multiple pregnancy and cerebral palsy

There is an increased risk of cerebral palsy among children of multiple pregnancies compared with singleton pregnancies. The prevalence rate among twins is six times higher than the rate in singletons, and among triplets the risk is increased approximately 20-fold[39–41] (Table 2.3). This is almost completely accounted for by their increased risk of preterm birth.

It has been noted that the risk of cerebral palsy in a monochorionic twin is further increased, up to 15-fold, when the co-twin dies *in utero*.[42] This may be due to a hypoxic-ischemic insult which results in the death of one twin and ischemic brain damage in the other. Alternatively, the death of one twin may cause severe circulatory changes resulting in compromise of the cerebral circulation of the surviving twin. This may be acute or chronic. These observations have led to a hypothesis that cerebral palsy in some 'singleton' births may have resulted from the very early fetal death of a co-twin.[43] This needs further testing by review of early fetal ultrasound examinations and by careful placental examination. If this hypothesis is sustained, the 'vanishing twin' could account for a proportion of cerebral palsy whose etiology is at present unclear.

The numbers of multiple births are increasing in many countries, largely as a result of the increasing use of methods of assisted conception and ovarian stimulants, and from time to time selective feticide is used to reduce fetal number. The impact of these new technologies on the rate and numbers of children with cerebral palsy will need to be monitored.

Table 2.2 Comparison of prevalence rates of cerebral palsy by birthweight group in four populations in the 1980s

Geographical area	Birth year	Rate of cerebral palsy per 1000 survivors		
		<1500 g	1500–2499 g	≥2500 g
Northern region (UK)[5]	1984–88	75.9	9.7	1.3[a]
	1989–93	80.0	11.8	1.3[a]
Oxford (UK)[29]	1984–87	73.5	12.1	1.4
	1988–90	84.3	10.5	1.4
Sweden[8,38]	1983–86[31]	49.8	14.4	1.5
	1987–90[6]	68.2	13.9	1.4
Mersey[20 b]	1984–86	75.5	11.8	1.6
	1987–89	96.7	11.7	1.3
Scotland[20 b]	1984–86	55.1	8.9	0.9
	1987–89	58.6	9.5	0.9
W. Australia[33]	1985–89	59.0	9.9	1.5
	1990–94	60.8	7.9	1.6

[a] Expressed as rate per 1000 survivors.

[b] Data from authors.[14]

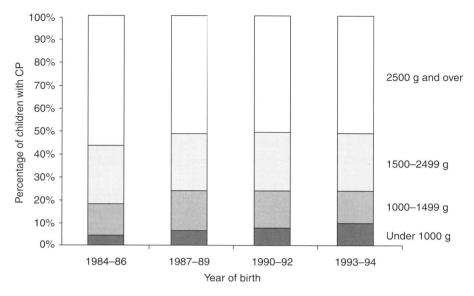

Figure 2.6   Low birthweight babies as a percentage of all children with cerebral palsy (CP; excluding cerebral palsy of a postneonatal origin).

Table 2.3 Prevalence rate per 1000 survivors of cerebral palsy (95% CI) among single and multiple births

Geographic location	Birth years	Singleton rate (95% CI)	Twin rate (95% CI)	Triplet rate (95% CI)
Mersey[6]	1982–89	2.3 (2.1–2.5)	12.6 (9.7–16.1)	44.8 (16.6–94.9)
W. Australia[40]	1980–89	1.6 (1.4–1.8)	7.3 (4.9–9.7)	27.9 (10.3–59.8)
California[41]	1983–85	1.1 (1.0–1.3)	6.7 (4.2–11)	–
Avon[28]	1984–88	1.9 (1.5–2.2)	8.4 (4.2–15.1)	–
Oxford[29]	1984–94	2.1 (2.0–2.3)	7.5 (5.7–9.3)	–

2.4.5.4 Sex of child and cerebral palsy

There are more males than females in all reports of geographically defined populations of children with cerebral palsy (RR = 1.4; 95% CI 1.2–1.6).[29] The frequency of antepartum hemorrhage, pre-eclampsia, and delayed fetal growth is also increased among mothers of male fetuses compared with female fetuses. As these are risk factors for cerebral palsy it is possible that these might be contributing to the higher rate of cerebral palsy among boys. A similar sex difference is also present in spontaneous abortion rates, perinatal mortality rates, and in the rates of a number of fetal malformations, however, suggesting that there are other sex-linked biological factors in early development, which are poorly understood.

2.4.5.5 Socio-economic factors and cerebral palsy

As there is a strong association between low birthweight and socio-economic deprivation, and as low birthweight is a risk factor for cerebral palsy, it might be expected that there would be a relationship between socio-economic deprivation and cerebral palsy. In 1990, Dowding and Barry[44] showed that there was an increased risk of cerebral palsy with decreasing social class (measured using paternal occupation). Somewhat surprisingly this was present only among children with a birthweight over 2500 g and not, as had been expected, among the low birthweight cerebral palsy population. Dolk and co-workers, using data from the Northern Ireland register, were unable to demonstrate a relationship between cerebral palsy and deprivation as measured using the Townsend index of socio-economic deprivation derived from census data.[45] However, further work on data from the Oxford area has confirmed Dowding's original findings, demonstrating an upward trend of cerebral palsy prevalence with increasing deprivation among normal birthweight babies but not among LBW babies.[46] This raises interesting etiologic issues, suggesting that some risk factors for normal birthweight cerebral palsy are more prevalent or more severe with increasing deprivation, and are likely to be exerting their effect prenatally.

We have considered some of the social and biological risk factors for cerebral palsy that can be studied in large population registers using readily available data. Further study of risk factors usually involves specially mounted studies with separate data collection, often from hospital notes. In recent years interest has particularly focused on the association of cerebral palsy and maternal infection,[47,48] pre-eclampsia,[47,49] and thyroid dysfunction.[50] These, however, are all areas that will be dealt with in Chapter 3.

2.5 SEVERE LEARNING DISABILITY

Learning disability is the commonest type of disability seen in childhood. Severe learning disability (IQ < 50) occurs in 3.5 per 1000 livebirths and more than half of these are attributed to genetic causes.[51] The prevalence may be higher in less-developed countries, possibly because nutritional, traumatic, and infective risk factors are more frequent. In some areas there is an increase in autosomal recessive disease associated with consanguinity.

Although low socio-economic status is a strong predictor of mild learning disability, there is little or no association with severe learning disability. So, to what extent is severe learning disability a manifestation of recognized prenatal and neonatal brain injury? Genetic, metabolic, nutritional, and infective factors are dealt with elsewhere and account for the majority of the known causes of severe learning disability. However, a few observations arising from epidemiological studies can be made about the relationship of severe learning difficulty, brain injury around the time of birth and other clinical manifestations of perinatal hypoxic-ischemic injury.

- When severe learning disability is associated with perinatal risk factors, cerebral palsy is also present.[52]
- It is common for infants with learning disability of prenatal origin to demonstrate clinical signs suggestive of 'birth asphyxia', for example those with microcephaly.
- Cerebral palsy among low birthweight survivors became not only more prevalent in the 1980s but there was also a higher frequency of associated severe learning disability.[6]
- It has been predicted that with prenatal diagnosis and the option of termination, there will be a reduction in the numbers of children with severe learning disability due to genetic causes. In future, children with both severe learning disability and cerebral palsy will contribute a greater proportion to the population of children in the community with severe learning disabilities.[53]

2.6 SPECIFIC LEARNING AND EDUCATIONAL PROBLEMS

There is little evidence to suggest that there is an association between specific learning difficulties and brain injury occurring before or around the time of birth. Although preterm birth is a risk factor for later school difficulties,[54] the relationship of adverse perinatal events in term babies, particularly clinical signs which appear to reflect a hypoxic-ischemic event, and educational problems is less clear. Studies of the follow-up of children with neonatal encephalopathy (as a marker of intrapartum hypoxic-ischemia) from one center have suggested that there is a relationship between mean IQ and grade of neonatal encephalopathy.[55,56] From this work, it seems possible that milder degrees of hypoxic-ischemic injury can cause cognitive delay without evidence of motor disability. More well-designed prospective follow-up studies of children with evidence of fetal and neonatal brain injury, preferably based on neuro-imaging, are needed in order to understand the range of disability following such injury.

It is likely that in the future further understanding of the causes and mechanisms of brain injury will come from evidence provided by cellular biologists, neuropathologists, physiologists, and neuro-radiologists. However, the epidemiologists will still have a role in study and experimental design and indeed a multidisciplinary approach will be needed, particularly in testing interventions which may prevent or reduce the effects of hypoxic injury.

2.7 REFERENCES

1 Blair E. A research definition for 'birth asphyxia'. *Developmental Medicine and Child Neurology* 1993; **35**: 449–55.
2 MacLennan A. For the International Cerebral Palsy Task Force. A template for defining a causal relation between acute intrapartum events and cerebral palsy: international consensus statement. *British Medical Journal* 1999; **319**: 1054–9.

3 Bakketeig LS. Only a minor part of cerebral palsy cases begin in labour. *British Medical Journal* 1999; **319**: 1016–17.

4 Johnson A, King R. A regional register of early childhood impairments: a discussion paper. *Journal of Public Health Medicine* (formerly *Community Medicine*) 1989; **11**: 352–63.

5 Colver AF, Gibson M, Hey EN, Jarvis SN, Mackie PC, Richmond S. Increasing rates of cerebral palsy across the severity spectrum in north east England 1964–1993. *Archives of Disease in Childhood Fetal and Neonatal Edition* 2000; **83**: F7–F12

6 Pharoah P, Platt MJ, Cooke T. The changing epidemiology of cerebral palsy. *Archives of Disease in Childhood* 1996; **75**: F169–F173.

7 Mutch L, Ronald E. *The Scottish Register of children with a motor deficit of central origin 1990–1992.* Glasgow: Report to the Office of the Chief Scientist, 1992.

8 Hagberg B, Hagberg G, Olow I, v Wendt L. The changing panorama of cerebral palsy in Sweden V11. Prevalence and origin in the birth year period 1987–90. *Acta Paediatrica* 1996; **85**: 954–60.

9 Topp M, Uldall P, Langhoff-Roos J. Trend in cerebral palsy birth prevalence in eastern Denmark: birth year period 1979–86. *Paediatric Perinatal Epidemiology* 1997; **11**: 451–60.

10 Stanley FJ, Watson L. Trends in perinatal mortality and cerebral palsy in Western Australia 1967–1985. *British Medical Journal* 1992; **304**: 1658–62.

11 Grether JK, Cummins SK, Nelson KB. The California Cerebral Palsy Project. *Pediatric and Perinatal Epidemiology* 1992; **6**: 339–51.

12 Johnson A. Use of registers in child health. *Archives of Disease in Childhood* 1995; **72**: 474–7.

13 Paneth N. Neonatal care and patterns of disability in the community in obstetrics in the 1990s: current controversies. In: Chard T, Richards MPM eds. *Clinics in developmental medicine* Nos 123–4. London: MacKeith Press, 1992: 232–41.

14 Stanley F, Blair E, Alberman E. Causal pathways to the cerebral palsies: a new aetiological model. In: *Cerebral palsies: epidemiology and causal pathways.* London: MacKeith Press, 2000: 40.

15 Johnson A. Randomised controlled trials in perinatal medicine: 3. Identifying and measuring endpoints in randomised controlled trials. *British Journal of Obstetrics and Gynaecology* 1997; **104**: 768–71.

16 Bax M. Terminology and classification of cerebral palsy. *Developmental Medicine and Child Neurology* 1964; **6**: 295–7.

17 Badawi N, Watson L, Pettersen B *et al*. What constitutes cerebral palsy? *Developmental Medicine and Child Neurology* 1998; **40**: 520–7.

18 SCPE Collaborative Group. Surveillance of Cerebral Palsy in Europe: a European collaboration of cerebral palsy surveys and registers. *Developmental Medicine and Child Neurology* 2000; **42**: 816–24.

19 Evans P, Johnson A, Mutch L, Alberman E. A standard form for recording clinical findings in children with a central motor deficit. *Developmental Medicine and Child Neurology* 1989; **31**: 119–27.

20 Pharoah POD, Cooke T, Johnson A, King R, Mutch L. The epidemiology of cerebral palsy in England and Scotland 1984–89. *Archives of Disease in Childhood* 1998; **79**: F21–F25.

21 Nelson KB. Prenatal origin of hemiparetic cerebral palsy. *Pediatrics* 1991; **88**: 1059–62.

22 Palisano R, Rosenbaum P, Walter S, Russell D, Wood E, Galuppi B. Development and reliability of a system to classify gross motor function in children with cerebral palsy. *Developmental Medicine and Child Neurology* 1997; **39**: 214–23.

23 Colver A, Jessen C. Measurements of health status and quality of life in neonatal follow-up studies. *Seminars in Neonatology* 2000; **5**: 149–58.

24 Hutton JL, Cooke T, Pharoah POD. Life expectancy in children with cerebral palsy. *British Medical Journal* 1994; **309**: 431–5.

25 Evans PM, Evans SJW, Alberman E. Cerebral palsy: why we must plan for survival. *Archives of Disease in Childhood* 1990; **65**: 1329–33.

26 Barabus G, Matthews W, Lumoff P. Care-load for children and young adults with severe cerebral palsy. *Developmental Medicine and Child Neurology* 1992; **34**: 979–84.

27 Stanley F, Blair E, Alberman E. How common are the cerebral palsies? In: *Cerebral palsies: epidemiology and causal pathways*. London: MacKeith Press, 2000: 22.

28 Macgillivray I, Campbell DM. The changing pattern of cerebral palsy in Avon. *Paediatric and Perinatal Epidemiology* 1995; **9**: 146–55.

29 Oxford Register of Early Childhood Impairments. *Annual report*. Oxford: National Perinatal Epidemiology Unit, 1999.

30 Cussen GH, Barry JE, Moloney AM, Crowley MJ. Cerebral palsy in southern Ireland – a population based study 1966–1990. *Paediatric and Perinatal Epidemiology* 1996; **10**: A3.

31 Dolk H, Hill AE, Parkes J. The prevalence of cerebral palsy in Northern Ireland. *Paediatric and Perinatal Epidemiology* 1996; **10**: A3.

32 Topp M, Langhoff-Roos J, Uldall P. Validation of the cerebral palsy register in Denmark. *Paediatric and Perinatal Epidemiology* 1996; **10**: A2.

33 Report of W Australia Cerebral Palsy Register 1999. TVW Telethon Institute for Child Health Research, Perth, Australia.

34 Meberg A, Broch H. A changing pattern of cerebral palsy: declining trend for incidence of cerebral palsy in a 20 year period 1970–89. *Journal of Perinatal Medicine* 1995; **23**: 395–402.

35 Lallo D, Miceli M, Mastroiacovo P, Schirripa G, Perucci CA. Cerebral palsy register in Central Italy: methodology and preliminary results. *Paediatric and Perinatal Epidemiology* 1996; **10**: A1.

36 Kavcic A, Perat MV. Cerebral palsy in Slovenia: an epidemiological overview in children born

1981–1990. *Paediatric and Perinatal Epidemiology* 1996; **10**: A1.

37 Pharoah P, Cooke J, Cooke RW, Rosenbloom L. Birthweight specific trends in cerebral palsy. *Archives of Disease in Childhood* 1990; **65**: 602–6.

38 Hagberg B, Hagberg G, Olow I. The changing panorama of cerebral palsy in Sweden V1. Prevalence and origin in the birth year period 1983–86. *Acta Paediatrica* 1993; **82**: 387–93.

39 Pharoah POD, Cooke T. Cerebral palsy and multiple births. *Archives of Disease in Childhood* 1996; **75**: F174–F177.

40 Petterson B, Nelson KB, Watson L, Stanley FW. Twins, triplets and cerebral palsy in births in Western Australia in the 1980s. *British Medical Journal* 1993; **307**: 1239–42.

41 Grether JK, Nelson KB, Cummins SK. Twinning and cerebral palsy: experience in four northern California counties, births 1983 through 1985. *Pediatrics* 1993; **92**: 854–8.

42 Pharoah POD, Adi Y. Consequnces of in-utero death in a twin pregnancy. *Lancet* 2000; **355**: 1597–602.

43 Pharoah POD, Cooke RWI. A hypothesis for the aetiology of spastic cerebral palsy – the vanishing twin. *Developmental Medicine and Child Neurology* 1997; **39**: 292–6.

44 Dowding VM, Barry C. Cerebral palsy: social class differences in prevalence in relation to birthweight and severity of disability. *Journal of Epidemiology and Community Health* 1990; **44**: 191–5.

45 Dolk H, Parkes J, Hill AE. Cerebral palsy prevalence in relation to socioeconomic deprivation in Northern Ireland. *Paediatric and Perinatal Epidemiology* 1996; **10**: A4.

46 Vrijheid M, Dolk H, Stone D, Abramsky L, Alberman E, Scott JE. Socioeconomic inequalities in risk of congenital anomaly. *Archives of Disease in Childhood* 2000; **82**: 349–52.

47 Murphy DJ, Sellers S, Mackenzie IZ, Yudkin PL, Johnson A. Case-control study of antenatal and intrapartum risk factors for cerebral palsy in very preterm singleton babies. *Lancet* 1995; **346**: 1449–54.

48 Grether JK, Nelson KB. Maternal infection and cerebral palsy in infants of normal birthweight. *Journal of the American Medical Association* 1997; **278**: 207–11.41.

49 Gaffney G, Sellers S, Flavell V, Squier M, Johnson A. Case control study of intrapartum care, cerebral palsy and perinatal death. *British Medical Journal* 1994; **308**: 743–50.

50 Reuss ML, Paneth N, Pinto-Martin JA, Lorenz JM, Susser M. The relation of transient hypothyroxinemia in preterm infants to neurologic development at two years of age. *New England Journal of Medicine* 1996; **334**: 821–7.

51 McLaren J, Brysen SE. Review of recent epidemiological studies of mental retardation: prevalence, associated disorders and etiology. *American Journal of Mental Retardation* 1987; **92**: 243–54.

52 Susser M, Hauser WA, Keily JL. Quantitative estimates of prenatal and perinatal risk factors for perinatal mortality, cerebral palsy, mental retardation and epilepsy. In: Freeman JM ed. *Prenatal and perinatal factors associated with brain disorder*. NIH publication no. 85–1149. Bethesda: US Department of Health and Human Services, Public Health Service, NIH, 1985: 359–432.

53 Nicholson A, Alberman E. Cerebral palsy, an increasing contributor to severe mental retardation. *Archives of Disease in Childhood* 1992; **67**: 1050–5.

54 Middle C, Johnson A, Alderdice F, Petty T, Macfarlane A. Birthweight and health and development at the age of seven years. *Child: Care, Health and Development* 1996; **22**: 55–71.

55 Robertson CM, Finer NN. Term infants with hypoxic-ischaemic encephalopathy: outcome at 3–5 years. *Developmental Medicine and Child Neurology* 1985; **27**: 473–84.

56 Robertson CM, Finer NN, Grace MG. School performance of survivors of neonatal encephalopathy associated with birth asphyxia at term. *Journal of Pediatrics* 1989; **114**: 753–60.

3 Etiology of fetal and neonatal brain damage

Geraldine Gaffney

The evolution of perinatal brain damage remains a perplexing question for those involved in perinatal care. It is of fundamental importance to determine when and how damage to the developing brain occurs. Traditionally, the times at which brain injury has been acquired have been divided into the prenatal, intrapartum, and postnatal periods. This classification still remains useful if somewhat limited.

Unfortunately, brain damage which has potentially been acquired during labor has, until relatively recently, received the greatest attention. This is doubly unfortunate because this approach has deflected attention away from the other times during development when cerebral injury can occur, in addition to encouraging defensive obstetric clinical practice with prohibitive rates of litigation. Historically, the reason for emphasis on the intrapartum period as the time when cerebral injury is most likely to occur is partly due to the fact that the examination of the fetal brain during the prenatal period was almost impossible until the introduction of ultrasound. Thus, the evidence for prelabor or prenatal brain injury could only be made by inference. Despite this limitation, as early as 1897 Freud suggested that prenatal influences might play a role in the development of cerebral impairment when he stated that 'Since the process of birth

frequently produces no effect…diplegia still might be of congenital origin. Difficult birth in itself in certain cases is merely a symptom of deeper effects that influenced the development of the fetus.'

Therefore, it is logical to suppose that the prenatal period might be a likely time of origin of cerebral injury, particularly when a comparison is made between the long period of time of gestation in which intrauterine cerebral development occurs and the relatively short time that the fetus is exposed to the forces of labor.

The feasibility of direct examination of the brain of both the preterm fetus and preterm neonate was assisted by parallel developments in obstetrics and pediatrics, in particular the development of ultrasound imaging of the fetal and neonatal brain. As expertise was gained in the use of cerebral ultrasound, it was appreciated that the brains of the preterm fetus and neonate differed from those of the term infant and, in particular, injury produced a different pattern of hemorrhagic and ischemic cerebral lesions. Concurrently, epidemiological studies began to show that not all perinatal brain injury could be attributed to insults during labor. Other work demonstrated that prenatal exposure to a variety of noxious substances could adversely alter brain development. Ultimately, the notion that brain injury may occur both prior to and independent of the intrapartum period became accepted.

Bax used the following definition of cerebral palsy, which gives a key to understanding the development of perinatally acquired cerebral injury: 'Cerebral palsy is an umbrella term which covers a group of non-progressive, but often changing, motor impairment syndromes secondary to lesions or abnormalities of the brain arising early in its development.'[1]

Thus, the developing brain should be viewed as being in a state of constant change, subject to a constantly changing environment that may be either adverse or beneficial. Clearly, the brain is vulnerable to injury throughout this process, but the type of injury that results will depend on when and how that injury occurred.[2] Consequently, the pattern of impairment may give clues to the likely time of origin of the original insult. For example, spastic diplegia is commonly associated with preterm infants where ischemic injury to the periventricular area leads to damage of the motor tracts to the lower limbs. Pathological or radiological examination of the brains of fetuses who later develop signs of cerebral injury may be of enormous help in determining etiology.[3]

Not all children with brain injury acquired in the perinatal period will be amenable to either radiological or pathological examination. Furthermore, examination may not reveal any cause for injury. An alternative approach to identifying fetuses at risk of perinatal cerebral injury is to examine the associated features of pregnancies from which children have later evidence of cerebral injury. It is important that the limitations of association are taken into account, in particular that association does not imply causation. However, in demonstrating factors associated with brain injury a line of inquiry may be opened which may lead to later proof of causation.

The clinical manifestations of perinatally acquired cerebral injury may be very diverse. In the following discussion antecedent factors that have been identified are related to the later development of cerebral palsy. While cerebral palsy is a clear manifestation of cerebral injury acquired during the perinatal period, it is not the only one. Perinatal injury may be so severe as to lead to death *in utero* or in the early neonatal period, or conversely, so slight that it may produce only subtle neurological changes in later life. Equally, some of the syndromes leading to later intellectual and motor impairment may result from injury to the developing fetal brain, yet these syndromes may be excluded from the definition of cerebral palsy.

This classification is under constant change, however, as a number of clinical syndromes previously categorized as cerebral palsy have been shown to have a genetic or metabolic basis. The genetics of cerebral palsy will be discussed in Chapter 5, but these genetically based syndromes could be viewed as a form of injury to the programming of cerebral development at the earliest possible stage.

3.1 ASSESSMENT OF INTRAUTERINE ETIOLOGY

Adverse effects on the prenatal intrauterine environment may be responsible for early brain injury. It is a reasonable assumption that children with cerebral injury of perinatal origin are more likely to have been born following pregnancies that were more complicated than children with normal development. However, direct evidence of intrauterine injury may be difficult to obtain apart from in a minority of cases. Furthermore, some individuals have greater predisposition to obstetric complications because of pre-existing disease, making their pregnancies more susceptible to adverse prenatal influences. Studies that have addressed this issue have found several associated factors, which have emerged consistently as being associated with cerebral palsy.

The largest of the prospective epidemiological studies to address the question of risk factors for cerebral palsy was the National Collaborative Perinatal Project (NCPP) of the National Institute of Neurological and Communicative Disorders and Stroke which examined over 57 000 pregnancies. This study examined approximately 400 maternal characteristics, and features found to be positively associated with cerebral palsy were subjected to both univariate and multivariate analysis.[4,5] Naeye analysed a subgroup of the data from the Collaborative Perinatal Study (CPS) of the National Institute of Neurological and Communicative Disorders and Stroke, confining his analysis to 43 437 term pregnancies.[6] In a study of 19 044 children monitored in California, cerebral palsy was identified in 0.2 percent. These children were compared with the rest of the group in order to identify clinical antecedents.[7] In these studies, which examined children born at all gestational ages, adjustment was made for the increased risk of low birthweight. However, some of these studies do not differentiate between low birthweight that occurs as a consequence of prematurity and low birthweight that occurs as a consequence of intra-uterine growth retardation. A failure to make this distinction may confound any true associations that have been found.[8]

Large prospective studies are an ideal method in theory, but in practice they are hindered by the long time required for follow-up. Therefore retro-spective case–control studies may provide a more amenable alternative. Furthermore, case–control studies allow specific groups to be examined in more detail – term infants only, for example. A number of case–control studies exist that look at risk factors for specific groups of children with cerebral palsy. Children with spastic cerebral palsy in Western Australia were examined for ante-cedent factors and a variety of factors were identi-fied as being more frequent among the 315 children with cerebral palsy.[9] Using cases identi-fied by the Oxford Register of Cerebral Palsy, 141 term infants with cerebral palsy were examined in a matched case–control study for antecedent and intrapartum factors.[10] In order to address the associated features of prematurity, 59 children born before 33 weeks gestation with cerebral palsy were examined for antenatal and postnatal antecedents.[11,12] A number of characteristics have been found based on the findings of these studies that are associated with cerebral palsy. These will be discussed in the following sections.

3.2 MATERNAL FACTORS

It might be expected that mothers of children with cerebral palsy might differ in some way that predisposes their children to intrauterine cerebral injury. This may be addressed from both a patho-logical and environmental perspective. Does pre-existing maternal disease contribute to a poor intrauterine environment or are some mothers more prone to experiencing adverse external influ-ences that may predispose to poor intrauterine conditions?

3.2.1 Family history

Familial patterns among children with cerebral palsy have contributed to and initiated the concept that there might be a genetic basis for cerebral palsy. It has been estimated that about 2 percent of cases of cerebral palsy may have an underlying genetic mechanism.[13] The genetics of cerebral palsy syndromes will be dealt with in detail in Chapter 5 and therefore will not be entered into in great detail here. However, it is worth considering familial groups of cerebral palsy briefly.

Ataxic cerebral palsy accounts for a small pro-portion of cerebral palsy – approximately 6.4 per-cent in the Oxford region.[14] However, between a third and a half of cases of ataxic cerebral palsy may show a familial pattern, usually with reces-sive inheritance but occasionally with a dominant and X-linked pattern.[15] A variety of syndromes are represented among cases of ataxic cerebral palsy, such as Joubert's, Marinesco-Sjögren, Gillespie's, and Behr's, familial cerebellar ataxia, and mental retardation or as part of a metabolic disorder such as metachromatic leukodystrophy.

Familial groups with either spastic diplegia or quadriplegia occur less frequently. A recurrence risk of approximately 10 percent has been esti-mated and familial grouping is more likely in those in whom there are additional problems such as mental handicap, seizure disorder, consanguin-ity, and asymmetrical motor signs. Consanguinity may be particularly important for some sections of the community, in particular in those ethnic groups where consanguineous marriage is cus-tomary. Sinha and colleagues estimated individual rates of cerebral palsy within the Bradford area of the UK.[16] Rates of cerebral palsy for Asian families differed significantly from those for non-Asian families (5.48 per 1000 versus 3.18 per 1000). The Asian families had a 51.7 percent rate of consan-guineous marriage, and 31 percent had a sibling or first-degree relative who was affected by a motor disorder. Finally, in an interesting study by Foley it was found that 93 percent of the children born to a parent with cerebral palsy had normal develop-ment and that obstetric complications did not occur more frequently among the mothers with cerebral palsy.[17] None of the large prospective studies was able to report a familial association with cerebral palsy. However, intellectual impair-ment was found to occur more frequently among the mothers and siblings of those with cerebral palsy.[4,7]

In the Oxford Register of children with cerebral palsy, there were 41 term infants born between 1984 and 1987 who were excluded from the case–control study because of a presumed prenatal cause for cerebral palsy based on the presence of a major associated congenital anomaly, a known pattern of inheritance, or family history of cerebral palsy. There were two sibling pairs among these 41 children. A further six children were felt to have a probable genetic foundation for their cerebral

Table 3.1 List of 15 children in whom there was a possible genetic component for cerebral palsy

1	Adrenoleukodystrophy[a]
2	Adrenoleukodystrophy[a]
3	Non-ketotic hyperglycinemia[a]
4	Non-ketotic hyperglycinemia[a]
5	Autosomal recessive microcephaly
6	Autosomal recessive microcephaly
7	X-linked microcephaly
8	Autosomal dominant spastic paraplegia
9	Incontinentia pigmenti (X-linked dominant)
10	X-linked spastic quadriplegia
11	Batten's disease
12	Phosphoglycerate kinase deficiency
13	Pyridoxine-dependent seizure disorder
14	Angelman's syndrome
15	Aicardi syndrome

[a]Sibling pairs.

palsy based on a Mendelian pattern of inheritance. Finally, there were a further five children in whom a specific genetic defect was known, giving a total of 15 out of 41 (37 percent) in whom a possible or proven genetic component was present (Table 3.1). Consanguinity or a family history of mental handicap was not more frequent among this small group.

3.2.2   Reproductive performance

Lilienfield and Pasamanick introduced the phrase 'the continuum of reproductive casualty' which included cerebral palsy as part of the spectrum from early pregnancy loss to perinatal death.[18] They suggested that this spectrum of reproductive loss was the consequence of the same disease process. Thus, the previous reproductive history and reproductive interval were of interest as potential etiological factors in those who had children with cerebral palsy.

The assumption that previous poor outcomes from pregnancy precede a pregnancy resulting in cerebral palsy supports the notion of a hostile intrauterine environment. It is important, however, that a consistent definition of previous poor pregnancy outcome is used. Most studies that have examined this question have defined previous poor obstetric performance as pregnancies that have led to intrauterine fetal loss, neonatal death, or the birth of siblings with cerebral impairment. However, many of these conditions may occur as a consequence of a multiplicity of etiological factors and it is possible that these families are victims of unfortunate coincidence rather than of a single mechanism that leads to reproductive casualty. Another

problem which may confound the definition of poor reproductive performance is the inclusion of women in this group who have experienced one or more previous first trimester spontaneous abortions. Many early spontaneous abortions are undetected or unreported and thus precise ascertainment of early pregnancy loss may not be possible. Studies examining the association of subfertility with cerebral palsy may have been conducted at a time when there was limited medical help available for those with fertility problems. Consequently, this definition may not carry much weight by present-day standards. Other reproductive factors that have been examined are the interval between pregnancies, maternal age at the time of the affected pregnancy, and a history of subfertility.

Bearing the limitations of these possible associated characteristics in mind, a number of associations have been found between reproductive performance and later cerebral palsy. Women whose children developed cerebral palsy were more likely to have 'unusual pregnancy intervals' defined as being either less than 3 months or greater than 3 years between pregnancies.[7] An association was also found between cerebral palsy and maternal menstrual cycles of more than 36 days.[7] This association persisted when subjected to multivariate analysis. The NCPP also demonstrated an association between abnormally long menstrual cycles and cerebral palsy.[5] Poor reproductive performance manifest as previous spontaneous abortion and intrauterine fetal death was found to be more frequent among the mothers of children with cerebral palsy in the NCPP study.[5]

In the Oxford case–control study of 141 term singleton infants with cerebral palsy, poor obstetric history was defined as a previous intrauterine death, previous spontaneous abortion at greater than or equal to 15 weeks gestation, two or more spontaneous abortions at any gestation, previous neonatal death, previous live child with disability or handicap related to perinatal asphyxia, or previous premature delivery. No increased incidence of subfertility or previous poor obstetric history was found among the mothers of children with cerebral palsy in comparison with their matched controls.[10]

3.2.3   Pre-existing maternal disease

Maternal disease present during pregnancy may create an adverse environment that may impair fetal development and lead to direct or indirect injury to the fetus. Nelson found that maternal mental retardation, seizures, and hyperthyroidism occurred more frequently among mothers of children with cerebral palsy.[4] Furthermore, prenatal exposure to thyroid and estrogen hormones, and in particular exposure to both, was also found to be associated with cerebral palsy on univariate analysis. More recently, both maternal hypothyroidism and hyperthyroidism have been associated with the development of neonatal encephalopathy.[19] The possible mechanism for this association has been postulated to be similar to the effects of congenital hypothyroidism on intellectual development.[20]

However, when these associations were subjected to multivariate analysis the only characteristic which remained significant was maternal mental retardation.[5] This may reflect an underlying genetic predisposition to neurological dysfunction, or alternatively may reflect the fact that mothers with mental handicap are more likely to experience social disadvantage and are thus more prone to preterm delivery with higher rates of neurological impairment.

These associations were not demonstrated among either term or preterm infants in the Oxford study of cerebral palsy.[10] However, this may be accounted for by the fact that individually, these factors occurred with relative infrequency among the mothers of the children in this group. In order to overcome the problem of various characteristics occurring infrequently, a number of maternal diseases were grouped together and defined by existing maternal disease at the time of the index pregnancy as 'chronic hypertension, renal disease with abnormal biochemical, radiological features, diabetes or other chronic disease'. Using this definition it was found that 'existing maternal disease' was more frequent among mothers with cerebral palsy children born at term, but not those with cerebral palsy born preterm.[10,11] Using a similar definition, 'existing maternal disease' was also found to occur more frequently in the study of children with cerebral palsy born in California.[7]

3.2.4 Maternal infection during pregnancy

The association between infection and the development of cerebral injury has not yet been fully elucidated but is proving to be an extremely fertile area of enquiry. The evidence for an association between maternal infection during pregnancy and cerebral injury has been supported by epidemiological and pathological evidence. A proportion of pregnancies that result in intrauterine or early neonatal death will show postmortem evidence of fetal prenatal white matter ischemic damage.[21–24] This has been shown to occur in between 8 and 20 percent of pregnancies examined. When the clinical antecedents of prenatal white matter damage are examined, a strong association is shown between both maternal infection during pregnancy and neonatal infection in those that survived until after delivery.[21,23]

A similar study of clinical antecedents of a series of babies with prenatally acquired ischemic white matter damage was unable to confirm this association with either maternal or neonatal infection.[25] In addition, among the Oxford cohort of term infants with cerebral palsy no association was found between maternal or neonatal infection and cerebral palsy.[10] The lack of association with infection in this group may have been due to the diversity of both the type and severity of infection in these mothers and the relative infrequency of maternal infection. However, when the clinical antecedents of the group of preterm infants who formed part of the Oxford group were examined, a number of characteristics connected with prenatal infection were found to be associated with cerebral palsy: prolonged premature rupture of membranes, chorioamnionitis, and maternal infection.[11] Furthermore, neonatal sepsis was also found to be present more frequently among the cases of cerebral palsy than their age-matched controls, independent of the presence of antenatal infection.[12] An increased exposure to intrauterine infection has also been shown to occur in children of both low and normal birthweight who develop cerebral palsy among cases on the Southern Californian register.[26,27]

Several authors have postulated a mechanism for the development of white matter cerebral damage associated with infection.[28–30] Infection leads to a release of inflammatory cytokines which, in turn, leads to release of prostaglandins that stimulate the myometrium and lead to preterm labor. Cerebral white matter damage or periventricular leukomalacia is the most significant form of associated cerebral injury and is estimated to carry an 80 percent chance of later permanent neurological impairment.[31] The inflammatory cytokines have been implicated in the development of cerebral injury, especially in the development of white matter cerebral injury. Evidence for cytokine-mediated damage is both indirect and direct. Astrocytes are the precursors of glial cells, the scar-forming tissue of the developing brain. Astrocyte activation occurs almost universally in response to cerebral injury but the mechanism of activation is only partially understood. Selmaj and co-workers demonstrated astrocyte proliferation *in vivo* as a consequence of stimulation by interleukins.[32] Mice that are genetically interleukin 6 (IL-6) deficient do not produce activated astrocytes in response to injury.[33]

Increased levels of the inflammatory cytokines, especially IL-6, have been found in maternal blood, amniotic fluid, and the placental tissue of infants with chorioamnionitis and preterm labor.[34] Postmortem examination of the brain of infants has shown increased expression of tumor necrosis factor and IL-6 in those with evidence of periventricular leukomalacia.[35] Furthermore, elevated IL-6 levels have been demonstrated in the amniotic fluid and umbilical cord blood of preterm neonates with ultrasound evidence of white matter damage.[36,37] There was evidence of neurodevelopmental delay among these preterm infants at the age of one year. However, due to small numbers studied the findings failed to reach statistical significance. IL-6 is the cytokine that correlates best with later perinatal events, but the behavior of the other cytokines in perinatal infection and preterm delivery varies. Not all of the inflammatory cytokines lead to cerebral injury and indeed some cytokines may exert a protective role on the developing brain. Interleukin-1 receptor antagonist (IL-1ra) has been shown to protect against ischemic cerebral injury in animal studies.[38,39] IL-1ra is not elevated in the cord blood of preterm neonates who develop white matter injury.[40]

This association of infection and later cerebral injury is of interest as debate exists about the value of treating women with both preterm labor and preterm rupture of membranes with prophylactic antibiotics. Systematic review by the Cochrane collaboration of trials of antibiotics in preterm labor or following premature rupture of membranes has demonstrated benefit in terms of prolongation of pregnancy but not in terms of neonatal morbidity and mortality.[41,42] The ORACLE multicenter randomized controlled trial has completed and shows that there is no evidence to support the use of prophylactic antibiotics in premature labor with intact membranes, but that erythromycin may offer benefit where there has been prelabor preterm rupture of membranes.[43,44] The trial will go on to evaluate long-term cerebral development amongst the babies of study participants.

An understanding of the role of infection and the inflammatory mediators produced by infection in the development of cerebral palsy in the preterm infant will undoubtedly lead to greater understanding of the mechanism of causation of cerebral injury and may lead to the ability to devise preventative strategies. However, will it be sufficient to treat amniotic fluid infection with antimicrobial treatment to eliminate the neurological effects of infection? This pertinent question was asked in a recent editorial in the *Journal of the American Medical Association* where it was also suggested that treatment to suppress the immunological effects of infection might also be required.[45] The editorial questioned the effect of the large immunosuppressive doses of antenatal steroids that are administered to the fetus at risk of preterm delivery in suppressing these inflammatory mediators. Certainly, there is evidence that neonates born following antenatal steroids have better neurological outcomes than their untreated counterparts, but the assumption is that this is through the consequent reduction in respiratory distress syndrome.[46]

3.3 OBSTETRIC FACTORS

Just as the presence of adverse maternal conditions may lead to a hostile intrauterine environment, conditions specific to pregnancy could also contribute to the development of poor intrauterine conditions. In this section conditions specific to pregnancy which have been examined in relation to the development of cerebral palsy will be discussed. Adverse events that might occur during labor and delivery will not be considered in this section.

3.3.1 Multiple pregnancy

The possibility of multiple pregnancy leading to cerebral injury during intrauterine life has much to support it in terms of biological and epidemiological plausibility. The rate of cerebral palsy among twins on the Western Australian register was increased eight-fold among twin pregnancies and was increased by a factor of 47 among triplet pregnancies.[47] An increased rate was also found among twins born in the North East Thames Region of the UK where the rate of cerebral palsy was 7.6 per 1000 infant survivors compared with 1.0 per 1000 singleton infant survivors.[48] In Merseyside the rate among twins was 12.6 per 1000 infant survivors compared with 1.0 per 1000 singleton survivors.[49]

Multiple pregnancy predisposes to an increased rate of preterm delivery, lower than average birthweight and more complicated labor and delivery, all of which are independent risk factors for the development of cerebral palsy. However, additional characteristics specific to multiple pregnancy found to occur more frequently among multiples who develop cerebral palsy are monochorionicity, the presence of abnormal vascular placental connections and the death of one twin *in utero*.[47,50] Abnormal placentation may also lead to developmental abnormalities of the umbilical cord and the development of arteriovenous or arterioarterial anastomoses.[51] These risk factors – monochorionicity, abnormal vascular anastomoses, death *in utero* of one twin – may, in reality, represent different manifestations of the same pathology, twin-to-twin or fetofetal transfusion syndrome.

Monochorionic twins represent 1 percent of all twin pregnancies and 15 percent of these will develop abnormal vascular anastomoses leading to the twin-to-twin or fetofetal transfusion syndrome.[52] Here, blood is shunted from the donor twin to the recipient causing potential problems in both. The donor twin becomes anemic and growth retarded and the recipient twin polycythemic with polyhydramnios. If this progresses to the worst end of the spectrum – the 'stuck twin' syndrome – a high untreated mortality rate occurs. Here, the donor twin exhibits almost complete anhydramnios and is extremely growth retarded; the recipient has polyhydramnios and ascites. The most effective treatment for this condition is debated; traditionally, large-volume serial amniocentesis is used to alleviate polyhydramnios in the recipient and, through adjustment of intra-amniotic pressures, the liquor volume between both gestation sacs is equated. The treated survival rate of 'stuck twins' was found to be 69 percent using serial amniocentesis compared with an untreated survival rate of 16 percent.[53] More recently, laser ablation of placental vascular connections between the twins has been promoted.[54] The incidence of neurological morbidity occurring as a consequence of twin-to-twin transfusion syndrome is difficult to estimate. Clearly, confounding factors such as the gestation at which delivery occurs and the effect of any intrauterine treatment must be considered.

The introduction of early pregnancy ultrasound has established that many singleton pregnancies were, in fact, early twin pregnancies in which spontaneous intrauterine death of one twin has occurred. A suggestion that this 'vanishing twin' phenomenon may also be accompanied by additional neurological morbidity is currently under investigation.[55]

Children with cerebral palsy from multiple pregnancies are relatively rare; there were only two such children on the Oxford Register from the period 1984–1987. An international register of twin pregnancies where at least one twin has developed cerebral impairment has been instituted by Petterson and her colleagues in Western Australia. This should help considerably in addressing the specific issues that relate to this group of children.

3.3.2 Antepartum hemorrhage

Antepartum hemorrhage may occur from a low-lying placenta, from placental separation or, rarely, from abnormally sited vessels in the placenta – vasa praevia. In practice, the cause of bleeding during pregnancy is often unknown. However, there is a tendency, which may or may not be justified, to regard pregnancies with small recurrent bleeds as carrying extra risk of adverse outcome. The underlying theory is that small recurrent bleeds may represent clinically undetectable placental separation that may compromise placental function.

Precise definition is a problem when categorizing antepartum hemorrhage. It is notoriously difficult to estimate accurately the amount of blood lost at the time of hemorrhage, therefore attempts to classify hemorrhage into categories such as moderate and severe must be dogged by inaccuracy. In the Oxford Register study of term infants antepartum hemorrhage was classified as being either simply present or sufficient to require maternal resuscitation. No association was demonstrated between either of these two categories of antepartum hemorrhage and later cerebral palsy. However, Torfs found that premature placental separation was almost eight times more frequent among children who developed cerebral palsy.[7] Dale and Stanley also found an association between antepartum hemorrhage and cases of cerebral palsy in Western Australia.[9]

3.3.3 Intrauterine growth retardation and oligohydramnios

Intrauterine growth restriction (IUGR) is defined as a birthweight of less than 2 standard deviations below the mean. Traditionally, IUGR is classified as being either symmetric or asymmetric, the latter being associated with placental insufficiency. Symmetric growth restriction is thought to reflect early influences on fetal growth and is more commonly associated with congenital abnormality, intrauterine infection, or early exposure to toxins.

In order to detect intrauterine growth problems during pregnancy, fetal growth is estimated from measurements of the fetal head circumference, abdominal circumferences, and the femur length. Standardized growth charts have been derived, such as those appropriate for the UK.[56] Fetuses below the 5th percentile or who deviate from their initial percentile are assumed to have IUGR. However, the most concrete estimate of IUGR is the actual birthweight, as prenatal estimates are made by inference and may be inaccurate due to intra- and inter-observer measurement error.

A number of problems beset the diagnosis of IUGR. First, as discussed above, the diagnosis is based on assessment of fetal growth by ultrasound using parameters that may be subject to measurement error. Secondly, it is important that assessment of fetal size takes constitutional and ethnic influences into account. Thirdly, when placental insufficiency is severe, both symmetric and asymmetric reduction of the fetal head and abdominal circumference may occur. Finally, fetal growth parameters may be normal or above average initially but growth impairment may develop later, still remaining above the 5th percentile, and may thus be overlooked.

Problems exist for the studies that attempt to relate IUGR and neurodevelopmental outcome. Many early studies of fetal growth in relation to cerebral palsy failed to differentiate low birthweight of prematurity from true IUGR where the fetus is small for gestational age. It is also possible to miss the diagnosis of IUGR, as at present there is no useful antenatal screening test widely accepted for the detection of fetuses with IUGR. Thus, detection is a matter of clinical suspicion, previous reproductive performance, and opportunism.

Oligohydramnios is usually seen in conjunction with IUGR due to placental insufficiency. Here, impaired fetal circulation leads to poor fetal renal perfusion and reduced fetal urinary output in combination with impaired placental production of amniotic fluid. Oligohydramnios is defined as a measurement of a pool of amniotic fluid of less than 2 cm on ultrasound examination.

Fetuses with IUGR are thought to be at greater risk of death *in utero* and other obstetric complications, such as fetal distress in labor. IUGR and pre-eclampsia frequently occur together as a manifestation of poor placental function. Pre-eclampsia occurs secondary to abnormal development of the placental vasculature that leads to both systemic maternal and fetal vascular endothelial injury.[57] This causes a reduction in the supply of oxygenated blood to the fetus and impairment of fetal growth results. However, IUGR may also

occur in isolation. Fetuses with IUGR are also more prone to preterm delivery, including iatrogenic preterm delivery undertaken because of severe accompanying maternal disease. Thus, when addressing the question of whether IUGR is an independent factor in the development of fetal cerebral injury it is important that the confounding variables of prematurity and coexisting maternal disease are addressed. It may be difficult, particularly in older studies, to obtain accurate data regarding gestational age, especially before there was routine early ultrasound to help confirm or readjust inaccurate menstrual data.

It is biologically plausible that IUGR should be associated with fetal cerebral injury. Fetuses with IUGR have been shown to be both hypoxic and acidotic on analysis of fetal blood samples obtained *in utero*. Limited data support a reduced developmental quotient in these infants at 18 months of age.[58] Doppler velocimetry of the cerebral circulation of fetuses with IUGR has shown that the fetus initially compensates for this state of relative hypoxia by increasing cerebral blood flow.[59] Ultimately, when the fetus can no longer compensate for its adverse environment, the cerebral circulation becomes one of high resistance, presumably with hypoperfusion of the fetal circulation. Among our own study of the clinical antecedents of prenatal white matter ischemic damage found at postmortem, those with white matter damage were more likely to have had a birthweight less than 2 standard deviations below the mean for gestational age.[25]

Among children with cerebral palsy in Sweden, the association between intrauterine growth retardation and cerebral palsy was found among term (greater than or equal to 37 weeks) and moderately preterm infants (34–36 weeks), but not among preterm infants (28–33 weeks).[60] Among children born in Western Australia there was an increased risk of the birthweight being below both the 3rd and 10th percentiles among children with cerebral palsy. When examined by gestational age this association persisted for term infants, was strongest for infants born between 34 and 37 weeks gestation but was lost among those infants born at less than 34 weeks gestation.[61] In the Oxford studies, children with cerebral palsy born at term were more likely to have had IUGR. This was defined as a birthweight of less than 2500 g in term infants, which occurred in 10 percent of cases and less than 2 percent of controls.[10] However, no association was found in children with cerebral palsy who were born at less than 32 completed weeks of gestation in Oxford between a birthweight of less than 2 standard deviations for gestational age and cerebral palsy.[11]

We speculated whether the association between cerebral palsy and growth retardation among term infants might reflect different etiological pathways among this group of children with cerebral palsy. We hypothesized that those children whose cerebral palsy might have originated in the prenatal period due to chronic intrauterine compromise might be more likely to exhibit IUGR as a manifestation of this compromise. These children were more likely to have had an uncomplicated intrapartum and neonatal course. In contrast, children who experienced neonatal or hypoxic-ischemic encephalopathy at the time of delivery were more likely to have had an acute intrapartum origin for cerebral palsy and thus were unlikely to have growth problems as a manifestation of the insult that they had experienced. We compared the birthweight and head circumference of these two groups but were unable to support the hypothesis as no difference was found between them. Among 141 cases with cerebral palsy, 41 children had evidence of neonatal encephalopathy, 100 children did not. A birthweight of less than the 10th percentile for gestation age was found among 8 of 41 (19.5 percent) of those who had encephalopathy – cerebral palsy and 18 of 100 (18 percent) of those who did not, which was not statistically different. Nor was there a statistical difference between a head circumference of less than the 10th percentile which was found in 9 of 41 (22.0 percent) of those with encephalopathy and 19 of 100 (19.0 percent) of those with no encephalopathy.[62] Thus we were unable to support this hypothesis with the data from our cohort of term infants with cerebral palsy.

In conclusion, children with cerebral palsy are more likely to be growth retarded at birth than children without at gestational ages of greater than 34 weeks. This is true for a child with cerebral palsy in whom major congenital anomaly has been excluded. This association is lost in infants with cerebral palsy who are born at an earlier gestational age. The mechanism by which cerebral palsy develops in the growth-retarded fetus is unclear, although mechanisms that lead to chronic intrauterine hypoxia are implicated.

3.3.4 Pre-eclampsia and magnesium sulfate

In contrast to the association of IUGR with cerebral palsy, a number of studies have shown a protective effect of maternal pre-eclampsia against cerebral palsy. In the Oxford case–control study of children with cerebral palsy who were born before 32 completed weeks of gestation there was a negative association between cerebral palsy and pre-eclampsia. This was also found by Nelson and co-workers among cases of cerebral palsy born prematurely in Southern California.[63] In this study, this finding was attributed to maternal exposure to magnesium sulfate used to treat pre-eclampsia. However, magnesium sulfate was not used to treat pre-eclampsia at the time that the Oxford cases were born, therefore an alternative explanation for the possible protective effect of maternal pre-eclampsia must be sought. This is particularly pertinent as pre-eclampsia frequently produces fetal compromise manifest as IUGR, which is associated with cerebral palsy. One possible explanation is that these infants were born after a period of maternal hospitalization, which permitted administration of antenatal steroids to promote fetal lung maturity. The administration of antenatal steroids has been shown to have a negative association with later cerebral palsy.[46] Furthermore, it is likely that the infants of mothers with pre-eclampsia had timed elective delivery by cesarean section. Delivery before the onset of labor was found to carry a protective effect against cerebral palsy among the preterm infants born in the Oxford study.[11] However, this explanation is purely supposition and does not explain the conflicting associations with cerebral palsy of different manifestations of the same disease process.

In contrast, among term infants, pre-eclampsia was found to occur more frequently among mothers whose children developed cerebral palsy in the Oxford term infant study.[10] Severe pre-eclampsia was defined as the presence of significant proteinuria, an untreated diastolic blood pressure of 110 mmHg or abnormal liver biochemistry. Severe pre-eclampsia occurred in 8.6 percent of cases and only 2.4 percent of controls, almost four times more frequently among cases. Severe proteinuria was also identified by Nelson in the NCPP study as being significantly associated with babies of over 2500 g with cerebral palsy on both univariate and multivariate analysis.[4,5]

3.4 FETAL FACTORS

Much of the early epidemiological work on cerebral palsy concentrated on the effect of external influences on the fetus and, in particular, the influence of labor on the fetus. Recently, there has been greater awareness of the fact that many fetuses become neurologically abnormal during intrauterine

Table 3.2   List of children with a prenatal cause for cerebral palsy

1		**Circulatory disorders**
	i	Vein of Galen aneurysm
	ii	Hydranencephaly
	iii	Gross cerebral hemiatrophy
	iv	Basilar artery occlusion
	v	Hydrocephalus secondary to cerebral infarction
	vi	Porencephalic cyst
	vii	Porencephalic cyst
2		**Syndromes**
	viii	Joubert's syndrome
	ix	Joubert's syndrome
	x	Walker-Clodius syndrome
	xi	Prune belly syndrome
	xii	Cerebral palsy with associated imperforate anus, renal and vertebral anomalies (VATER variant)
3		**Congenital infection**
	xiii	Cytomegalovirus
	xiv	Cytomegalovirus
	xv	Varicella
4		**Structural cerebral anomalies**
	xvi	Neuronal migration disorder
	xvii	Walker-Warburg syndrome
	xviii	Common ventricular system with cerebral atrophy
	xix	Absent corpus callosum
	xx	Microcephaly
	xxi	Hydrocephalus secondary to aqueduct stenosis
	xxii	Hydrocephalus with shunt
	xxiii	Occipital encephalocele
	xxiv	Meningomyelocele with hydrocephalus
	xxv	Meningomyelocele with hydrocephalus
5		**Miscellaneous**
	xxvi	Congenital oligodendroma

development. The improved ability to identify underlying disorders in children with cerebral palsy has been due to advances in the understanding of genetic and metabolic disorders, and not least to the contribution of more accurate neuroimaging in identifying cerebral abnormality which has been previously only amenable to postmortem examination.

The range of underlying disorders that may be found in a single population of cerebral palsy is enormous and, with continuing improvements in the accuracy of diagnosis, is likely to increase. Consequently, there are a number of disorders that probably should no longer remain included on registers of cerebral palsy. However, as diagnosis of these disorders is inconsistent between populations of children with cerebral palsy, the removal of these conditions in an erratic way from registers of cerebral palsy could lead to distortion of the rates of cerebral palsy within populations. Thus, in an attempt to maintain consistency of case ascertainment, the Western Australia cerebral palsy register has published an extensive list of cases which should and should not be included on registers of cerebral palsy.[64]

In Oxford, within the population of term infants with cerebral palsy, there were 41 children who were felt to have a 'prenatal' cause for their disorder. A description of 15 of these 41 cases is outlined in Table 3.1. The remaining 26 cases are described in Table 3.2. The cases have been grouped roughly into arbitrary subcategories that will be discussed to indicate the principal types of fetal disorder found.

3.4.1   Circulatory disorders in the fetus

Prenatal cerebral injuries secondary to circulatory disturbance and vascular malformations have been well described in the fetus.[65-71] A variety of lesions have been reported, including parenchymal hemorrhage, intraventricular and choroid plexus hemorrhage, subdural hemorrhage, and porencephaly. Few definite precipitating causes can be identified for fetal intracranial hemorrhage. These include fetal hemorrhagic problems such as allo-immune thrombocytopenia or exposure to maternal drugs such as warfarin and aspirin. Cerebrovascular accident has also been well described in the first few days of life, although often in association with trauma or asphyxia during delivery.[72–74] Many of the precipitating factors for prenatal circulatory disorders are not known, and these events may have occurred following single, short-lived episodes of maternal or fetal hypoperfusion.

Vergani and colleagues described six cases of fetal intracranial hemorrhage diagnosed by prenatal ultrasound and reviewed a further 36 cases identified from the literature.[75] They reported a variety of intracerebral lesions: parenchymal hemorrhage, choroid plexus hemorrhage and porencephaly. They attempted to ascribe a prognosis on the basis of the type of hemorrhage found and found that parenchymal hemorrhage was associated with poor outcome, whereas intraventricular hemorrhage had a reasonably good outcome with survivors developing normally or with minimal neurological impairment.

Among the 41 term infants with cerebral palsy and associated congenital anomaly on the Oxford Register, seven children were felt to have had an underlying vascular cause responsible for cerebral palsy. These seven children are described further in Table 3.2 (cases i–vii). Most of the underlying causes are rare and occur in isolation.

Vascular occlusive events were felt to be responsible for cerebral palsy in three cases. Here, the affected occluded vessel was determined from the resulting area of cerebral damage. The area of cerebral damage corresponds to the territory supplied by the vessel and the degree of subsequent cerebral impairment will depend on the importance of the vessel that has been occluded. The second case was one of hydranencephaly, which is felt to occur from obstruction of the carotid vessels early in gestation leading to secondary disruption of the developing cerebral hemispheres. In the third case gross cerebral hemiatrophy may have also occurred as a consequence of early vascular disruption. In the fourth case, the cerebral tissue loss corresponded to the distribution of the basilar artery. The precipitating events for these vaso-occlusive phenomena in early pregnancy are not understood. There were two cases of porencephalic cysts among the seven cases of circulatory disorder (cases vi and vii). Porencephalic

cysts occur as a consequence of cavitation of necrotic cerebral tissue following an ischemic insult. They are differentiated from other cystic lesions by being single, unilateral, and unlikely to disappear.[76]

Other forms of ischemic injury may occur prenatally. Periventricular leukomalacia (PVL) is the classic form of white matter ischemic injury that occurs typically in the preterm neonate.[77] PVL covers a spectrum from mild gliosis or scarring to multicystic encephalopathy. The latter carries an almost inevitable outcome of neurological handicap, but the outcome for milder forms is not so clear.[78–80] Conventionally, PVL was thought to occur solely in the postnatal period. However, in a retrospective study of children with cerebral palsy, infants born at term without a history of birth asphyxia were shown to have lesions typical of PVL on magnetic resonance imaging.[81] The lesions in these children must have occurred prenatally as injury at term does not produce lesions typical of PVL.

3.4.2   Infection

The effects of maternal infection on the preterm fetus, including amniotic fluid infection as a possible mechanism for the development of white matter injury, have been discussed in detail in Section 3.2.4. However the developing brain itself may be subject to primary early intrauterine infection which is known to cause developmental abnormalities with residual neurological damage.

3.4.2.1   Intrauterine infection

In this section congenital intrauterine infection which may lead to permanent cerebral injury and impairment will be discussed. These intrauterine infections often occur in the absence of appreciable maternal signs. The TORCH group of infections (TOxoplasma, Rubella, Cytomegalovirus, and Herpes) is most often cited, but varicella and human immunodeficiency virus (HIV) have also been associated with permanent fetal cerebral injury. Maternal infection during pregnancy with rare infectious agents such as Venezuelan equine encephalitis virus may also lead to permanent cerebral impairment.

Since 1941 when Gregg, an Australian ophthalmologist, correctly associated the development of childhood cataract with prenatal exposure to the rubella virus, it has been appreciated that

Table 3.3 Intracerebral sequelae following congenital infection with TORCH, HIV, and varicella

Toxoplasma	Microcephaly
	Hydrocephaly
	Chorioretinitis
	Calcifications
	Psychomotor retardation
	Seizures
	Microphthalmia
Rubella	Sensorineural deafness
	Post-encephalitic cerebral palsy
	Cataracts
	Microphthalmia
Cytomegalovirus	Spasticity
	Seizures
	Calcifications
	Microcephaly
Herpes	Microcephaly
	Calcification
	Chorioretinitis
	Hydranencephaly
Human immunodeficiency virus	Microcephaly
Varicella	Cortical atrophy
	Microcephaly
	Ventriculomegaly
	Microphthalmia
	Developmental delay
	Cataracts

intrauterine infection might cause permanent developmental effects. Furthermore, as seen with rubella infection during pregnancy, the stage at which intrauterine infection occurs is critical to the type of impairment that will ensue. Almost all rubella infection before 12 weeks gestation will lead to congenital damage with one or more defects, about 17 percent of infection between 13 and 16 weeks will lead to retinopathy and deafness and only a minority will develop problems if infection occurs after 17 weeks of gestation.[82] The most severe sequelae of varicella and *Toxoplasma* are the consequence of infection occurring in the first half of pregnancy.

With this group of agents the transmission of maternal infection does not cause universal fetal infection; maternal cytomegalovirus (CMV) infection will infect 40 percent of fetuses. Furthermore, not all fetal infection leads to neurological impairment, as only 5 percent of infected fetuses will develop CMV disease, of which 20 percent will have permanent neurological impairment.[83] With perinatal varicella infection only a quarter of maternal infection will lead to fetal infection.

The principal intracerebral findings associated with each of the congenital infections are listed in

Table 3.3. Some of these features are amenable to prenatal diagnosis. Treatment *in utero* is possible for fetal *Toxoplasma* infection when maternal spiromycin is used.[84] In the remainder, treatment, if available, is commenced after delivery. Perinatal herpes may respond to acyclovir or vidarabine, and antiviral treatment may also be indicated for Varicella. Passive immunization with varicella-zoster immune globulin (VZIG) may be helpful if given to the mother following contact during pregnancy.[85] Congenital infection may also lead to a high rate of premature delivery and death *in utero*.

Among the Oxford series of children with prenatally acquired cerebral palsy three children had evidence of intrauterine infection. Of these three, two had intrauterine CMV infection and the third had congenital infection due to varicella (Table 3.2).

3.4.2.2 *Postnatal infection*

Perinatal or postnatally acquired infection may also lead to serious cerebral impairment. This is not surprising as cerebral development continues well into childhood and the immature neonatal brain is extremely vulnerable to insult. In the preterm infant neonatal sepsis has been found to be associated with the development of later cerebral palsy.[12] Among term infants, central nervous system infection is associated with high rates of mortality. However, infection of the central nervous system may contribute to appreciable later morbidity. During the period 1984–1987 there were 27 term infants who had cerebral palsy of postnatal origin identified by the Oxford Register. Infection was the most common cause for cerebral palsy affecting this group (Table 3.4). It was responsible for 12 cases of cerebral palsy, which consisted of seven cases of meningitis and five cases of encephalitis. The median age of onset of infection was 3 months. The infective agent was known in only a few of these cases, but where this has been identified, *Haemophilus influenzae*

Table 3.4 Causes for cerebral palsy of postnatal onset

Cause	n	Age at onset (months)
CNS infection	12	3
Trauma	6	28
Cerebrovascular accident	3	24
Post-operative	3	36
Miscellaneous	3	13
Total	27	

type B was most frequently found. It remains to be seen whether the widespread introduction of the *Haemophilus influenzae* B vaccine will lead to a reduction in the number of cases of long-term neurological impairment resulting from meningitis.

3.4.3   Toxins

Intrauterine exposure to external toxins may have either a direct or an indirect effect on later neurological development. A number of substances have been clearly documented as being capable of causing later cerebral palsy. Outbreaks of fetal Minamata disease were reported in Japan in children born between 1953 and 1971; an outbreak was also reported in Iraq. Toxicity occurred secondary to maternal ingestion of fish contaminated with methyl mercury.[86] Cerebral manifestations of methyl mercury exposure *in utero* include ataxia, and swallowing, speech, and gait disturbances due to cerebellar deposition of mercury. Thyroid dysfunction has been previously mentioned as being associated with the development of cerebral palsy. In the 1960s Pharoah observed the effect of administration of iodine to pregnancy women in New Guinea in reducing the incidence of endemic cretinism with accompanying motor impairment.[87] A number of other toxins, such as lead, have been associated with milder forms of developmental delay.

Transplacental passage of certain drugs may also cause toxic effects on fetal cerebral development. Maternal administration of warfarin in the first trimester of pregnancy causes a distinct warfarin embryopathy with facial abnormalities and a skeletal abnormality similar to chondrodysplasia punctata. In the second trimester warfarin administration is felt to be safer, but there have been reports of fetal intracranial hemorrhage.[88] Intracranial hemorrhage in the fetus has also been reported following maternal ingestion of salicylate.[89] Reports of the development of intracranial anomalies such as hydranencephaly and lissencephaly have been seen following exposure of the fetus to retinoids. The administration of anticonvulsant medication such as phenobarbitone, phenytoin, and carbamazepine may cause fetal liver enzyme induction leading to a reduction in the available amount of vitamin K and predisposing to hemorrhagic disease of the newborn which may lead to intracranial hemorrhage.[90]

Illegal drug exposure during pregnancy, in particular to cocaine, may also lead to adverse effects on fetal neurological development. A fetal cocaine syndrome has been described with evidence of seizures and intracranial hemorrhage after delivery.[91] The vasoconstrictive effect of cocaine on the fetal vessels has been associated with disorders of neuronal migration.[92] Excessive alcohol consumption during pregnancy is a well-known teratogen, causing a variety of defects that may include neurodevelopmental delay.[93]

3.4.4   Neoplasia

Congenital cerebral neoplasia is a rare occurrence. Among children with prenatal cerebral palsy on the Oxford Register there was only one child who developed long-term neurological impairment secondary to a congenital oligodendroma (Table 3.2).

A variety of congenital tumors have been described in the literature. Haddad and colleagues have reviewed their experience with congenital tumors in 22 children over 11 years. Among these children, seven had astrocytomas, six had primitive neuroectodermal tumors, and the remaining nine had various other diagnoses such as papilloma of the choroid plexus, teratoma, embryonal rhabdomyosarcoma and dermoid tumors. Not surprisingly, the outlook for these children carried an appreciable mortality and morbidity despite treatment.[94]

3.4.5   Trauma

Traditionally, trauma at delivery was felt to be responsible for a considerable amount of fetal intracranial injury. It is not within the remit of this chapter to discuss birth trauma and asphyxia but suffice to say that serious cerebral trauma which occurs as a consequence of assisted vaginal delivery with either forceps or the Ventouse extractor is extremely rare. The infrequency of lethal perinatal trauma in present-day obstetric practice has been confirmed by reviews of perinatal mortality such as the confidential Enquiry into Deaths in Stillbirths and Infancy (CESDI).[95] While it is true that soft-tissue injury is not infrequent following assisted vaginal delivery, there is no suggestion that it is likely to be associated with any accompanying intracerebral injury giving rise to long-term neurological impairment.

Direct trauma to the fetal brain during the prenatal period has been reported from a range of causes, all fortunately occurring infrequently. Cases of invasive intrauterine procedures, such as amniocentesis, leading to fetal intracranial injury have been described.[96] Specific injuries such as porencephaly and third nerve palsies have been described as a consequence of direct fetal trauma from amniocentesis.[97,98] Prenatal maternal abdominal trauma has led to secondary fetal intracranial injury. Baethmann and colleagues have reported a series of nine women who experienced severe abdominal trauma during pregnancy. Seven women sustained their injuries following road accidents, two following blunt abdominal trauma. The outcome was variable: two had hydrocephalus, three had movement disorders, one had convulsions, one had cerebral palsy and two survived unscathed.[99]

3.5   CONCLUSION

Cerebral palsy is not a single etiological entity but the final outcome of a number of diverse disease pathways. In a few instances these pathways have been fully elucidated, but in the majority of cases they are being slowly unraveled. In Table 3.5 a comparison is shown between some of the etiological groups that were found among the cohort of 338 children born with cerebral palsy in the Oxford region between 1984 and 1987 and children born with cerebral palsy from 1983 to 1986 in Western Sweden. A remarkable similarity in the frequency of the different etiological groups within these two different populations is seen.[100] It can also be seen from this table that a large proportion of cerebral palsy is still of unknown etiology.

Prenatal cerebral injury is likely to explain the development of cerebral palsy in an increasing proportion of affected children. The diagnosis of prenatal cerebral palsy has been helped by improved understanding of cerebral developmental pathology in addition to improved methods of neuroimaging of the neonatal and pediatric brain. Furthermore, improved understanding of the genetic basis of disease has shown that some cerebral malformation may have a genetic basis for causation.

Table 3.5 Comparison of etiological groups of children with cerebral palsy born in Oxford between 1984 and 1987 and born in Sweden between 1983 and 1986

	Oxford 1984–1987 n (%)	Sweden 1983–1986 n (%)
Preterm	123 (40)	69 (39)
Perinatal	41 (13.4)	27 (15)
Prenatal	41 (13.4)	30 (17)
Unknown	100 (33)	51 (29)
	305 (100)	177 (100)

Where no cause is known for the development of cerebral injury however, initial clues may be identified from the study of antecedent events. These factors may be maternal in nature, specific to pregnancy or occur as a consequence of fetal exposure to adverse environmental features.

Maternal characteristics that have been identified as being positively associated with the development of cerebral palsy are maternal thyroid disease and abnormal menstrual and reproductive intervals. Factors specific to pregnancy which are associated with cerebral palsy are antepartum hemorrhage, intrauterine growth retardation after 34 weeks of gestation and the presence of pre-eclampsia or proteinuria at term. In both the term and preterm infant, maternal infection, preterm prolonged premature rupture of the membranes, and chorioamnionitis are associated with the development of cerebral palsy. Postnatal sepsis is also a risk factor for cerebral palsy.

Structural developmental anomaly may account for a number of cases of cerebral palsy. It is not clear whether this type of abnormality is genetically determined or if it occurs secondary to early intrauterine exposure to adverse environmental effects. Early intrauterine exposure to specific toxins such as mercury, alcohol, infective agents, and prescribed and illegal drugs may also lead to early cerebral injury.

Gestational age and weight at birth are the factors that have the strongest relationship with the development of cerebral palsy. However, clearly not all premature or small-for-gestational age infants have later neurodevelopmental problems. It is important that these subgroups of children are studied separately to identify the features among the individual groups that might make brain injury more likely.

3.6   REFERENCES

1 Bax M. Terminology and classification of cerebral palsy. *Developmental Medicine and Child Neurology* 1964; **6**: 295–307.
2 Kuban KB, Leviton A. Cerebral palsy. *New England Journal of Medicine* 1994; **330**: 188–95.
3 Kendall BE, Damaerel P. Imaging of pediatric and congenital brain disease. *Current Opinion in Radiology* 1992; **4**: 28–37.
4 Nelson KB, Ellenberg JH. Antecedents of cerebral palsy. Univariate analysis of risk. *American Journal of Diseases of Children* 1985; **139**: 1031–8.
5 Nelson KB, Ellenberg JH. Antecedents of cerebral palsy. Multivariate analysis of risk. *New England Journal of Medicine* 1986; **315**: 81–6.

6 Naeye RL, Peters EC, Bartholemew M, Landis R. Origins of cerebral palsy. *American Journal of Diseases of Children* 1989; **143**: 1154–61.

7 Torfs CP, Van den Berg BJ, Oechsli FW, Cummins S. Prenatal and perinatal factors in the aetiology of cerebral palsy. *Journal of Paediatrics* 1990; **116**: 615–19.

8 Stanley FJ, Alberman E. Birthweight, gestational age and the cerebral palsies. In: *The epidemiology of the cerebral palsies*. Philadelphia: JB Lippincott, 1984: 57–68.

9 Dale A, Stanley FJ. An epidemiological study of cerebral palsy in Western Australia 1956–1975. *Developmental Medicine and Child Neurology* 1980; **22**: 13–25.

10 Gaffney G, Sellers S, Flavell V, Squier M, Johnson A. Case-control study of intrapartum care, cerebral palsy and perinatal death. *British Medical Journal* 1994; **308**: 743–50.

11 Murphy DJ, Sellers S, MacKenzie IZ, Yudkin P, Johnson AM. Case-control study of antenatal and intrapartum risk factors for cerebral palsy in very preterm singleton babies. *Lancet* 1995; **346**: 1449–53.

12 Murphy DJ, Hope PL, Johnson A. Neonatal risk factors for cerebral palsy in very preterm babies: case-control study. *British Medical Journal* 1997; **314**: 404–8.

13 Hughes I, Newton R. Genetic aspects of cerebral palsy. *Developmental Medicine and Child Neurology* 1992; **34**: 80–6.

14 Oxford Regional Register of Early Childhood Impairment. *Annual report*. Oxford: Anglia and Oxford Regional Health Authority, 1996.

15 Gustavson KH, Hagberg B, Sanner G. *Acta Paediatrica Scandinavica* 1969; **58**: 330–40.

16 Sinha G, Corry P, Subesinghe D, Wild J, Levene MI. Prevalence and type of cerebral palsy in a British ethnic community: the role of consanguinity. *Developmental Medicine and Child Neurology* 1997; **39**: 259–62.

17 Foley J. The offspring of people with cerebral palsy. *Developmental Medicine and Child Neurology* 1992; **34**: 972–8.

18 Lilienfield AM, Pasamanick B. The association of maternal and fetal factors with the development of cerebral palsy and epilepsy. *American Journal of Obstetrics and Gynecology* 1955; **70**: 93–101.

19 Badawi N, Kurinczuk JJ, Keogh JM *et al*. Maternal thyroid disease in pregnancy and newborn encephalopathy in the term infant. *Paediatric and Perinatal Epidemiology* 1996; **10**: A14.

20 Ackerman-Liebrich U, Alberman E, Moessinger A *et al*. Conference summary, The epidemiology of cerebral palsies – Berne 14–15 March 1996. *Paediatric and Perinatal Epidemiology* 1996; **10**: 355–7.

21 Gilles FH, Leviton A, Dooling EC. *The developing human brain: growth and epidemiologic neuropathology*. Boston: John Wright, 1983.

22 Sims ME. Brain injury and intrauterine death. *American Journal of Obstetrics and Gynecology*. 1985; **151**: 721–3.

23 Ellis WG, Goetzman BW, Lindenberg JA. Neuropathological documentation of prenatal brain damage. *American Journal of Diseases of Children* 1988; **142**: 858–66.

24 Squier M, Keeling JW. The incidence of prenatal brain injury. *Neuropathology and Neurobiology* 1992; **17**: 29–38.

25 Gaffney G, Squier MV, Sellers S, Flavell V, Johnson A. Clinical associations of prenatal ischaemic white matter damage. *Archives of Disease in Childhood* 1994; **70**: F101–6.

26 Grether JK, Nelson KB. Maternal infection and cerebral palsy in infants of normal birth weight. *Journal of the American Medical Association* 1997; **278**: 207–11.

27 Grether JK, Nelson KB, Emery ES, Cummins SK. Prenatal and perinatal factors and cerebral palsy in very low birth weight infants. *Journal of Pediatrics* 1996; **128**: 407–14.

28 Leviton A. Preterm birth and cerebral palsy: is tumor necrosis factor the missing link? *Developmental Medicine and Child Neurology* 1993; **35**: 553–8.

29 Dammann O, Leviton A. Maternal intrauterine infection, cytokines and brain damage in the preterm infant. *Pediatric Research* 1997; **42**: 1–8.

30 Adinolfi M. Infectious diseases in pregnancy, cytokines and neurological handicap: an hypothesis. *Developmental Medicine and Child Neurology* 1993; **35**: 549–53.

31 Kuban K. White matter disease of prematurity, periventricular leukomalacia and ischaemic lesions. *Developmental Medicine and Child Neurology* 1998; **40**: 571–3.

32 Selmaj KW, Farooq M, Norton WT, Raine CS, Brosna CE. Proliferation of astrocytes in vitro in response to cytokines. A primary role for tumor necrosis factor. *Journal of Immunology* 1990; **144**: 129–35.

33 Klein MA, Moller JC, Jones LL, Bleuthmann H, Kreutzberg GW, Raivich G. Impaired neuroglial activation in interleukin-6 deficient mice. *GLIA* 1997; **19**: 227–33.

34 Andrews WW, Hauth JC, Goldenberg RL, Gomez R, Romero R, Cassell GH. Amniotic fluid interleukin-6: correlation with upper genital tract microbial colonization and gestational age in women delivered after spontaneous labour versus indicated delivery. *American Journal of Obstetrics and Gynecology* 1995; **173**: 606–12.

35 Yoon BH, Romero R, Kim CJ *et al*. High expression of tumor necrosis factor-alpha and interleukin-6 in periventricular leukomalacia. *American Journal of Obstetrics and Gynecology* 1997; **177**: 406–11.

36 Yoon BH, Romero R, Yang SH *et al*. Interleukin-6 concentrations in umbilical cord plasma are elevated in neonates with white matter lesions associated with periventricular leukomalacia. *American Journal of Obstetrics and Gynecology* 1996; **174**: 1433–9.

37 Yoon BH, Jun JK, Romero R *et al*. Amniotic fluid inflammatory cytokines (interleukin-6, interleukin-1 beta and tumor necrosis factor-alpha), neonatal brain

white matter lesions and cerebral palsy. *American Journal of Obstetrics and Gynecology* 1997; **177**: 19–26.

38 Relton JK, Rothwell NJ. Interleukin-1 receptor antagonist inhibits ischaemic and excitotoxic neuronal damage in the rat. *Brain Research Bulletin* 1992; **29**: 243–6.

39 Martin D, Chinookswong N, Miller G. The interleukin-1 receptor antagonist (rhIL-1ra) protects against cerebral infarction in a rat model of hypoxia-ischaemia. *Experimental Neurology* 1994; **130**: 362–7.

40 Romero R, Sepulveda W, Mazor M *et al*. The natural interleukin-1 receptor antagonist in term and preterm parturition. *American Journal of Obstetrics and Gynecology* 1992; **167**: 863–72.

41 King J, Flenady V. Antibiotics in preterm labour with intact membranes. In: Neilson JP, Crowther CA, Hodnett ED, Hofmeyr GJ, eds. *Pregnancy and childbirth module of the Cochrane Database of Systematic Reviews* (updated 02 December 1997). *Cochrane Collaboration*, Issue 1. Oxford: Update Software, 1988.

42 Kenyon S, Boulvain M. Antibiotics for preterm premature rupture of membranes (Cochrane Review). In: *The Cochrane Library*, Issue 4. Oxford: Update Software, 1998.

43 Kenyon SL, Taylor DJ, Tarnow-Mordi W, for the ORACLE Collaborative Group. Broad-spectrum antibiotics for preterm, prelabour rupture of fetal membranes: the ORACLE I randomised trial. *Lancet* 2001; **357**: 979–88.

44 Kenyon SL, Taylor DJ, Tarnow-Mordi W, for the ORACLE Collaborative Group. Broad-spectrum antibiotics for spontaneous preterm labour: the ORACLE II randomised trial. *Lancet* 2001; **357**: 989–94.

45 Eschenbach DA. Amniotic fluid infection and cerebral palsy. Focus on the fetus. (Editorial) *Journal of the American Medical Association* 1997; **278**: 247–8.

46 Salakorpi T, Sajaniemi N, Halliback H, Kari A, Rita H, von Wendt L. Randomised study of the effects of antenatal dexamethasone on growth and development of premature children at the corrected age of 2 years. *Acta Paediatrica* 1997; **86**: 294–8.

47 Petterson B, Nelson KB, Watson L, Stanley FJ. Twins, triplets and cerebral palsy in births in Western Australia in the 1980s. *British Medical Journal* 1993; **307**: 1239–43.

48 Williams K, Hennessy E, Alberman E. Cerebral palsy, effects of twinning, birthweight and gestational age. *Archives of Disease in Childhood Fetal Neonatal Edition* 1996; **75**: F178–82.

49 Pharoah PO, Cooke T. Cerebral palsy and multiple births. *Archives of Disease in Childhood Fetal Neonatal Edition* 1996; **75**: F174–7.

50 Rhydstrom H, Ingemarsson I. Prognosis and long-term follow-up of a twin after antenatal death of the co-twin. *Journal of Reproductive Medicine* 1993; **38**: 142–6.

51 Benriscke K. The biology of the twinning process: how placentation influences outcome. *Seminars in Perinatology* 1995; **19**: 542–50.

52 Nicolaides K, Petterson H. Fetal therapy. *Current Opinion in Obstetrics and Gynaecology* 1994; **6**: 486–91.

53 Mahony BS, Petty CN, Nyberg DA, Luthy DA, Hickok DE, Hirsch JH. The 'stuck twin' phenomenon: ultrasonographic findings, pregnancy outcome and management with serial amniocentesis. *American Journal of Obstetrics and Gynecology* 1990; **163**: 1513–22.

54 De Lia JE, Cruikshank DP, Keye WR. Fetoscopic neodymium:YAG laser occlusion of placental vessels in severe twin-to-twin transfusion syndrome. *Obstetrics and Gynecology* 1990; **75**: 1046–53.

55 Pharoah PO, Cooke RW. A hypothesis for the aetiology of spastic cerebral palsy – the vanishing twin. *Developmental Medicine and Child Neurology* 1997; **39**: 292–6.

56 Altman DG, Chitty LS. Charts of fetal size: 1. Methodology. *British Journal of Obstetrics and Gynaecology* 1994; **101**: 29–34.

57 Sargent IL, Smarason AK. Immunology of pre-eclampsia; current views and hypothesis. In: Kurpisz M, Fernandez N eds. *Immunology of human reproduction*. Oxford: Bios Scientific, 1995: 355–70.

58 Soothill PW, Ajayi RA, Campbell S, Ross DCA, Snijders RM, Nicolaides KH. Relationship between fetal acidemia at cordocentesis and subsequent neurodevelopment. *Ultrasound in Obstetrics and Gynaecology* 1992; **2**: 80–3.

59 Vyas S, Nicolaides KH, Bower S, Campbell S. Middle cerebral artery flow velocity waveforms in fetal hypoxaemia. *British Journal of Obstetrics and Gynaecology* 1990; **97**: 797–803.

60 Uvebrandt P, Hagberg G. Intrauterine growth in children with cerebral palsy. *Acta Paediatrica* 1992; **81**: 407–12.

61 Blair E, Stanley F. Intrauterine growth and spastic cerebral palsy. I. Association with birth weight and gestational age. *American Journal of Obstetrics and Gynecology* 1990; **162**: 29–37.

62 Gaffney G, Johnson A, Squier MV, Sellers S. Cerebral palsy and neonatal encephalopathy. *Archives of Disease in Childhood* 1994; **80**: F195–200.

63 Nelson KB, Grether JK. Can magnesium sulfate reduce the risk of cerebral palsy in very low birthweight infants? *Pediatrics* 1995; **95**: 263–9.

64 Anonymous. The origins of cerebral palsy – a consensus statement. The Australian and New Zealand Perinatal Societies. *Medical Journal of Australia* 1995; **162**(2): 85–90.

65 Stoddart RA, Clark SL, Minton SD. In utero ischemic injury: sonographic diagnosis and medicolegal implications. *American Journal of Obstetrics and Gynecology* 1990; **159**: 23–5.

66 Stirling HF, Hendry M, Brown JK. Prenatal intracranial haemorrhage. *Developmental Medicine and Child Neurology* 1989; **31**: 807–15.

67 Bondurant S, Boehm FH, Fleischer AC, Machin JE. Antepartum diagnosis of fetal intracranial hemorrhage by ultrasound. *Obstetrics and Gynecology* 1984; **63**: 255–75.

68 Bejar P, Wozniak P, Allard M *et al*. Antenatal origin of neurologic damage in newborn infants. *American*

Journal of Obstetrics and Gynecology 1988; **159**: 357–63.

69 Jennett RJ, Daily WJ, Tarby TJ, Manwaring KH. Prenatal diagnosis of intracerebellar haemorrhage: case report. *American Journal of Obstetrics and Gynecology* 1990; **162**: 1472–4.

70 Reiss I, Gortner L, Moller J, Gehl HB, Baschat AA, Gembruch U. Fetal intracerebral haemorrhage in the second trimester: diagnosis by sonography and magnetic resonance imaging. *Ultrasound in Obstetrics and Gynecology* 1996; **7**: 49–51.

71 Kirkinen P, Partanen K, Rynanen M, Orden MR. Fetal intracranial haemorrhage. Imaging by ultrasound and magnetic resonance imaging. *Journal of Reproductive Medicine* 1997; **42**: 467–72.

72 Roessmann U, Miller RT. Thrombosis of the middle cerebral artery associated with birth trauma. *Neurology* 1980; **30**: 889–92.

73 Mannino FL, Trauner DA. Stroke in neonates. *Journal of Pediatrics* 1983; **102**: 605–10.

74 de Vries LS, Groenendaal F, Eken P, van Haastert IC, Rademaker KJ, Meiners LC. Infarcts in the vascular distribution of the middle cerebral artery in preterm and fullterm infants. *Neuropediatrics* 1997; **28**: 88–96.

75 Vergani P, Strobelt N, Locatelli A *et al.* Clinical significance of fetal intracranial hemorrhage. *American Journal of Obstetrics and Gynecology* 1996: 536–43.

76 Volpe JJ. *Neurology of the newborn*, 2nd edn. Philadelphia: WB Saunders, 1987.

77 Banker BQ, Larroche JD. Periventricular leukomalacia of infancy: a form of neonatal encephalopathy. *Archives of Neurology* 1962; **7**: 32–50.

78 Weindling AM, Rochefort MJ, Calvert SA, Fok TF, Wilkinson A. Development of cerebral palsy after detection of periventricular cysts in the newborn. *Developmental Medicine and Child Neurology* 1985; **27**: 800–6.

79 Fawer CL, Calame A, Perentes E, Andregg A. Periventricular leukomalacia and neurodevelopmental outcome in preterm infants. *Archives of Disease in Childhood* 1987; **62**: 30–6.

80 Volpe JJ. Current concepts of injury in the premature infant. *American Journal of Radiology* 1989; **153**: 243–51.

81 Krageloh-Mann I, Hagberg B, Petersen D, Riethmuller J, Gut E, Michaelis R. Bilateral spastic cerebral palsy – pathogenetic aspects from MRI. *Neuropediatrics* 1992; **23**: 46–8.

82 Sutherland S. (ed.) **TORCH** *screening reassessed*. Public Health Laboratory Service. Shaftesbury: The Blackmore Press, 1993.

83 Becker LE. Infections of the developing brain. *American Journal of Neuroradiology* 1992; **13**: 537–49.

84 Stray-Pedersen B. Toxoplasmosis in pregnancy. *Baillières Clinical Obstetrics and Gynaecology* 1993; **7**: 107–37.

85 Buyse ML. (ed.) *Birth defects encyclopedia*. Massachusetts: The Center for Birth Defects Information Service/Blackwell Scientific, 1990.

86 Stanley F. Prenatal risk factors in the study of the cerebral palsies. In: Stanley FJ, Alberman E, eds. *The epidemiology of the cerebral palsies*. Philadelphia: JB Lippincott, 1984: 87–97.

87 Pharoah PO, Butfiels IH, Hetzel BS. Neurological damage in the fetus resulting from severe iodine deficiency during pregnancy. *Lancet* 1971; **1**: 308–10.

88 Ville Y, Jenkins E, Shearer MJ, *et al.* Fetal intraventricular haemorrhage and maternal warfarin. *Lancet* 1993; **341**(8854): 1211.

89 Karlowicz MG, White LE. Severe intracranial hemorrhage in a term neonate associated with maternal acetylsalicylic acid ingestion. *Clinical Pediatrics Philadelphia* 1993; 740–3.

90 Moslet U, Hansen ES. A review of vitamin K, epilepsy and pregnancy. *Acta Neurologica Scandinavica* 1992; **85**: 39–43.

91 Kapur RP, Shaw CM, Shepherd TH. Brain haemorrhages in cocaine-exposed human fetuses. *Teratology* 1991; **44**: 11–18.

92 Dominguez R, Vila-Coro AA, Slopis JM, Bohan TP. Brain and ocular abnormalities in infants with in utero exposure to cocaine and other street drugs. *American Journal of Diseases of Children* 1991; **145**: 688–94.

93 Pietrantoni M, Knuppel RA. Alcohol use in pregnancy. *Clinical Perinatology* 1991; **18**: 93–111.

94 Haddad SF, Menezes AH, Bell WE, Godersky JC, Afifi AK, Bale JF. Brain tumors occurring before 1 year of age: a retrospective review of 22 cases in an 11 year period (1977–1987). *Neurosurgery* 1991; **29**: 8–13.

95 Confidential Enquiries into Stillbirths and Deaths in Infancy. *Fifth annual report*. London: Maternal and Child Health Research Consortium, 1998.

96 Squier MV, Chamberlain P, Zaiwalla Z, *et al.* Five cases of brain injury following amniocentesis in midterm pregnancy. *Developmental Medicine and Child Neurology* 2000; **42**: 554–60.

97 Eller KM, Kuller JA. Porencephaly secondary to fetal trauma during amniocentesis. *Obstetrics and Gynecology* 1995; **85**: 865–7.

98 Patel CK, Taylor DS, Russell-Eggitt IM, Kriss A, Demaerel P. Congenital third nerve palsy associated with mid-trimester amniocentesis. *British Journal of Ophthalmology* 1993; **77**: 530–3.

99 Baethmann M, Kahn T, Lenard HG, Voit T. Fetal CNS damage after exposure to maternal trauma during pregnancy. *Acta Paediatrica* 1996; **85**: 1331–8.

100 Hagberg B, Hagberg G, Olow I. The changing panorama of cerebral palsy in Sweden IV: prevalence and origin during the birth period 1983–1986. *Acta Paediatrica* 1993; **82**: 387–93.

4 Asphyxia and the developing brain

Alistair J Gunn, Peter D Gluckman, and Laura Bennet

The fetus is highly adapted to intrauterine conditions, which include low partial pressures of oxygen and relatively limited supply of other substrates, compared with postnatal life. The key fetal adaptations are left shift of the oxygen dissociation curve, increased organ blood flow, greater anaerobic capacity in many tissues, and increased oxygen extraction. These adaptations provide a margin of safety for events such as labor that may compromise uteroplacental gas exchange. In addition, fetal cardiovascular adaptations to acute asphyxia help to preserve oxygen delivery to vital organs such as the brain.

The effectiveness of these adaptations is such that the concept of 'birth asphyxia' itself has been questioned.[1] However, many studies have shown that infants with clinical evidence of birth asphyxia and a precipitating episode in the immediate peripartum period have evidence of acute evolving cerebral injury[2-4] with long-term cognitive or functional sequelae.[3]

One seminal concept, derived from basic clinical studies and *in vitro* and *in vivo* models, is that asphyxia may not cause immediate neuronal death but may precipitate a complex series of biochemical events leading to cell death many hours or even days later. The final outcome of an asphyxial injury is modulated by complex interactions between a number of factors: the severity, duration, and pattern (single or repeated) of the insult in relation to the compensatory mechanisms of the fetus, and factors that may sensitize the fetus. Critical sensitizing factors include gestational age (including the maturational status of both heart and brain), maternal temperature, and pre-existing metabolic disturbances such as intrauterine growth retardation (IUGR) and possibly fetal glucose and lactate levels.

A variety of classical patterns of cerebral damage have been described, for example parasagittal, cortical or 'watershed' injury, periventricular leukomalacia, and status marmoratus.[5,6] Until recently the factors that might make certain regions more vulnerable to injury were not understood, but experimental studies are providing insights into these patterns of injury.

The present chapter will discuss the neural responses of the developing brain to hypoxic-ischemic injury, the factors that modulate neuronal death, the systemic adaptations of the fetus to asphyxia, and recent evidence linking different patterns of asphyxial insult to particular histological patterns of damage.

4.1   THE PATHOGENESIS OF CELL DEATH

4.1.1   Primary and secondary phases of cell death

The seminal concept that has evolved regarding asphyxial brain injury is that neuronal and glial cell death occurs not only during the insult (primary cell death) but may continue to develop for hours and days after restoration of cerebral perfusion (secondary cell death). Some neurons and glia die during the asphyxial insult itself: the longer and more severe the insult, then the greater the proportion of primary neural injury.[7,8] After focal ischemic injury with permanent vessel occlusion the secondary phase is relatively small. There is a dense ischemic core in which primary cell death with pan-necrosis occurs. This core is surrounded by an ischemic 'penumbra', which has some residual blood supply.[9] Damage extends from the core out to the penumbra over a few hours under experimental conditions.[10] The evolution of damage in the penumbra has been associated with waves of depolarization that deplete remaining cellular energy reserves.[11]

In contrast, a distinct secondary phase of delayed neuronal death is well described after transient global hypoxia-ischemia. Magnetic resonance spectroscopic studies of hypoxic-ischemic injury in piglets suggest that after the primary phase of energy failure during hypoxia, cerebral metabolism may transiently recover, but then deteriorate 6–48 hours later.[12] Similarly, Roth and co-workers found that some infants with evidence of moderate to severe asphyxia had normal cerebral oxidative metabolism shortly after birth, but then went on to develop secondary energy failure, associated with high mortality. In survivors, the degree of secondary energy failure at 24–48 hours accurately predicted neurodevelopmental outcome at 18 months and 4 years of age.[3]

Many of the pathophysiological events associated with secondary injury have been characterized in a model of cerebral ischemia in the chronically instrumented fetal sheep, studied *in utero*.[7,13] Such fetal preparations allow detailed evaluation of responses to prenatal ischemia under stable conditions,[13] avoiding the significant neural effects of anesthesia.[14,15]

The primary and secondary phases of injury seen in this model are illustrated in Fig. 4.1. During carotid artery occlusion (the primary phase) the electroencephalogram (EEG) shows an immediate

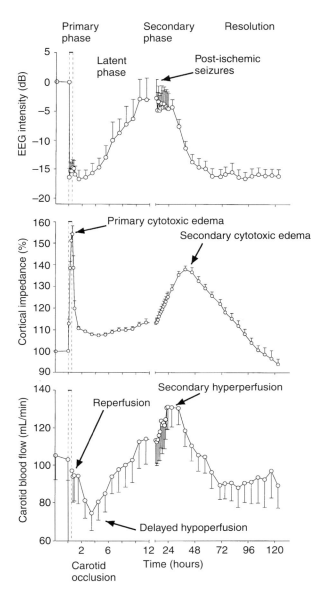

Figure 4.1   An illustration of the pathophysiological phases of injury after 30 minutes of global cerebral ischemia in fetal sheep (*n* = 7). Data derived from Gunn *et al.* (1997).[13] The insult (*primary* phase) with profound suppression of the EEG and increased cortical impedance (a measure of cytotoxic edema) is marked by the dashed lines. Although the EEG remains suppressed for many hours after this, cortical impedance rapidly resolves within 30 minutes, with only a small residual elevation. Delayed, secondary hypoperfusion occurs, associated with suppressed oxidative metabolism during this *latent* phase. The *secondary* phase is shown by an abrupt increase in EEG activity (corresponding with intense epileptiform activity) which starts approximately 6–8 hours after the insult, with an associated rise in cytotoxic edema and carotid blood flow. The peak cytotoxic edema occurs after resolution of seizures. The final EEG intensity is very low, reflecting severe neuronal loss with laminar necrosis in the underlying parasagittal cortex.

loss of amplitude, becoming isoelectric after 30 seconds. After 30 minutes of occlusion, the EEG remains suppressed for 5–8 hours (the latent period), during which there is secondary hypoperfusion reflecting depressed cerebral metabolism.[13] The secondary phase starts 6–9 hours after injury and is marked by an abrupt onset of seizure activity, with an increase in cerebral blood flow and cytotoxic edema.[13,16] The delayed seizure activity peaks rapidly at approximately 12 hours, then progressively resolves over 1–2 days. The residual EEG intensity after resolution of seizures is directly related to the amount of neuronal death in the underlying cortex.[7] Cytotoxic edema or cell swelling (measured by cortical impedance[17]) occurs rapidly during ischemia, and almost completely resolves over 30–60 minutes of reperfusion. A secondary phase of cytotoxic edema, initiated after the onset of seizures, peaks much later and takes 2–3 days to resolve. If seizures are abolished by infusion of a selective glutamate antagonist, the secondary phase of edema is delayed rather than aborted,[18] suggesting that the edema is not a direct consequence of seizures but reflects primary ongoing encephalopathic processes. The timing of secondary edema is consistent with that of secondary energy failure.[3,12]

Histological analysis after 3 days' recovery shows that 30 minutes of ischemia causes consistent injury of the parasagittal cortex and dorsal hippocampus. As shown in the control cases in Fig. 4.2, there is at least 75–90 percent neuronal death in the parasagittal cortex, with lesser loss in other areas.[13] The depths of the sulci tend to show greater damage than the adjacent gyri. This pattern of predominant parasagittal and sulcal injury closely mimics a common pattern in asphyxiated term neonates.[5]

4.1.2 Mechanisms of cell death: apoptosis and necrosis

Although neurons (and glia) may initially recover from the primary injury, processes initiated by asphyxial brain injury have been shown in clinical and experimental studies to lead to cell death hours or days later.[8,19–21] Two morphological patterns of cell death have been described: necrosis and apoptosis.[8,22] Necrosis is defined by loss of plasma membrane integrity associated with a random pattern of DNA degradation. Typically there is swelling of the cytoplasm and organelles, with lysis of the nucleus. Eventually the shrunken cell breaks into small, rounded, basophilic fragments. The classic microscopic picture of apoptosis is karyorrhexis: condensation of chromatin leading to a dark, shrunken nucleus associated with cyto-

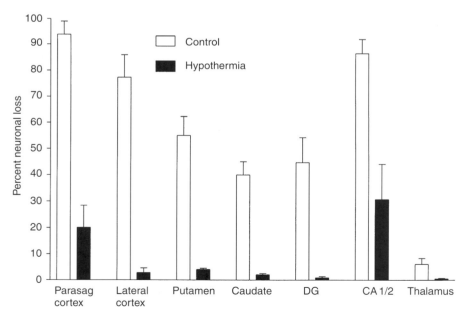

Figure 4.2 Effect of 72 hours cerebral cooling started 90 minutes after reperfusion on microscopically assessed neuronal loss in different brain regions at 5 days after ischemia. A significant reduction ($p < 0.001$) in neuronal loss was seen in all regions in fetuses treated with moderate selective cerebral cooling (closed bars) compared with sham cooled fetuses (open bars). In the hypothermia group, only fetuses in which the extradural temperature was maintained below 34 °C for the first 12 hours are shown. CA 1/2, cornu ammonis subfields 1 and 2; DG, dentate gyrus. Data derived from Gunn *et al.* (1997).[13] Mean ± SEM.

plasmic shrinkage. DNA is actively degraded by endonucleases which cleave the chromatin at internucleosomal points, leading to fragments of fixed size, with a characteristic laddered appearance on chromatography.[23]

By analogy with the active process of developmental loss of excess cells (including neurons), it is suggested that an apoptotic morphology reflects active or 'programmed' cell death, involving a cascade of 'suicide' processes.[8,24] In contrast, necrosis is suggested to reflect biophysical damage to the cell.[8,22] Both types have been clearly described in infants dying after perinatal asphyxia.[25,26] Apoptosis may be initiated by several intracellular pathways involving alterations in the balance of intracellular factors such as Bcl, which inhibits apoptosis[27] and Bax which promotes apoptosis,[28] and amplified by a family of proteases related to ICE (interleukin-converting enzyme), known as caspases.[29]

Recently, it has become clear that the underlying processes of cell death may not be as clearly separated as was originally thought. Hypoxic cell death *in vitro* appears to include a combination of both apoptotic and necrotic processes, with one or the other being more prominent depending on factors such as maturity.[30,31] The concept of delayed cell death remains an important one, since if neuronal and glial cell death is an active response, mediated by activation of second and third messengers, then it should logically be possible to interrupt these events and modify the effects of acute hypoxia.

4.1.3 Mechanisms of primary cell death

A variety of closely interrelated mechanisms have been implicated in the primary phase of injury. The key mechanisms are cytotoxic edema leading to cell lysis, excitotoxicity, free radical mediated cytotoxicity, and intracellular calcium accumulation.

Hypoxia-induced failure of energy-dependent mechanisms such as the Na^+/K^+ ATP-dependent export leads to loss of intracellular homeostasis. Depolarization occurs, with calcium and sodium entry into cells. This in turn favors further cation and water entry, leading to intracellular edema. If sufficiently severe this may cause immediate neuronal lysis,[32] but the swollen neurons may recover if the hypoxia is reversed or the osmotic environment is manipulated. Finally, hypoxia is associated with failure of energy-dependent re-uptake of excitatory amino acids (EAAs), such as glutamate, which are endogenous neurotransmitters.

The hypoxic rise in intracellular calcium induces free radical production, kinase activities, and hydroxyapatite precipitation which are all cytotoxic processes.[33] It is generally believed that free radicals play a particular role in the immediate reperfusion phase, when tissue oxygen levels abruptly recover.[34,35]

4.1.4 Mechanisms of delayed cell death

The events promoting or sustaining the apoptotic cascade after reperfusion are not known. Mitochondrial calcium overload after hypoxia-ischemia appears to be one of the critical steps initiating delayed death.[33,36] Other proposed damaging factors include loss of trophic growth factor support[37] and free radical release.[34] In addition, there is a close temporal and possibly causal association between microglial activation and apoptosis.[8,38] Microglia are the macrophages resident in the brain, but other macrophages may also cross from the circulation and play a role in the activation of the neuroimmune system after asphyxial injury.

In the secondary phase, *in vivo* microdialysis shows that both glutamate and nitric oxide (NO) are induced.[39] Elevated extracellular glutamate is associated with seizures.[39,40] In the human neonate, seizure activity is a strong prognostic indicator of bad outcome,[41] and in fetal sheep it has been definitively shown that post-asphyxial seizures in part extend the area of brain injury.[18]

NO is a volatile, rapidly regulated gas, which plays an important role in many areas, including as a neuromodulator in the brain, in regulating arterial vasodilatation, and in macrophage activity. Three different types of NO synthase (NOS) mediate these key. Endothelial NO is a vasodilator which, under physiological conditions, plays an important role in the regulation of cerebral blood flow (CBF) and the control of platelet aggregation and adhesion.[42] In contrast, iNOS mediates the release by activated macrophages of very highly concentrated killing bursts of NO, which may contribute to reperfusion injury.[43]

4.1.5 Endogenous protective mechanisms

Many of the endogenous responses of the brain act to limit injury. These responses include release of neuromodulators/inhibitory neurotransmitters, induction of neurotrophic factors and intracellular anti-apoptotic systems, and, postnatally, spontaneous cerebral hypothermia. Additionally, as discussed below, the cerebrovascular responses to asphyxia are clearly protective, since they tend to maintain preferential oxygen delivery to organs such as the brain and heart.

4.1.5.1   Inhibitory neuromodulators

Ischemia is typically associated with a large increase in inhibitory neuromodulators such as gamma aminobutyric acid (GABA),[39] adenosine,[44] and cerebral opioids.[45] These factors may reduce cerebral metabolic demand by reducing neural activity and antagonizing the receptor-mediated effects of the excitatory neurotransmitters.[46]

Microdialysis studies in the fetal lamb after 30 minutes of ischemia show that, in contrast to studies in adult species, there is a disproportionately large release of GABA relative to excitotoxins during the primary phase.[39] GABAergic agonists may be neuroprotective.[46] It is interesting to note that adults of species such as the turtle that are very tolerant to hypoxia also show a very elevated GABA response to anoxia.[47]

The inhibitory neuromodulator adenosine is elevated after perinatal asphyxia.[48] This endogenous adenosine may be neuroprotective since its inhibition by theophylline in the post-asphyxial period exacerbates delayed neuronal death.[46] Adenosine A1 (and A3) neuronal receptors are inhibitory and act to reduce glutamate release, while the vascular A2 receptor mediates local vasodilatation.[49] Pretreatment with adenosine A1 agonists can markedly reduce damage associated with global and focal brain ischemia.[46,49] This effect is highly receptor specific since agonists of the adenosine A3 receptor markedly worsen outcome.[49]

4.1.5.2   Cellular factors

Biochemical responses within cells may also help to reduce damage. Increased expression of anti-apoptotic proteins such as Bcl-2 following mild ischemia limits neuronal loss.[50] Transient increase in the expression of the calcium-binding protein calbindin D28k after ischemia is postulated to buffer increased intracellular free calcium.[51] A significant protective role for calbindin is supported by the differential expression of calbindin across different neuronal populations. Mature cell populations that are very resistant to ischemic injury, such as the granule cells in the dentate gyrus of the hippocampus, express high levels of calbindin.[52]

In their immature state these cells do not express calbindin, and are as susceptible to ischemia as other populations.[53] The neuroprotective actions of some neurotrophic factors have been related to induction of calbindin expression.[54,55]

4.1.5.3   Endogenous neurotrophic factors

Nieto-Sampedro and colleagues showed many years ago that neurotrophic activity was dramatically increased after wounding of the rat cortex and that this response was considerably greater in the juvenile than in the adult brain.[56] However, the neurotrophins involved have only recently been identified. Extensive studies have examined changes in these factors in the 'Levine' model of unilateral hypoxic-ischemic injury in the immature rat. One carotid artery is ligated, causing ischemia in the middle cerebral artery territory, but both hemispheres are subjected to hypoxia, providing an internal control for the effect of hypoxia alone. Such studies suggest that there are two phases of neurotrophin production after hypoxic-ischemic injury.

Shortly after the end of hypoxia, there is minimal induction of messenger RNAs (mRNAs) coding for members of the early-immediate genes (c-fos, c-jun) and the nerve growth factor family (nerve growth factor β, brain-derived growth factor, neurotensin 3). Such induction is restricted to the hippocampus of the non-injured side and has been shown to be induced by post-asphyxial seizures rather than hypoxia itself.[57] In contrast, broadly acting growth factors were expressed more slowly, but intensely and for prolonged periods in injured regions of the brain. For example, insulin-like growth factor 1 (IGF-1) mRNA is maximally induced at 3–5 days after hypoxia-ischemia by injured glia in a dose-related manner.[37]

In view of its known anti-apoptotic effects,[58,59] the therapeutic effects of exogenous IGF-1 have been tested. In both the adult rat and the fetal lamb a single dose of intraventricular IGF-1 was associated with reduced secondary neuronal death.[37,60] In the rat, cortical infarction and selective neuronal loss were reduced.[37] In the fetal lamb partial protection was obtained, with improved recovery of EEG activity and reduced neuronal loss in most regions of the brain.[60]

Basic fibroblast growth factor (bFGF) is induced after injury in a more limited manner and is reported to be neuroprotective in some but not all studies.[61] There is one report suggesting that its actions are mediated by IGF-1 induction.[62] Finally, transforming growth factor β (TGFβ) and activin are two members of a large evolutionarily related family of growth factors that are induced after injury.[63] TGFβ₁ also may reduce delayed neuronal death at appropriate doses.[63]

4.1.5.4 Cerebrovascular responses in the secondary phase

A secondary phase of hyperperfusion or 'luxury perfusion' is well described after perinatal asphyxia.[64,65] Delayed cerebral hyperperfusion occurs after 30 minutes of cerebral ischemia in the fetal sheep, and peaks well after the peak in seizure activity, suggesting that it is only partly related to increased cerebral metabolism.[16] This delayed rise is mediated in part by endothelial NO synthase; NO blockade aggravates injury, suggesting that the increase in CBF may be beneficial for injured tissue.[66] Prostacyclin may also play a role in mediating the late increase in cerebral blood flow – this may be one further reason for concern with respect to the use of indomethacin, which inhibits prostacyclin, in fetal compromise.[67] Agents which depress blood pressure and thus impair cerebral blood flow in the post-asphyxial period aggravate brain injury. This has been demonstrated experimentally with calcium channel blockers[68] and is supported by clinical observation.[69]

4.1.5.5 Cerebral temperature

There is now good evidence that small changes in post-insult cerebral temperature can critically modulate encephalopathic processes initiated during hypoxia-ischemia.[70–72] Mild (2–3 °C) cerebral cooling, started immediately after hypoxic-ischemic injury and continued through the whole of the secondary phase (3 days) prevented the evolution of cortical infarction in the infant rat.[73] Conversely, prolonged mild hyperthermia during the secondary phase is deleterious.[70,71] Thirty minutes of moderate cerebral hypothermia starting 1.5–5.5 hours after ischemia and continuing until 72 hours after injury in the fetal sheep prevented secondary cytotoxic edema with a corresponding substantial reduction in neuronal loss (Fig. 4.2).[72] The mechanism is unknown but is likely to involve inhibition of delayed cell death.[74]

These data, which highlight the importance of small changes in cerebral temperature, suggest that the physiological cooling at birth (core temperature normally falls by 0.5–0.7 °C after delivery) may be an important natural protective process, augmented by greater cooling of the surface of the brain.[75] This has significant implications, since

infant care practices such as nursing asphyxiated infants under an overhead heater may adversely affect the normal gradient between core temperature and the brain.[75] Therapeutic use of hypothermia, however, requires considerable caution, as prolonged systemic hypothermia is associated with a number of potential adverse effects.[76]

4.1.6 Effect of maturation on neural sensitivity to injury

Surprisingly little work has been done to explore the effects of maturity on sensitivity to injury. This is of critical importance for two reasons. First, in recent years improvements in obstetric and pediatric management have resulted in significantly increased survival of preterm infants, which has been associated with a moderate rise in later cerebral palsy.[77] Secondly, there is increasing evidence that many infants may sustain neural injuries well before birth.[78]

4.1.6.1 Characteristics of preterm neural injury

The characteristic patterns of cerebral injury in the preterm fetus differ from those seen at term or after birth. Typical patterns in the immature brain include periventricular leukomalacia (PVL) and periventricular-intraventricular hemorrhage (PVH-IVH).[79] PVL is the major cause of neurodevelopmental handicap in surviving preterm infants.[6,80] The neurodevelopmental morbidity is directly correlated with the degree of parenchymal damage.[79] A proportion of infants with hemiplegia show diencephalic lesions, variably associated with PVL, cortical or subcortical lesions, and ventricular dilatation with clear evidence of a prenatal etiology.[81–83] Clinical imaging data suggest that profound asphyxia before 32 weeks gestation is associated with consistent injury to subcortical structures, particularly diencephalon (including the thalamus), basal ganglia, and brainstem.[84]

4.1.6.2 Pathogenesis of preterm injury

The pathogenesis of PVL and PVH-IVH has been related to several potential mechanisms. PVL occurs in areas that are postulated to represent arterial end zones or border zones.[79] Prolonged hypoperfusion potentially exposes these areas to severe ischemia. Further, there is evidence of prolonged loss of cerebrovascular autoregulation post-asphyxia which may leave the fetal brain vulnerable to fluctuations in blood pressure and thus cerebral blood flow; this is proposed to be a key mechanism in the pathogenesis of IVH.[79] Other factors that may contribute to IVH include the fragility of immature germinal matrix capillaries,[79,85] deficient vascular support,[86,87] and a limited vasodilatory capacity, impairing perfusion during asphyxia.[88]

It is postulated that immature white matter is intrinsically vulnerable to injury via several mechanisms. The midgestation period marks an important time for glial proliferation, differentiation, and myelination.[89] Actively differentiating cells have an increased metabolic demand and are sensitive to substrate limitation,[90] and developing oligodendroglia are very sensitive to the excitatory neurotransmitter glutamate and to free radical-mediated toxic mechanisms.[91,92]

Finally, recent compelling evidence has linked prenatal inflammation or infection to later cerebral palsy.[93] Exposure to maternal or placental infection is associated both with increased risk of preterm birth and also with brain lesions associated with cerebral palsy.[94] Increased neonatal levels of interleukins 1, 8 and 9, tumor necrosis factor α, and the interferons have been associated with other indicators of inflammation and with spastic diplegia.[95,96]

4.1.6.3   Maturation of neurotransmission

The importance of local maturational changes in neurotransmitter receptor function has been shown in a mouse model where vulnerability to excitotoxic neuronal death was assessed by microinjections of ibotenic acid, a glutaminergic agonist, to the cortex. When injected at birth, when only the first (supragranular) phase of neuronal migration is complete, ibotenate induced neuronal depopulation of layers V–VI and an abnormal sulcation of the overlying supragranular layers.[97] When injected after completion of all neuronal migration (P5–P10) ibotenate produced severe neuronal loss in layers II, III, IV, V, and VI. Periventricular white matter lesions were observed after ibotenate injection at P2–P10, with a peak of occurrence at P5. Interestingly, local magnesium therapy (which acts to inhibit the N-methyl-D-aspartate (NMDA) receptor) was protective only after P5, with the developmental acquisition of two properties of the excitotoxic cascade, namely the coupling of the massive calcium influx with NMDA-receptor overstimulation and the predominance of magnesium-blockable calcium channels.[98]

In fetal sheep at 0.65 gestation (96 days), a maturation comparable to the 28-week gestation human fetus, 30 minutes of cerebral ischemia induced by reversible carotid occlusion led to the development of infarction involving the deeper layers (V and VI) of the cortex and underlying white matter tracts.[99] In contrast, the same insult in the near-term fetal sheep leads to neuronal loss which is greatest in the superficial layers (II, III, and IV) of the cortex. The greater sensitivity of white matter and the deeper, more mature layers of the cortex to ischemic injury in the midgestational period may be related to transient expression of glutamate receptors as discussed above.[97] Finally, maturational changes in neuronal metabolism may also be important, with immature, migrating neurons primarily using anaerobic pathways.[100] This is an area requiring considerably greater attention.

4.1.7   Metabolic status

While the original studies of factors influencing the degree and distribution of brain injury, primarily by Myers,[101] focused on metabolic status, the influence of metabolic status remains controversial. It has been suggested, for example, that hyperglycemia is protective against hypoxia-ischemia in the infant rat[102] but not in the piglet.[103] The extreme differences between these neonatal species in the degree of neural maturation and activity of cerebral glucose transporters may underlie the different outcomes.[104] The most common metabolic disturbance of the fetus is IUGR associated with placental dysfunction. There is reasonable clinical presumption that IUGR leads to a greater sensitivity to brain injury.[105] However, it is not known whether such increased sensitivity is related to greater systemic compromise, as discussed in Section 4.2.3.4, or to altered neural development.

Neural maturation is markedly altered in IUGR, with some aspects delayed and others advanced,[106,107] and this may also influence the response to asphyxia and postnatal development. There may be reduced cerebral myelination and altered synaptogenesis[108] and smaller brain size.[109] Retardation of the EEG spectra occurs in the rat subjected to protein deprivation,[110] with perturbations of neurotransmitter activity.[111] Other possible effects include alterations in the neurotrophic milieu – for example expression of IGFs and their binding proteins is altered in tissues of growth-retarded fetuses, although the brain has not been studied.[112]

4.2 SYSTEMIC AND CARDIOVASCULAR ADAPTATION TO ASPHYXIA

In addition to the above studies of the purely cellular or neural responses to hypoxic-ischemic injury, the responses of the fetus to whole body asphyxia are also critical to outcome. Although the focus of most of the classic studies in this area was to delineate the cardiovascular and cerebrovascular responses, more recently the relationship between particular patterns of asphyxia and neurological outcome has been examined. The great majority of studies of the pathophysiology of asphyxia have been performed in the chronically instrumented fetal sheep, studied *in utero*.

4.2.1 Etiology of asphyxia

Systemic fetal asphyxia may be of fetal, placental, or maternal origin. Fetal causes include decreased fetal hemoglobin (e.g. hemolysis or feto-maternal hemorrhage), cord prolapse, cord compression, cord entanglements, and true knots in the cord. Placental causes include placenta previa, vasa previa, and placental abruption. Maternal causes include systemic hypoxia and reduced uteroplacental blood flow due to hypotension, vasospasm accompanying hypertension, and uterine hyperactivity.

Clearly the different etiological factors lead to different patterns of asphyxia, which may be acute, chronic, or acute on the background of chronic impairment. In labor, fetal asphyxia will most commonly be brief but frequently repeated, as placental blood flow is reduced by the rise in intrauterine pressure during contractions.[113] Conversely, catastrophic events such as cord prolapse or abruption will cause a single, profound and immediate insult. After placental abruption fetal blood loss further potentiates the direct effects of hypoxia on the fetus.

4.2.2 Hypoxia

The response of the fetal sheep to moderate, stable maternal hypoxia has been extensively characterized.[114] Fetal PaO_2 is typically reduced to 10–12 mmHg, where normal is 20–25 mmHg, by manipulating the maternal inspired fraction of oxygen. This technique of manipulating maternal FIO_2 alone can allow the components of asphyxia (hypoxia, hypercapnia, and acidemia) to be studied separately. As the severity of hypoxia is increased, progressive changes in the fetal cardiovascular responses can be distinguished.

In the late-gestation fetus, mild to moderate hypoxia is associated with an initial transient, moderate bradycardia followed by tachycardia, and a rise in blood pressure (Fig. 4.3). There is an overall increase in cardiac output and increased flow to essentially all organs.[115] With increasing severity of hypoxia there is redistribution of blood flow with further increases in blood flow to vital organs, the brain, heart, and adrenals, at the expense of peripheral organs.[114] This phenomenon

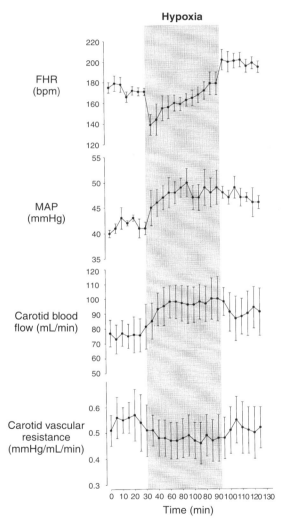

Figure 4.3 Cerebrovascular responses in the near-term fetal sheep to moderate isocapnic hypoxia for 60 minutes, induced by altering the maternal inspired gas mixture, showing changes in fetal heart rate (FHR), mean arterial blood pressure (MAP), carotid blood flow and carotid vascular resistance. During hypoxia there is a transient fetal bradycardia that gradually resolves, accompanied by sustained fetal hypertension. Carotid artery blood flow is increased throughout the hypoxic period, thus maintaining oxygen delivery to the brain. This is mediated partly by the rise in MAP, but also by a small reduction in vascular resistance (bottom panel). Data derived from Bennet *et al.* (1998).[163]

is termed 'centralization' of the circulation. Cerebral oxygen consumption is little changed even if arterial oxygen content falls as low as 1 mmol/L due to compensating increases in both cerebral blood flow and oxygen extraction.[115,116] Within the brain there is a greater increase in blood flow to the brainstem compared with the cerebrum, such that oxygen delivery is fully maintained to the brainstem, but not to the cerebrum.[115,116] Nitric oxide has been shown to play a role in mediating the local increase in cerebral blood flow.[117] These adaptations are illustrated in Fig. 4.3, which shows the combination of increased mean arterial pressure, reduced cerebral vascular resistance and sustained increase in carotid blood flow.

These changes in fetal heart rate (FHR) and cardiac output are reflexly mediated, in part by muscarinic (parasympathetic) pathways, and by α-adrenergic stimulation. The adrenergic input is derived partly from the sympathetic neural system and partly by circulating catecholamines released from the adrenal medulla. The rise in blood pressure during asphyxia is at least partly mediated by vasopressors including the catecholamines, arginine vasopressin (AVP), and angiotensin II (AII).[114,118] There is also a large adrenocorticotropic (ACTH) and cortisol response to hypoxia. The role of ACTH in the cardiovascular response to hypoxia is unclear, but cortisol has been shown to modulate the actions of other vasopressors,[119] and to help maintain blood pressure in stressed premature newborns.[120]

4.2.2.1 Prolonged hypoxia

The effect of prolonged hypoxemia on cerebral metabolism in near-term fetal sheep has been studied during step-wise reductions of maternal FIO_2.[121] Until the fetal arterial oxygen saturation was reduced to less than 30 percent of baseline, cerebral oxidative metabolism remained stable. At the lowest inspired oxygen concentration (with 3 percent CO_2) a progressive metabolic acidemia was induced. Initially, cerebral blood flow increased, thus maintaining cerebral oxygen delivery. As the pH fell below 7.15, hypotension developed, with corresponding impairment of CBF, and ultimately a fall in cerebral oxygen consumption to less than 50 percent of control values.

With chronic hypoxemia there is a gradual decrease in oxygen consumption which is at least in part related to a reduction in growth and altered activity.[122] In one study where fetal sheep were exposed to a 10 mmHg decrease in PaO_2 for up to 28 days, tissue oxygen delivery was supported by increased hemoglobin synthesis, mediated by greater erythropoietin release.[123] The increase was such that ultimately fetal oxygen content was unchanged from control. Values of mean arterial pressure and heart rate did not differ from controls and at term their body weights were normal. Epinephrine also increased moderately and remained elevated throughout the study.

4.2.2.2 Maturational changes in responses to hypoxia

The cardiovascular response to fetal hypoxia is age related. In the premature fetal sheep before 100 days (0.7) gestation isocapnic hypoxia[124] and hemorrhagic hypotension[125] are not associated with hypertension, bradycardia, or peripheral vasoconstriction. Thus it has been suggested that peripheral vasomotor control starts to develop at 0.7 gestation, coincident with maturation of neurohormonal regulators and chemoreceptor function.[126] As will be discussed in the section on asphyxia, however, in interpreting these results it is also important to consider the degree of hypoxia in relation to the much greater anaerobic capacity of the premature fetus. It is likely that the degree of hypoxia attained in these studies did not reduce tissue oxygen availability below critical levels for this developmental stage.

4.2.3 Asphyxia

Asphyxia, by definition, consists of impaired respiratory gas exchange (with hypoxia and respiratory acidosis) accompanied by the development of metabolic acidosis. The most common approaches to induce experimental asphyxia in the fetal sheep are reduced uterine perfusion or occlusion of the umbilical cord. In the first method an occluder is placed around the common internal iliac artery (which supplies both uterine horns) to manipulate uterine blood flow. The ovarian vessels must be ligated to prevent anastomotic flow. In the second, an inflatable occluder is attached around the umbilical cord. The results of these approaches have been comparable where similar degrees and patterns of asphyxia were induced.

Both approaches may be considered to represent physiological situations. Uterine perfusion is linearly compromised by increased uterine pressure.[113] The buffer effects of amniotic fluid protect the umbilical cord during early uterine contractions,[127] but when the amount of amniotic fluid is reduced, e.g. in IUGR, oligohydramnios, or after rupture of the amniotic membranes, physiologic uterine contractions may compress the umbilical cord and compromise the fetus.[127,128]

Brief, total clamping of the uterine artery or umbilical cord leads to a rapid reduction of fetal oxygenation within a few minutes, associated with massive hemodynamic changes and rapid metabolic deterioration.[129,130] In contrast, prolonged gradual clamping induces a slow fetal metabolic deterioration without the acute fetal cardiovascular responses of bradycardia and hypertension which are seen during acute short clamping.[131]

The responses to moderate asphyxia are similar to those described above for hypoxia, with redistribution of blood flow to the brain, heart, and adrenals.[132] During profound asphyxia, corresponding with a reduction of uterine blood flow to 25 percent or less, with fetal arterial oxygen contents of less than 1 mmol/L, the cardiovascular responses of the normal fetus are substantially different. Bradycardia is sustained and blood flow to the cerebrum no longer rises or may even fall despite initially increased fetal blood pressure. There is a generalized vasoconstriction involving essentially all organs.[132] Within the brain, blood flow during asphyxia is preferentially redirected to the brainstem, which maintains autonomic function at the expense of the cerebrum.[133] Furthermore, the reduced oxygen content limits oxygen extraction from the blood. The combination of these two factors, restricted cerebral blood flow and reduced oxygen extraction, leads to a profound fall in cerebral oxygen consumption.[134] During such an insult, as illustrated in Fig. 4.4, blood pressure initially increases markedly but this rise is not sustained and as asphyxia proceeds the fetus becomes hypotensive.

The sustained bradycardia and increased peripheral resistance in the late gestation fetus during asphyxia are mediated by the carotid chemoreceptors; a logarithmic rise in circulating catecholamine levels further augments the peripheral vasoconstriction.[116] The subsequent hypotension is primarily related to asphyxial impairment of myocardial contractility,[135] due to a direct inhibitory effect of profound acidosis[136] and depletion of myocardial glycogen stores.[137] Once glycogen is depleted, there is rapid loss of high-energy metabolites such as ATP in mitochondria.[138] During a shorter episode (e.g. 5 minutes) of asphyxia, the fetus may not become hypotensive. If the insult is repeated before myocardial glycogen can

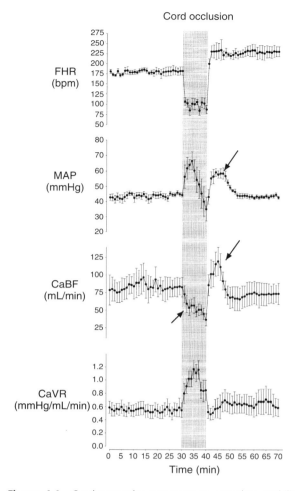

Figure 4.4 Cerebrovascular responses to complete umbilical cord occlusion for 10 minutes in the near-term fetal sheep. In contrast to the response to moderate hypoxia, there is a profound fetal heart rate (FHR) deceleration maintained throughout the occlusion. Fetal mean arterial blood pressure (MAP) is initially elevated but then falls to below normal just prior to release. Carotid blood flow (CaBF) is significantly reduced from the start of occlusion, but falls further once MAP begins to fall. This initial paradoxical response is mediated by an increase in carotid vascular resistance (CaVR). Data derived from Bennet et al. (1998).[163]

be replenished, successive periods of asphyxia will be associated with increasing duration of hypotension.[139,140]

Another possible factor leading to impaired contractility is myocardial injury, which has been found after severe birth asphyxia and congenital heart disease in limited case series.[141] Myocardial cell death may not be necessary for dysfunction to occur; studies in adult animals have shown that there may be a significant delay in recovery of cardiac contractility after reperfusion from brief ischemia in the absence of necrosis. This delayed recovery has been termed 'myocardial stunning'.[142]

There is evidence that 'stunning' may contribute to progressive myocardial dysfunction during repeated asphyxia in the fetal lamb.[143]

4.2.3.1 Progressive asphyxia

During gradually induced asphyxia, even to arterial oxygen contents of less than 1 mmol/L, fetal adaptation may be closer to that seen with hypoxia. Progressive reduction of uterine perfusion over a 3 to 4-hour period in near-term fetal sheep led to a mean pH <7.00, serum lactate levels >14 mmol/L, with a fetal mortality of 53 percent. Surviving animals remained normotensive and normoglycemic, and cerebral blood flow was more than doubled. Cerebrospinal fluid metabolite concentrations, including lactate, hypoxanthine, and xanthine, increased by two- to five-fold.[144]

Interestingly, in surviving fetuses, neuronal damage was limited to selective loss of cerebellar Purkinje cells.[131]

4.2.3.2 Brief repeated asphyxia

In normal human labor, uterine contractions are relatively brief (typically less than 1 or 2 minutes). The effects of total umbilical cord occlusions have been studied in fetal lambs near term at frequencies consistent with active labor, either 1 minute out of every 2.5 minutes or 2 minutes out of every 5 minutes, continued for many hours until fetal hypotension (<20 mmHg) occurred.[139,145] There was an initial sustained rise in blood pressure during early occlusions followed after 15 minutes by the appearance of a biphasic pattern. At this time fetal blood pressure would rise with each occlusion, but then begin to fall. From then on a progressive fall in the nadir of fetal arterial blood pressure occurred with each occlusion.

At a pH between 7.04 and 6.85 in individual fetuses, the recovery of arterial blood pressure after each occlusion became markedly delayed. The rapid decompensation associated with this sustained hypotension could not in the majority of cases be detected by changes in the shape of FHR decelerations, which highlights the poor diagnostic value of FHR monitoring to identify the compromised fetus.[139] Cerebral edema progressively developed during occlusions and remained present for a mean of 11 hours after the final occlusion. Mild seizure-like activity was present for 5–10 hours after the final insult. Histologic analysis demonstrated the presence of focal neuronal damage in the parasagittal cortex, the thalamus, and the cerebellum, while the hippocampus and striatum were almost wholly spared.[145]

4.2.3.3 Maturational changes in fetal responses to asphyxia

The premature lamb fetus at 0.6 gestation (equivalent to the 26–28-week human fetus) can tolerate extended periods of up to 20 minutes of umbilical cord occlusion without neuronal loss.[146] The very prolonged cardiac survival (up to 30 minutes)[147] corresponds with the maximal levels of cardiac glycogen which are seen in the very premature fetus.[137] Interestingly, in contrast to the limited effects of moderate hypoxia,[124] the pattern of the cardiovascular response during asphyxia was similar to that seen in more mature fetuses, with sustained bradycardia, accompanied by initial hypertension, then a progressive fall in pressure to very low levels after 15 minutes.[147]

Even before the onset of hypotension there is evidence of limited redistribution of cardiac output to the brain during the initial part of asphyxia. Cerebral blood flow is maintained, but does not increase despite increased blood pressure.[147] The mechanism of this remains speculative. As shown in Fig. 4.5, CBF then falls in parallel with the fall blood pressure. Post-asphyxia, a brief period of arterial hypertension and hyperperfusion is followed by a prolonged period of hypoperfusion despite normalization of blood pressure.[147] Near infrared spectroscopy suggests that not only is the period of cerebral hypoperfusion accompanied by a fall in cerebral blood volume but also that there is a relative reduction in oxygen availability to the brain, with a fall in oxyhemoglobin during the first few hours of hypoperfusion (Fig. 4.6, p.68).[147] These data suggest that this phase of hypoperfusion and reduced oxygen delivery may be related to the pathogenesis of cerebral injury or may represent a period of increased vulnerability to secondary insults.

4.2.3.4 Chronic asphyxia and intrauterine growth retardation

In addition to its impact on neurodevelopment, chronic asphyxia may also adversely affect the ability of the fetus to adapt to acute insults. In experimental animals chronic placental damage produced by microsphere embolism leads to fetal arterial hypertension and myocardial hypertrophy with increased umbilical artery resistance.[148]

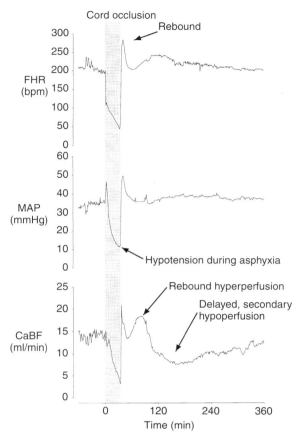

Figure 4.5 An example of the cerebrovascular responses of a premature (0.6 gestation) fetal sheep to complete umbilical cord occlusion for 30 minutes. The overall response of the premature fetus is similar to that of the near-term fetus, with initial hypertension, followed by hypotension. After reperfusion, the premature fetus shows initial hyperperfusion followed by a prolonged phase of secondary hypoperfusion consistent with marked suppression of cerebral metabolism. The ability of the premature fetus to survive profound asphyxia for such a prolonged period is likely to be related to its very elevated cardiac glycogen levels and enhanced anaerobic reserve. CaBF, carotid blood flow; FHR, fetal heat rate; MAP, mean aterial blood pressure. Data derived from Bennet *et al.* (1999).[147]

Experimentally growth-retarded fetuses exhibit sustained elevation of plasma catecholamines,[148] cortisol, and PGE_2,[149] with a significant fall in corticotropin,[150] and have a blunted rise in plasma catecholamines and cardiovascular response to further acute hypoxic challenges.[151] Similar observations have been made in newborn rats exposed to chronic hypoxia *in utero*,[152] and in the llama, a species adapted to the hypoxemia of high altitude.[153] Human growth-retarded fetuses have increased catecholamine levels in amniotic fluid.[154] These data suggest that growth-retarded fetuses may be unable to mount an appropriate sympathetic nervous system response to acute hypoxia.

4.3 PATHOPHYSIOLOGICAL DETERMINANTS OF ASPHYXIAL INJURY

4.3.1 The role of hypotension

The data discussed above lead to the concept that one of the key factors precipitating cerebral damage during acute asphyxia is the occurrence and duration of hypotension during the insult. Clearly some white or gray matter injury may still occur even when significant hypotension is not seen,[131,155] particularly when hypoxia is very prolonged.[156,157] Nevertheless, there is a strong correlation between hypotension and neuronal loss both within individual studies of acute asphyxia,[145,155,158] and between similar paradigms causing severe fetal acidosis, manipulated to either cause fetal hypotension,[155,158] or to prevent it.[131] For example, in fetal lambs exposed to prolonged severe partial asphyxia significant neuronal loss occurred only in those in whom one or more episodes of acute hypotension occurred.[158] In contrast, where an equally 'severe' insult was induced gradually and titrated to maintain normal or elevated blood pressure throughout the insult no neuronal loss was seen outside the cerebellum.[131] Similarly, in adult cats exposed to 25 minutes of marked hypoxia, animals that maintained their blood pressure were cerebrally intact, whereas hypotensive animals showed severe neuronal necrosis.[159]

This crucial role for arterial pressure during hypoxia is likely to be related to the limited autoregulatory range of the fetal cerebrovasculature.[160] Since normal fetal blood pressure corresponds to the lower end of the autoregulatory range, CBF will be impaired by even mild hypotension.[147,161–163] As discussed earlier, during moderate hypoxia, with normal or raised blood pressure, centralization of blood flow with sustained hypertension allows the fetus to maintain sufficient oxygen delivery to the brain (Fig. 4.3). During severe asphyxia of rapid onset however, hypotension develops rapidly, and, once it is present, there is a linear reduction in cerebral perfusion (Figs 4.4 and 4.5). Interestingly, the phase of rapidly falling blood pressure during asphyxia has been related to failure of centralization, with increased blood flow to peripheral structures.[147,164]

4.3.2 The 'watershed' distribution of neuronal loss, and variants

A number of different patterns of histopathologically and radiologically defined cerebral injury

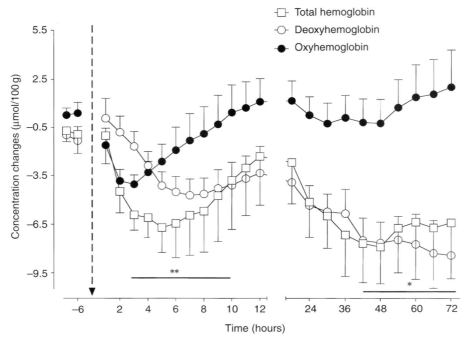

Figure 4.6 Changes in cerebral deoxyhemoglobin, oxyhemoglobin, and total hemoglobin (THb, an index of cerebral blood volume) measured by near-infrared spectroscopy, after 30 minutes of umbilical cord occlusion in the 0.6 gestation fetal sheep. There was a significant fall in THb between 2 and 8 hours post occlusion (** $p < 0.005$ compared to baseline) and again between 30 and 54 hours post occlusion (* $p < 0.05$ compared to baseline), consistent with the time course of secondary hypoperfusion indicated by the fall in carotid blood flow shown in Fig. 4.5. In addition, there was a marked fall in oxyhemoglobin between 2 and 5 hours, with the nadir at 3 hours post occlusion ($p < 0.005$), suggesting functional impairment of cerebral oxygen delivery. Mean ± SEM. Data derived from Bennet et al. (1999).[147]

have been reported in association with human perinatal asphyxia.[5,165] Recent experimental studies of asphyxia in the near-term fetal sheep have explored the relationship between the distribution of neuronal damage and the type of insult. In most paradigms, the data are consistent with the hypothesis that the overall distribution of damage is related to local cerebral perfusion.

After brief (1–2 minutes) episodes of repeated cord occlusions continued until severe hypotension (<20 mmHg) developed, patchy infarction and selective neuronal loss were localized to the parasagittal cortex, the thalamus and the cerebellar neocortex.[145] 'Watershed' zones are areas of tissue between the territory of supply of major cerebral arteries, where perfusion pressure is least.[166] Figure 4.7a shows the similarity of distribution of damage following asphyxia to that seen after reversible cerebral ischemia in the fetal sheep (Fig. 4.8). These data are consistent with other experimental studies in the fetal sheep including 10 minutes of cord occlusion,[130] and prolonged partial asphyxia,[155,158] although there are some

specific differences which are discussed below. In both human adults and neonates, lesions in the 'watershed' areas have generally been associated with systemic hypotension,[166] and are commonly observed after perinatal asphyxia at term.[5,165]

4.3.3 Hippocampal involvement

The dorsal hippocampus lies within the watershed zone between the middle cerebral artery and the anterior and posterior arteries, and is severely injured after a single profound episode of asphyxia or ischemia in the near-term fetal sheep.[7,130] Nevertheless, the hippocampus (dentate gyrus and cornu ammonis 1 and 2 (CA 1/2) fields of the hippocampus are shown in Fig. 4.7) was strikingly spared after both brief repeated asphyxia[145] and prolonged partial asphyxia.[158] Interestingly, *in vitro* studies suggest that acidosis can limit both hypoxic and excitotoxic neuronal injury in hippocampal neurons.[167,168] Very profound acidosis (pH 6.83 ± 0.03) during brief repeated cord occlusions was associated with

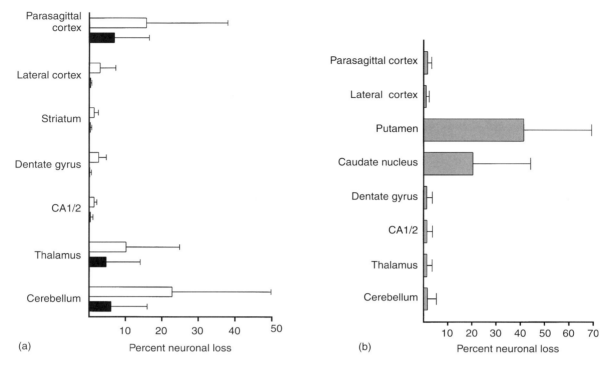

Figure 4.7 The distribution of neuronal loss assessed after 3 days recovery from two different patterns of prenatal asphyxia in near-term fetal sheep. (a) The effect of brief (1 or 2 minutes) cord occlusions repeated at frequencies consistent with established labor. Occlusions were terminated after a variable time, when the fetal blood pressure fell below 20 mmHg for two successive occlusions. This insult leads to a classic watershed distribution of cerebral damage.[145] CA 1/2 and the dentate gyrus are regions of the hippocampus. (b) The effect of 5-minute episodes of cord occlusion, repeated four times, at intervals of 30 minutes. This paradigm is associated with selective neuronal loss in the putamen and caudate nuclei of the striatum. Data derived from de Haan et al. (1997).[140] Mean ± SD.

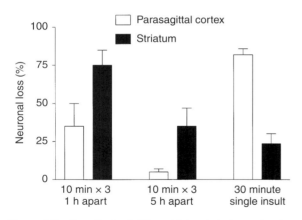

Figure 4.8 The effects of different intervals between insults on the distribution of cerebral damage after ischemia in fetal sheep. Cerebral ischemia was induced by carotid occlusion for 10 minutes repeated three times, at intervals of either 1 hour or 5 hours, compared with a single continuous episode of 30 minutes occlusion, on cortical and striatal neuronal loss in the late-gestation fetal sheep. The divided insults were associated with a preponderance of striatal injury, whereas a single episode of 30 minutes of carotid occlusion was associated with severe cortical neuronal loss. Increasing the interval to 5 hours nearly completely abolished cortical injury, but was still associated with significant neuronal loss in the striatum. Data derived from Mallard et al. (1993).[170] Mean ± SD.

sparing of the hippocampus.[145] In contrast, the relatively mild metabolic acidosis (after 5 minutes recovery the mean pH was >7.10) after 10 minutes of umbilical cord occlusion was associated with severe selective loss in the cornu ammonis fields of the hippocampus.[130]

4.3.4 Striatal damage

The one apparent exception to a general tendency to a 'watershed' distribution after global asphyxial insults near term is the selective neuronal loss in striatal nuclei (putamen and caudate nucleus, Fig. 4.7) after repeated but widely spaced episodes of complete cord occlusion.[140,169] Significant striatal involvement was also seen after prolonged partial asphyxia in which distinct episodes of bradycardia and hypotension occurred.[158] A study of repeated 10-minute episodes of cerebral ischemia in the near-term fetal sheep has shown that as the spacing between episodes of ischemia was increased, the amount of striatal damage increased relative to cortical neuronal loss, as illustrated in Fig. 4.8.[170]

It is thus likely that pathogenesis of striatal involvement is related to the precise timing of the relatively prolonged episodes of asphyxia and not to more severe local hypoperfusion since the striatum is not in a watershed zone but rather within the territory of the middle cerebral artery. The vulnerability of the striatum to this type of insult may be related to a greater release of glutamate after repeated insults compared with a single insult of the same cumulative duration.[171] Immunohistochemical techniques have shown that inhibitory striatal neurons were primarily affected.[169]

4.4   SUMMARY

Although it is possible that regional differences in the rate of maturation between the sheep and human may contribute to differences in brain damage, the experimental studies discussed in this chapter demonstrate that the exact pattern by which asphyxia is induced makes an important contribution to localization of the damage. It has become evident that the key factors determining the magnitude of perinatal brain damage are (1) cerebral perfusion pressure, as reflected by arterial blood pressure, during the event(s) and (2) the pattern of the insult, modified by fetal maturity, aerobic reserve and environmental temperature. As the critical events which lead to clinically significant perinatal hypoxic-ischemic encephalopathy are clarified by innovative experimental approaches our ability to recognize significant prenatal events and to intervene appropriately will also improve.

4.5   ACKNOWLEDGEMENTS

The authors' work reported in this review has been supported by USPHS R01 HD-32752, and by grants from the Health Research Council of New Zealand, the Auckland Medical Research Foundation and the Lottery Grants Board of New Zealand.

4.6   REFERENCES

1 Nelson KB, Leviton A. How much of neonatal encephalopathy is due to birth asphyxia? *American Journal of Diseases of Children* 1991; **145**: 1325–31.

2 Van Bel F, Dorrepaal CA, Benders MJ, Zeeuwe PE, van de Bor M, Berger HM. Changes in cerebral hemodynamics and oxygenation in the first 24 hours after birth asphyxia. *Pediatrics* 1993; **92**: 365–72.

3 Roth SC, Baudin J, Cady E *et al*. Relation of deranged neonatal cerebral oxidative metabolism with neuro-developmental outcome and head circumference at 4 years. *Developmental Medicine and Child Neurology* 1997; **39**: 718–25.

4 Westgate JA, Gunn AJ, Gunn TR. Antecedents of neonatal encephalopathy with fetal acidaemia at term. *British Journal of Obstetrics and Gynaecology* 1999; **106**: 774–82.

5 Volpe JJ. Hypoxic-ischemic encephalopathy: neuropathology and pathogenesis. In: *Neurology of the newborn*, 3rd edn. Philadelphia: WB Saunders, 1995: 279–313.

6 Volpe JJ. Brain injury in the premature infant – neuropathology, clinical aspects, pathogenesis, and prevention. *Clinical Perinatology* 1997; **24**: 567ff.

7 Williams CE, Gunn AJ, Mallard C, Gluckman PD. Outcome after ischemia in the developing sheep brain: an electroencephalographic and histological study. *Annals of Neurology* 1992; **31**: 14–21.

8 Beilharz EJ, Williams CE, Dragunow M, Sirimanne ES, Gluckman PD. Mechanisms of delayed cell death following hypoxic-ischemic injury in the immature rat: evidence for apoptosis during selective neuronal loss. *Molecular Brain Research* 1995; **29**: 1–14.

9 Memezawa H, Minamisawa H, Smith ML, Siesjö BK. Ischemic penumbra in a model of reversible middle cerebral artery occlusion in the rat. *Experimental Brain Research* 1992; **89**: 67–78.

10 Folbergrova J, Memezawa H, Smith ML, Siesjö BK. Focal and perifocal changes in tissue energy state during middle cerebral artery occlusion in normo- and hyperglycemic rats. *Journal of Cerebral Blood Flow Metabolism* 1992; **12**: 25–33.

11 Nedergaard M, Hansen AJ. Characterization of cortical depolarizations evoked in focal cerebral ischemia. *Journal of Cerebral Blood Flow Metabolism* 1993; **13**: 568–74.

12 Lorek A, Takei Y, Cady EB *et al*. Delayed ('secondary') cerebral energy failure after acute hypoxia-ischemia in the newborn piglet: continuous 48-hour studies by phosphorus magnetic resonance spectroscopy. *Pediatric Research* 1994; **36**: 699–706.

13 Gunn AJ, Gunn TR, de Haan HH, Williams CE, Gluckman PD. Dramatic neuronal rescue with prolonged selective head cooling after ischemia in fetal sheep. *Journal of Clinical Investigation* 1997; **99**: 248–56.

14 Warner DS, Ludwig PS, Pearlstein R, Brinkhous AD. Halothane reduces focal ischemic injury in the rat when brain temperature is controlled. *Anesthesiology* 1995; **82**: 1237–45.

15 Nakashima K, Todd MM. Effects of hypothermia, pentobarbital, and isoflurane on postdepolarization amino acid release during complete global cerebral ischemia. *Anesthesiology* 1996; **85**: 161–8.

16 Abi Raad R, Tan WK, Bennet L *et al*. Role of the cerebrovascular and metabolic responses in the delayed phases of injury after transient cerebral ischemia in fetal sheep. *Stroke* 1999; **30**: 2735–41.

17 Williams CE, Gunn A, Gluckman PD. Time course of intracellular edema and epileptiform activity follow-

ing prenatal cerebral ischemia in sheep. *Stroke* 1991; **22**: 516–21.

18 Tan WK, Williams CE, Gunn AJ, Mallard CE, Gluckman PD. Suppression of postischemic epileptiform activity with MK-801 improves neural outcome in fetal sheep. *Annals of Neurology* 1992; **32**: 677–82.

19 Petito CK, Feldmann E, Pulsinelli W, Plum F. Delayed hippocampal damage in humans following cardiorespiratory arrest. *Neurology* 1987; **37**: 1281–6.

20 Petito CK, Pulsinelli WA. Sequential development of reversible and irreversible neuronal damage following cerebral ischemia. *Journal of Neuropathology and Experimental Neurology* 1984; **43**: 141–53.

21 Andine P, Jacobson I, Hagberg H. Calcium uptake evoked by electrical stimulation is enhanced postischemically and precedes delayed neuronal death in CA1 of rat hippocampus: involvement of N-methyl-D-aspartate receptors. *Journal of Cerebral Blood Flow Metabolism* 1988; **8**: 799–807.

22 Dive C, Gregory CD, Phipps DJ, Evans DL, Milner AE, Wyllie AH. Analysis and discrimination of necrosis and apoptosis (programmed cell death) by multiparameter flow cytometry. *Biochimica Biophysica Acta* 1992; **1133**: 275–85.

23 Wyllie AH. Glucocorticoid-induced thymocyte apoptosis is associated with endogenous endonuclease activation. *Nature* 1980; **284**: 555–6.

24 Raff MC. Social controls on cell survival and cell death. *Nature* 1992; **356**: 397–400.

25 Edwards AD, Cox P, Hope PL, Azzopardi DV, Squier MV, Mehmet H. Apoptosis in the brains of infants suffering intrauterine cerebral injury. *Pediatric Research* 1997; **42**: 684–9.

26 Scott RJ, Hegyi L. Cell death in perinatal hypoxic-ischaemic brain injury. *Neuropathology and Applied Neurobiology* 1997; **23**: 307–14.

27 Larsen CJ. The BCL2 gene is the prototype of a gene family that controls programmed cell death (apoptosis). *Annals of Genetics Paris* 1994; **37**: 121–34.

28 MacGibbon GA, Lawlor PA, Sirimanne ES *et al.* Bax expression in mammalian neurons undergoing apoptosis, and in Alzheimer's disease hippocampus. *Brain Research* 1997; **750**: 223–34.

29 Gorman AM, Orrenius S, Ceccatelli S. Apoptosis in neuronal cells: role of caspases. *NeuroReport* 1998; **9**: R49–55.

30 Porteracailliau C, Price DL, Martin LJ. Excitotoxic neuronal death in the immature brain is an apoptosis-necrosis morphological continuum. *Journal of Comparative Neurology* 1997; **378**: 70–87.

31 Gottron FJ, Ying HS, Choi DW. Caspase inhibition selectively reduces the apoptotic component of oxygen-glucose deprivation-induced cortical neuronal cell death. *Molecular and Cellular Neuroscience* 1997; **9**: 159–69.

32 Rothman SM, Olney JW. Excitotoxicity and the NMDA receptor – still lethal after eight years. *Trends in Neurosciences* 1995; **18**: 57–8.

33 Choi DW. Calcium: still center-stage in hypoxic-ischemic neuronal death. *Trends in Neurosciences* 1995; **18**: 58–60.

34 Bagenholm R, Nilsson UA, Kjellmer I. Formation of free radicals in hypoxic ischemic brain damage in the neonatal rat, assessed by an endogenous spin trap and lipid peroxidation. *Brain Research* 1997; **773**: 132–8.

35 Kuroda S, Siesjo BK. Reperfusion damage following focal ischemia: pathophysiology and therapeutic windows. *Clinical Neuroscience* 1997; **4**: 199–212.

36 Kruman II, Mattson MP. Pivotal role of mitochondrial calcium uptake in neural cell apoptosis and necrosis. *Journal of Neurochemistry* 1999; **72**: 529–40.

37 Gluckman P, Klempt N, Guan J *et al.* A role for IGF-1 in the rescue of CNS neurons following hypoxic-ischemic injury. *Biochemical and Biophysical Research Communications* 1992; **182**: 593–9.

38 Lees GJ. The possible contribution of microglia and macrophages to delayed neuronal death after ischemia. *Journal of the Neurological Sciences* 1993; **114**: 119–22.

39 Tan WK, Williams CE, During MJ *et al.* Accumulation of cytotoxins during the development of seizures and edema after hypoxic-ischemic injury in late gestation fetal sheep. *Pediatric Research* 1996; **39**: 791–7.

40 During MJ, Spencer DD. Extracellular hippocampal glutamate and spontaneous seizure in the conscious human brain. *Lancet* 1993; **341**: 1607–10.

41 al Naqeeb N, Edwards AD, Cowan FM, Azzopardi D. Assessment of neonatal encephalopathy by amplitude-integrated electroencephalography. *Pediatrics* 1999; **103**: 1263–71.

42 Faraci FM, Brian JE. Nitric oxide and the cerebral circulation. *Stroke* 1994; **25**: 692–703.

43 Iadecola C, Zhang FY, Xu XH. Inhibition of inducible nitric oxide synthase ameliorates cerebral ischemic damage. *American Journal of Physiology* 1995; **37**: R286–92.

44 Rudolphi KA, Schubert P, Parkinson FE, Fredholm BB. Adenosine and brain ischemia. *Cerebrovascular and Brain Metabolism Reviews* 1992; **4**: 346–69.

45 Ting P, Xu S, Krumins S. Endogenous opioid system activity following temporary focal cerebral ischemia. *Acta Neurochirurgica Supplementum (Wien)* 1994; **60**: 253–6.

46 Shuaib A, Kanthan R. Amplification of inhibitory mechanisms in cerebral ischemia – an alternative approach to neuronal protection. *Histology and Histopathology* 1997; **12**: 185–94.

47 Nilsson GE, Lutz PL. Release of inhibitory neurotransmitters in response to anoxia in turtle brain. *American Journal of Physiology* 1991; **261**: R32–R37.

48 Irestedt L, Dahlin I, Hertzberg T, Sollevi A, Lagercrantz H. Adenosine concentration in umbilical cord blood of newborn infants after vaginal delivery and cesarean section. *Pediatric Research* 1989; **26**(2): 106–8.

49 von Lubitz DK. Adenosine and cerebral ischemia: therapeutic future or death of a brave concept? *European Journal of Pharmacology* 1999; **371**: 85–102.

50 Shimazaki K, Ishida A, Kawai N. Increase in bcl-2 oncoprotein and the tolerance to ischemia-induced neuronal death in the gerbil hippocampus. *Neuroscience Research* 1994; **20**: 95–9.

51 Lowenstein DH, Gwinn RP, Seren MS, Simon RP, Mcintosh TK. Increased expression of mRNA encoding calbindin-D28K, the glucose-regulated proteins, or the 72 kDa heat-shock protein in three models of acute CNS injury. *Molecular Brain Research* 1994; **22**: 299–308.

52 Waldvogel HJ, Faull RLM, Dragunow M. Differential sensitivity of calbindin and parvalbumin immuno-reactive cells in the striatum to excitotoxins. *Brain Research* 1991; **546**: 329–35.

53 Goodman JH, Wasterlain CG, Massarweh WF, Dean E, Sollas AL, Sloviter RS. Calbindin-D28k immuno-reactivity and selective vulnerability to ischemia in the dentate gyrus of the developing rat. *Brain Research* 1993; **606**: 309–14.

54 Nakao N, Kokaia Z, Odin P, Lindvall O. Protective effects of BDNF and NT-3 but not PDGF against hypoglycemic injury to cultured striatal neurons. *Experimental Neurology* 1995; **131**: 1–10.

55 Nieto-bona MP, Busiguina S, Torres-Aleman I. Insulin-like growth factor 1 is an afferent trophic signal that modulates calbindin-28kd in adult purkinje cells. *Journal of Neuroscience Research* 1995; **42**: 371–6.

56 Nietro P.60-Sampedro M, Lewis ER, Cotman CW et al. Brain injury causes a time-dependent increase in neurotrophic activity at the lesion site. *Science* 1982; **217**: 860–1.

57 Dragunow M, Beilharz E, Sirimanne E et al. Immediate-early gene protein expression in neurons undergoing delayed death, but not necrosis, following hypoxic-ischaemic injury to the young rat brain. *Molecular Brain Research* 1994; **25**: 19–33.

58 Yin QW, Johnson J, Prevette D, Oppenheim RW. Cell death of spinal motoneurons in the chick embryo following deafferentation: rescue effects of tissue extracts, soluble proteins, and neurotrophic agents. *Journal of Neuroscience* 1994; **14**: 7629–40.

59 Galli C, Meucci O, Scorziello A, Werge TM, Calissano P, Schettini G. Apoptosis in cerebellar granule cells is blocked by high KCl, forskolin, and IGF-1 through distinct mechanisms of action: the involvement of intracellular calcium and RNA synthesis. *Journal of Neuroscience* 1995; **15**: 1172–9.

60 Johnston BM, Mallard EC, Williams CE, Gluckman PD. Insulin-like growth factor-1 is a potent neuronal rescue agent following hypoxic-ischemic injury in fetal lambs. *Journal of Clinical Investigation* 1996; **97**: 300–8.

61 Cuevas P. Therapeutic prospects for fibroblast growth factor treatment of brain ischemia. *Neurological Research* 1997; **19**: 355–6.

62 Pons S, Torres-Aleman I. Basic fibroblast growth factor modulates insulin-like growth factor-1, its receptor, and its binding proteins in hypothalamic cell cultures. *Endocrinology* 1992; **131**: 2271–8.

63 Hughes PE, Alexi T, Walton M et al. Activity and injury-dependent expression of inducible transcription factors, growth factors and apoptosis-related genes within the central nervous system. *Progress in Neurobiology* 1999; **57**: 421–50.

64 Pryds O, Greisen G, Lou H, Friis-Hansen B. Vasoparalysis associated with brain damage in asphyxiated term infants. *Journal of Pediatrics* 1990; **117**: 119–25.

65 Levene MI, Fenton AC, Evans DH, Archer LN, Shortland DB, Gibson NA. Severe birth asphyxia and abnormal cerebral blood-flow velocity. *Developmental Medicine and Child Neurology* 1989; **31**: 427–34.

66 Marks KA, Mallard EC, Roberts I, Williams CE, Gluckman PD, Edwards AD. Nitric oxide synthase inhibition attenuates delayed vasodilation and increases injury following cerebral ischemia in fetal sheep. *Pediatric Research* 1996; **40**: 185–91.

67 Walton M, Sirimanne E, Williams C et al. Prostaglandin H synthase-2 and cytosolic phospholipase A2 in the hypoxic-ischemic brain: role in neuronal death or survival? *Brain Research and Molecular Brain Research* 1997; **50**: 165–70.

68 Gunn AJ, Williams CE, Mallard EC, Tan WKM, Gluckman PD. Flunarizine, a calcium channel antagonist, is partially prophylactically neuroprotective in hypoxic-ischemic encephalopathy in the fetal sheep. *Pediatric Research* 1994; **35**: 657–63.

69 Levene MI, Gibson NA, Fenton AC, Papathoma E, Barnett D. The use of a calcium channel blocker, nicardipine, for severely asphyxiated newborn infants. *Developmental Medicine and Child Neurology* 1990; **32**: 567–74.

70 Coimbra C, Drake M, Boris-Moller F, Wieloch T. Long-lasting neuroprotective effect of postischemic hypothermia and treatment with an anti-inflammatory/antipyretic drug. Evidence for chronic encephalopathic processes following ischemia. *Stroke* 1996; **27**: 1578–85.

71 Kuroiwa T, Bonnekoh P, Hossmann KA. Prevention of postischemic hyperthermia prevents ischemic injury of CA1 neurons in gerbils. *Journal of Cerebral Blood Flow Metabolism* 1990; **10**: 550–6.

72 Gunn AJ, Gunn TR. The 'pharmacology' of neuronal rescue with cerebral hypothermia. *Early Human Development* 1998; **53**: 19–35.

73 Sirimanne ES, Blumberg RM, Bossano D et al. The effect of prolonged modification of cerebral temperature on outcome after hypoxic-ischemic brain injury in the infant rat. *Pediatric Research* 1996; **39**: 591–7.

74 Edwards AD, Yue X, Squier MV et al. Specific inhibition of apoptosis after cerebral hypoxia-ischaemia by moderate post-insult hypothermia. *Biochemical and Biophysical Research Communications* 1995; **217**: 1193–9.

75 Gunn AJ, Gunn TR. Effect of radiant heat on head temperature gradient in term infants. *Archives of Disease in Childhood Fetal and Neonatal Edition* 1996; **74**: F200–3.

76 Schubert A. Side effects of mild hypothermia. *Journal of Neurosurgery and Anesthesiology* 1995; **7**: 139–47.

77 Bhushan V, Paneth N, Kiely JL. Impact of improved survival of very low birth weight infants on recent secular trends in the prevalence of cerebral palsy. *Pediatrics* 1993; **91**: 1094–100.

78 MacLennan A for The International Cerebral Palsy Task Force. A template for defining a causal relation between acute intrapartum events and cerebral palsy: international consensus statement. *British Medical Journal* 1999; **319**: 1054–9.

79 Perlman JM. White matter injury in the preterm infant: an important determination of abnormal neuro-development outcome. *Early Human Development* 1998; **53**: 99–120.

80 De Vries LS, Eken P, Groenendaal F, van Haastert IC, Meiners LC. Correlation between the degree of periventricular leukomalacia diagnosed using cranial ultrasound and MRI later in infancy in children with cerebral palsy. *Neuropediatrics* 1993; **24**: 263–8.

81 Truwit CL, Barkovich AJ, Koch TK, Ferriero DM. Cerebral palsy: MR findings in 40 patients. *American Journal of Neuroradiology* 1992; **13**: 67–78.

82 Steinlin M, Good M, Martin E, Banziger O, Largo RH, Boltshauser E. Congenital hemiplegia – morphology of cerebral lesions and pathogenetic aspects from MRI. *Neuropediatrics* 1993; **24**: 224–9.

83 Krageloh-Mann I, Hagberg G, Meisner C *et al.* Bilateral spastic cerebral palsy – a collaborative study between southwest Germany and western Sweden. III: Aetiology. *Developmental Medicine and Child Neurology* 1995; **37**: 191–203.

84 Barkovich AJ, Sargent SK. Profound asphyxia in the premature infant: imaging findings. *American Journal of Neuroradiology* 1995; **16**: 1837–46.

85 Takashima S, Tanaka K. Microangiography and vascular permeability of the subependymal matrix in the premature fetus. *Canadian Journal of Neurological Sciences* 1978; **5**: 45–50.

86 Gould SJ, Howard S. An immunohistochemical study of the germinal matrix layer in the late gestation human fetal brain. *Neuropathology and Applied Neurobiology* 1987; **13**: 421–37.

87 Hambleton G, Wigglesworth JS. Origin of intraventricular haemorrhage in the preterm infant. *Archives of Disease in Childhood Fetal and Neonatal Edition* 1976; **51**: 651–9.

88 Szymonowicz W, Walker AM, Cussen L, Cannata J, Yu VYH. Developmental changes in regional cerebral blood flow in fetal and newborn lambs. *American Journal of Physiology* 1988; **254**: H52–8.

89 Goldman JE. Regulation of oligodendrocyte differentiation. *Trends in Neurosciences* 1992; **15**: 359–62.

90 Azzarelli B, Caldemeyer KS, Phillips JP, DeMyer WE. Hypoxic-ischemic encephalopathy in areas of primary myelination: a neuroimaging and PET study. *Pediatric Neurology* 1996; **14**: 108–16.

91 Back SA, Gan X, Li Y, Rosenberg PA, Volpe JJ. Maturation-dependent vulnerability of oligodendrocytes to oxidative stress-induced death caused by glutathione depletion. *Journal of Neuroscience* 1998; **18**: 6241–53.

92 Laszkiewicz I, Mouzannar R, Wiggins RC, Konat GW. Delayed oligodendrocyte degeneration induced by brief exposure to hydrogen peroxide. *Journal of Neuroscience Research* 1999; **55**: 303–10.

93 Dammann O, Leviton A. Maternal intrauterine infection, cytokines, and brain damage in the preterm newborn. *Pediatric Research* 1997; **42**: 1–8.

94 Grether JK, Nelson KB. Maternal infection and cerebral palsy in infants of normal birth weight. *Journal of the American Medical Association* 1997; **278**: 207–11.

95 Grether JK, Nelson KB, Dambrosia JM, Phillips TM. Interferons and cerebral palsy. *Journal of Pediatrics* 1999; **134**: 324–32.

96 Nelson KB, Dambrosia JM, Grether JK, Phillips TM. Neonatal cytokines and coagulation factors in children with cerebral palsy. *Annals of Neurology* 1998; **44**: 665–75.

97 Marret S, Mukendi R, Gadisseux JF, Gressens P, Evrard P. Effect of ibotenate on brain development: an excitotoxic mouse model of microgyria and posthypoxic-like lesions. *Journal of Neuropathology and Experimental Neurology* 1995; **54**: 358–70.

98 Marret S, Gressens P, Gadisseux JF, Evrard P. Prevention by magnesium of excitotoxic neuronal death in the developing brain: an animal model for clinical intervention studies. *Developmental Medicine and Child Neurology* 1995; **37**: 473–84.

99 Reddy K, Mallard C, Guan J *et al.* Maturational change in the cortical response to hypoperfusion injury in the fetal sheep. *Pediatric Research* 1998; **43**: 674–82.

100 Hansen A. Extracellular potassium concentration in juvenile and adult rat brain cortex during anoxia. *Acta Physiologica Scandinavica* 1977; **99**: 412–20.

101 Myers RE. Experimental models of perinatal brain damage: relevance to human pathology. In: Gluck L ed. *Intrauterine asphyxia and the developing fetal brain.* Chicago: Year Book Medical, 1977: 37–97.

102 Vannucci RC, Mujsce DJ. Effect of glucose on perinatal hypoxic-ischemic brain damage. *Biology of the Neonate* 1992; **62**: 215–24.

103 LeBlanc MH, Huang M, Patel D, Smith EE, Devidas M. Glucose given after hypoxic ischemia does not affect brain injury in piglets. *Stroke* 1994; **25**: 1443–7.

104 Vannucci SJ, Maher F, Simpson IA. Glucose transporter proteins in brain: delivery of glucose to neurons and glia. *GLIA* 1997; **21**: 2–21.

105 Villar J, de Onis M, Kestler E, Bolanos F, Cerezo R, Bernedes H. The differential neonatal morbidity of the intrauterine growth retardation syndrome. *American Journal of Obstetrics and Gynecology* 1990; **163**: 151–7.

106 Stanley O, Fleming P, Morgan M. Abnormal development of visual function following intrauterine growth retardation. *Early Human Development* 1989; **19**: 87–101.

107 Cook CJ, Gluckman PD, Williams CE, Bennet L. Precocial neural function in the growth retarded fetal lamb. *Pediatric Research* 1988; **24**: 600–5.

108 Mallard EC, Rees S, Stringer M, Cock ML, Harding R. Effects of chronic placental insufficiency on brain development in fetal sheep. *Pediatric Research* 1998; **43**: 262–70.

109 Kramer MS, McLean FH, Olivier M, Willis DM, Usher RH. Body proportionality and head and length 'sparing' in growth-retarded neonates: a critical reappraisal. *Pediatrics* 1989; **84**: 717–23.

110 Morgane P, Austin K, Siok C, LaFrance R, Bronzino J. Power spectral analysis of hippocampal and cortical EEG following severe prenatal protein malnutrition in the rat. *Developmental Brain Research* 1985; **22**: 211–18.

111 Chanez C, Rabin O, Heroux M, Giguere JF. Cerebral amino acid changes in an animal model of intrauterine growth retardation. *Metabolic Brain Disease* 1993; **8**: 61–72.

112 Gallaher BW, Breier BH, Keven CL, Harding JE, Gluckman PD. Fetal programming of insulin-like growth factor (IGF)-I and IGF-binding protein-3: evidence for an altered response to undernutrition in late gestation following exposure to periconceptual undernutrition in the sheep. *Journal of Endocrinology* 1998; **159**: 501–8.

113 Janbu T, Nesheim BI. Uterine artery blood velocities during contractions in pregnancy and labour related to intrauterine pressure. *British Journal of Obstetrics and Gynaecology* 1987; **94**: 1150–5.

114 Giussani DA, Spencer JAD, Hanson MA. Fetal cardiovascular reflex responses to hypoxaemia. *Fetal and Maternal Medical Reviews* 1994; **6**: 17–37.

115 Peeters LL, Sheldon RE, Jones MDJ, Makowski EL, Meschia G. Blood flow to fetal organs as a function of arterial oxygen content. *American Journal of Obstetrics and Gynecology* 1979; **135**: 637–46.

115 Parer JT. Effects of fetal asphyxia on brain cell structure and function – limits of tolerance. *Comparative Biochemistry and Physiology Part A, Molecular and Integrative Physiology* 1998; **119**: 711–16.

117 Green LR, Bennet L, Hanson MA. The role of nitric oxide in the cardiovascular responses to acute hypoxia in the late gestation sheep fetus. *Journal of Physiology* 1996; **497**: 271–7.

118 Iwamoto HS, Rudolph AM. Effects of endogenous angiotensin II on the fetal circulation. *Journal of Developmental Physiology* 1979; **1**: 283–93.

119 Tangalakis K, Lumbers ER, Moritz KM, Towstoless MK, Wintour EM. Effect of cortisol on blood pressure and vascular reactivity in the ovine fetus. *Experimental Physiology* 1992; **77**: 709–17.

120 Bourchier D, Weston PJ. Randomised trial of dopamine compared with hydrocortisone for the treatment of hypotensive very low birthweight infants. *Archives of Disease in Childhood Fetal and Neonatal Edition* 1997; **76**: F174–8.

121 Richardson BS, Carmichael L, Homan J, Patrick JE. Cerebral oxidative metabolism in fetal sheep with prolonged and graded hypoxemia. *Journal of Developmental Physiology* 1993; **19**: 77–83.

122 Richardson BS, Bocking AD. Metabolic and circulatory adaptations to chronic hypoxia in the fetus. *Comparative Biochemistry and Physiology Part A, Molecular and Integrative Physiology* 1998; **119**: 717–23.

123 Kitanaka T, Alonso JG, Gilbert RD, Siu BL, Clemons GK, Longo LD. Fetal responses to long-term hypoxemia in sheep. *American Journal of Physiology* 1989; **256**: R1348–54.

124 Iwamoto HS, Kaufman T, Keil LC, Rudolph AM. Responses to acute hypoxemia in fetal sheep at 0.6–0.7 gestation. *American Journal of Physiology* 1989; **256**: H613–20.

125 Szymonowicz W, Walker AM, Yu VYH, Stewart ML, Cannata J, Cussen L. Regional cerebral blood flow after hemorrhagic hypotension in the preterm, near-term and newborn lamb. *Pediatric Research* 1990; **28**: 361–6.

126 Birk E, Iwamoto HS, Heymann MA. Hormonal effects on circulatory changes during the perinatal period. *Baillières Clinical Endocrinology and Metabolism* 1989; **3**: 795–815.

127 Shields LE, Brace RA. Fetal vascular pressure responses to nonlabor uterine contractions: dependence on amniotic fluid volume in the ovine fetus. *American Journal of Obstetrics and Gynecology* 1994; **171**: 84–9.

128 Golan A, Lin G, Evron S, Arieli S, Niv D, David MP. Oligohydramnios: maternal complications and fetal outcome in 145 cases. *Gynecologic and Obstetric Investigation* 1994; **37**: 91–5.

129 Block BS, Schlafer DH, Wentworth RA, Kreitzer LA, Nathanielsz PW. Intrauterine asphyxia and the breakdown of physiologic circulatory compensation in fetal sheep. *American Journal of Obstetrics and Gynecology* 1990; **162**: 1325–31.

130 Mallard EC, Gunn AJ, Williams CE, Johnston BM, Gluckman PD. Transient umbilical cord occlusion causes hippocampal damage in the fetal sheep. *American Journal of Obstetrics and Gynecology* 1992; **167**: 1423–30.

131 de Haan HH, Van Reempts JL, Vles JS, de Haan J, Hasaart TH. Effects of asphyxia on the fetal lamb brain. *American Journal of Obstetrics and Gynecology* 1993; **169**: 1493–501.

132 Yaffe H, Parer JT, Block BS, Llanos AJ. Cardiorespiratory responses to graded reductions of uterine blood flow in the sheep fetus. *Journal of Developmental Physiology* 1987; **9**: 325–36.

133 Rudolph AM. The fetal circulation and its response to stress. *Journal of Developmental Physiology* 1984; **6**: 11–19.

134 Field DR, Parer JT, Auslender RA, Cheek DB, Baker W, Johnson J. Cerebral oxygen consumption during asphyxia in fetal sheep. *Journal of Developmental Physiology* 1990; **14**: 131–7.

135 Rosen KG, Hrbek A, Karlsson K, Kjellmer I. Fetal cerebral, cardiovascular and metabolic reactions to intermittent occlusion of ovine maternal placental blood flow. *Acta Physiologica Scandinavica* 1986; **126**: 209–16.

136 Preziosi MP, Roig JC, Hargrove N, Burchfield DJ. Metabolic acidemia with hypoxia attenuates the hemodynamic responses to epinephrine during resuscitation in lambs. *Critical Care Medicine* 1993; **21**: 1901–7.

137 Dawes GS, Mott JC, Shelley HJ. The importance of cardiac glycogen for the maintenance of life in foetal lambs and new-born animals during anoxia. *Journal of Physiology* 1959; **146**: 516–38.

138 Pisarenko OI, Solomatina ES, Studneva IM, Kapelko VI. The relationship between the cardiac contractile function, adenine nucleotides and amino acids of cardiac tissue and mitochondria at acute respiratory hypoxia. *Pflugers Archiv* 1987; **409**: 169–74.

139 de Haan HH, Gunn AJ, Gluckman PD. Fetal heart rate changes during brief repeated umbilical cord occlusion do not reflect cardiovascular deterioration in fetal lambs. *American Journal of Obstetrics and Gynecology* 1997; **176**: 8–17.

140 de Haan HH, Gunn AJ, Williams CE, Heymann MA, Gluckman PD. Magnesium sulfate therapy during asphyxia in near-term fetal lambs does not compromise the fetus but does not reduce cerebral injury. *American Journal of Obstetrics and Gynecology* 1997; **176**: 18–27.

141 Donnelly WH. Ischemic myocardial necrosis and papillary muscle dysfunction in infants and children. *American Journal of Cardiovascular Pathology* 1987; **1**: 173–88.

142 Ferrari R. Metabolic disturbances during myocardial ischemia and reperfusion. *American Journal of Cardiology* 1995; **76**: 17B–24B.

143 Gunn AJ, Maxwell L, de Haan HH *et al.* Delayed hypotension and sub-endocardial injury after repeated umbilical cord occlusion in near-term fetal lambs. *American Journal of Obstetrics and Gynecology* 2000; **183**(6): 1564–72.

144 de Haan HH, Ijzermans ACM, de Haan J, Van Belle H, Hasaart THM. Effects of surgery and asphyxia on levels of nucleosides, purine bases, and lactate in cerebrospinal fluid of fetal lambs. *Pediatric Research* 1994; **36**: 595–600.

145 de Haan HH, Gunn AJ, Williams CE, Gluckman PD. Brief repeated umbilical cord occlusions cause sustained cytotoxic cerebral edema and focal infarcts in near-term fetal lambs. *Pediatric Research* 1997; **41**: 96–104.

146 Keunen H, Blanco CE, Van Reempts JL, Hasaart TH. Absence of neuronal damage after umbilical cord occlusion of 10, 15, and 20 minutes in midgestation fetal sheep. *American Journal of Obstetrics and Gynecology* 1997; **176**: 515–20.

147 Bennet L, Rossenrode S, Gunning MI, Gluckman PD, Gunn AJ. The cardiovascular and cerebrovascular responses of the immature fetal sheep to acute umbilical cord occlusion. *Journal of Physiology (London)* 1999; **517**: 247–57.

148 Murotsuki J, Challis JR, Han VK, Fraher LJ, Gagnon R. Chronic fetal placental embolization and hypoxemia cause hypertension and myocardial hypertrophy in fetal sheep. *American Journal of Physiology* 1997; **272**: R201–7.

149 Murotsuki J, Challis JRG, Johnston L, Gagnon R. Increased fetal plasma prostaglandin E(2) concentrations during fetal placental embolization in pregnant sheep. *American Journal of Obstetrics and Gynecology* 1995; **173**: 30–5.

150 Gagnon R, Challis J, Johnston L, Fraher L. Fetal endocrine responses to chronic placental embolization in the late-gestation ovine fetus. *American Journal of Obstetrics and Gynecology* 1994; **170**: 929–38.

151 Bennet L, Watanabe T, Spencer J, Hanson MA. Fetal reflexes in chronic hypoxaemia. *Advances in Experimental Medicine and Biology* 1994; **360**: 337–9.

152 Shaul PW, Cha C-JM, Oh W. Neonatal sympathoadrenal response to acute hypoxia: impairment after experimental intrauterine growth retardation. *Pediatric Research* 1989; **25**: 466–72.

153 Giussani DA, Riquelme RA, Moraga FA *et al.* Chemoreflex and endocrine components of cardiovascular responses to acute hypoxemia in the llama fetus. *American Journal of Physiology* 1996; **271**: R73–83.

154 Divers WA, Wilkes MM, Babaknia A, Hill LM, Quilligan EJ, Yen SS. Amniotic fluid catecholamines and metabolites in intrauterine growth retardation. *American Journal of Obstetrics and Gynecology* 1981; **141**: 608–10.

155 Ikeda T, Murata Y, Quilligan EJ *et al.* Physiologic and histologic changes in near-term fetal lambs exposed to asphyxia by partial umbilical cord occlusion. *American Journal of Obstetrics and Gynecology* 1998; **178**: 24–32.

156 Penning DH, Grafe MR, Hammond R, Matsuda Y, Patrick J, Richardson B. Neuropathology of the near-term and midgestation ovine fetal brain after sustained in utero hypoxemia. *American Journal of Obstetrics and Gynecology* 1994; **170**: 1425–32.

157 Rees S, Mallard C, Breen S, Stringer M, Cock M, Harding R. Fetal brain injury following prolonged hypoxemia and placental insufficiency: a review. *Comparative Biochemistry and Physiology Part A, Molecular and Integrative Physiology* 1998; **119**: 653–60.

158 Gunn AJ, Parer JT, Mallard EC, Williams CE, Gluckman PD. Cerebral histological and electrophysiological changes after asphyxia in fetal sheep. *Pediatric Research* 1992; **31**: 486–91.

159 de Courten-Myers GM, Kleinholz M, Wagner KR *et al.* Fatal strokes in hyperglycemic cats. *Stroke* 1989; **20**: 1707–15.

160 Papile L-A, Rudolph AM, Heymann MA. Autoregulation of cerebral blood flow in the preterm fetal lamb. *Pediatric Research* 1985; **19**: 159–61.

161 Cohn HE, Sacks EJ, Heymann MA, Rudolph AM. Cardiovascular responses to hypoxemia and acidemia in fetal lambs. *American Journal of Obstetrics and Gynecology* 1974; **15**: 817–24.

162 Jensen A, Berger R. Fetal circulatory responses to oxygen lack. *Journal of Developmental Physiology* 1991; **16**: 181–207.

163 Bennet L, Peebles DM, Edwards AD, Rios A, Hanson MA. The cerebral hemodynamic response to asphyxia and hypoxia in the near term fetal sheep as measured by near-infrared spectroscopy. *Pediatric Research* 1998; **44**: 951–7.

164 Bennet L, Quaedackers JS, Gunn AJ, Rossenrode S, Heineman E. The effect of asphyxia on superior mesenteric artery blood flow in the premature sheep fetus. *Journal of Pediatric Surgery* 2000; **35**: 34–40.

165 Kuenzle C, Baenziger O, Martin E *et al.* Prognostic value of early MR imaging in term infants with severe perinatal asphyxia. *Neuropediatrics* 1994; **25**: 191–200.

166 Torvik A. The pathogenesis of watershed infarcts in the brain. *Stroke* 1984; **15**: 221–3.

167 Tombaugh GC. Mild acidosis delays hypoxic spreading depression and improves neuronal recovery in hippocampal slices. *Journal of Neuroscience* 1994; **14**: 5635–43.

168 Giffard RG, Monyer H, Christine CW, Choi DW. Acidosis reduces NMDA receptor activation, glutamate neurotoxicity, and oxygen-glucose deprivation neuronal injury in cortical cultures. *Brain Research* 1990; **506**: 339–42.

169 Mallard EC, Waldvogel HJ, Williams CE, Faull RLM, Gluckman PD. Repeated asphyxia causes loss of striatal projection neurons in the fetal sheep brain. *Neuroscience* 1995; **65**: 827–36.

170 Mallard EC, Williams CE, Gunn AJ, Gunning MI, Gluckman PD. Frequent episodes of brief ischemia sensitize the fetal sheep brain to neuronal loss and induce striatal injury. *Pediatric Research* 1993; **33**: 61–5.

171 Lin B, Globus MYT, Dietrich WD, Busto R, Martinez E, Ginsberg MD. Differing neurochemical and morphological sequelae of global ischemia: comparison of single and multiple insult paradigms. *Journal of Neurochemistry* 1992; **59**: 2213–23.

5 Genetic causes of cerebral palsy

Michael A Patton

It is customary to recognize Gregor Mendel as the founding father of genetics, but his contribution was misunderstood when he first presented his work the nineteenth century. He basically showed that genetic traits could be inherited in a mathematically predictable manner and that traits were inherited independently. It is surprising that it was misunderstood since it provided an explanation for the very simple and universal observation that the distribution of males and females is equal! If his work had been applied to human genetics rather than peas it is likely it would have gained a more rapid acceptance. As it happened, the advances in genetics in the next 90 years were largely made in the field of plant and animal genetics and it was only in the 1950s that the subject began to develop applications in medicine. In 1956 the chromosome number in humans was identified for the first time and following this it was recognized that Down's syndrome was due to the presence of an extra chromosome, with 47 chromosomes instead of 46 chromosomes. At that stage chromosomes could not be identified individually and were classified into groups A–G with the sex chromosomes being identified individually. This period was followed by the recognition of other forms of mental handicap in which there were abnormalities in the chromosome number or shape.

The most recent advances have come from molecular genetics. When DNA (deoxyribonucleic acid) was first identified to be the source of genetic transmission there was no easy way of analyzing it, but since then numerous techniques have been developed which allow the DNA to be studied. The most ambitious research program is loosely labeled the Human Genome Project. This project is being carried out internationally in an attempt to sequence the entire genome. The first draft has been published already and all the DNA has been ordered in overlapping segments. All the estimated 60 000 genes will eventually be mapped to specific parts of the 23 pairs of chromosomes and the sequence of these genes will be decoded. Although this seemed an almost impossible task, the first draft was published well ahead of schedule and it is likely that the final target will be fully achieved in the near future.

The purpose of the gene mapping project is not simply as an academic exercise, but will lead to an enormous expansion in our understanding of human disease. From this understanding will also come advances in treatment including some examples of successful gene therapy. It is likely to aid our understanding not just of purely genetic disease but also of the genetic predisposition to a wide range of disorders.

5.1   GENETIC DISEASES: CLASSIFICATION

Genetic diseases may be divided into three groups: chromosomal, single gene, and multifactorial disorders.

The chromosomal disorders are those in which there is an imbalance in the amount of the chromosomal material. In addition to those conditions in which there is an abnormal chromosome number (aneuploidy), there are also conditions in which there are small deletions of chromosome material and other rearrangements, such as translocations where genetic material is exchanged between chromosomes. Chromosomal disorders frequently give rise to mental handicap, recurrent miscarriages, and infertility.

In single gene disorders the abnormality is confined to a 'spelling mistake' or mutation in a single gene. These mutations may be inherited in different ways. If the mutation is on the X chromosome it may give a sex-linked or X-linked pattern of inheritance in which females are carriers and males are affected. If the mutation is on one of the other chromosomes (which are called autosomes) the mutation can affect males and females equally and can be inherited in either a dominant or a recessive manner. Over 6000 single gene disorders have been identified and more are being described almost daily. They are, however, individually rare. The single gene disorders cover the whole spectrum of disease and can cause inherited forms of

spastic paraplegia and mental handicap resembling cerebral palsy.

The multifactorial diseases tend to be the common disorders like heart disease, isolated birth defects, and cancer. In all of these there is a combination between a genetic predisposition and environmental factors. Spina bifida is a good example of this. Family studies show there is genetic predisposition since there is an increased risk within families. However, this is not the whole story since the frequency of the defect varies widely. It was found that diet played an important part in the etiology and eventually it was found that folic acid was an important environmental factor. Fortunately it is possible to supplement the maternal diet with folic acid and to reduce the frequency of this nervous system malformation.

5.2   CHROMOSOME TESTING

It is vitally important in assessing any child with severe learning difficulties to ensure that the chromosomes have been tested with the most up-to-date and appropriate techniques. Chromosome abnormalities are the single largest cause of mental handicap. In order to understand whether the appropriate test has been carried out it is necessary to understand the basis of the laboratory techniques.

Chromosomes may be obtained from any tissue of the body but it is usual to use blood for most diagnostic purposes in childhood. The white cells are first separated from the blood and are set up for culture with a nutrient medium which contains a substance such as phytohemagglutinin to stimulate cell growth (Fig. 5.1). When the cells are growing well the cell growth may be arrested in metaphase using a spindle-blocking drug such as colchicine. Metaphase is the point in the cell cycle at which the chromosomes are maximally contracted and therefore most easily visualized. The cells are then lysed in hypotonic fluid and spread on a glass slide by dropping the cell suspension carefully with a glass pipette. The chromosome spread is fixed and stained so that it can be analyzed. Various stains can be used, but the commonest one is a Giemsa stain, which shows the chromosome as a banded structure and allows all the chromosomes to be identified individually by their length and banding pattern. Before reporting a chromosome result, up to 30 cells will be analyzed by an experienced cytogeneticist. It is worth pointing out that, unlike many other laboratory tests, this is not automated, and the

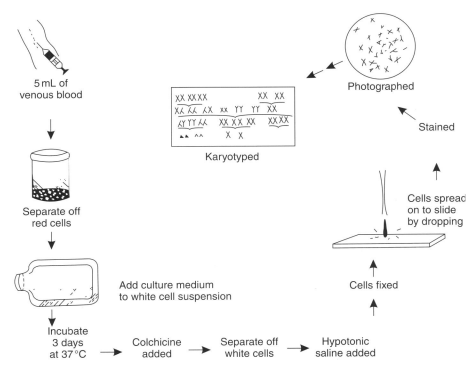

Figure 5.1   The preparation of a karyotype. (Reprinted from *Elements of Medical Genetics,* 5th edn, Emery, p. 55, 1979, by permission of the publisher Churchill Livingstone.)

result will depend on the experience and expertise of the scientist.

It is important to understand the improvement that has come over the last 20 years. Prior to 1974 when banding was introduced widely, it was difficult to identify individual chromosomes and minor deletions or rearrangements would almost certainly have been missed. The quality of a preparation is estimated by the number of bands visible. In good preparations today it is possible to identify around 400 bands on the chromosomes from one cell (the karyotype).

In medicolegal cases in the UK involving a minor with mental handicap it is possible to bring litigation at any stage up to adulthood. This may well mean that the chromosome test which was initially carried out is insufficient by today's standards to identify all chromosome abnormalities. Case 5.1 demonstrates how potential damages for obstetric negligence were avoided by repeating chromosome testing and the identification of a chromosome abnormality. This has been a frequent experience in the author's medicolegal practice and one in which the plaintiff's parents may also have the satisfaction of a clear explanation of their child's handicap.

It is possible to get greater resolution by extending the number of chromosome bands by stopping cell division just before metaphase (pro-metaphase). These preparations may be very difficult to analyze because the extended chromosomes are frequently overlapping and difficult to disentangle. A new development called fluorescent *in situ* hybridization (FISH) is revolutionizing the approach to chromosome testing. FISH involves taking a specific gene sequence from one chromosome and combining it with a fluorescent dye. When this sequence or probe is placed against the chromosome spread it will match up to the specific chromosome and the fluorescent dye makes that chromosome instantly recognizable. The aim of present research is to produce FISH paints with different colours for each chromosome and it is likely that this will soon be achieved.

FISH technology can also be used in other ways. It is possible to develop a fluorescent probe to specific genes that can be used to identify extremely small deletions which would not have been visible with conventional techniques. An example of this discussed below is the use of gene probes to detect deletions of chromosome 17 in the Miller-Dieker syndrome in which there is an underlying brain malformation.[1] As the number of FISH probes available commercially increases so the potential number of chromosome tests also increases, and it will no longer be possible to say that 'the chromosomes were looked at and they

---

Case 5.1

A boy is born to healthy parents after an emergency cesarean section. His Apgar scores are 2, 8, 10. He required brief intubation and oxygen but the pediatrician was present and administered this expertly. He went to the special care nursery for observation and had no further neonatal complications. When his motor delay was finally apparent the local pediatrician suggested that he might have a mild form of Cornelia de Lange syndrome on the basis of the developmental delay and his facial features. His parents came to accept this diagnosis but when he was in his early teens he was seen in a teaching hospital where they were told that he did not have Cornelia de Lange syndrome. As they no longer had an explanation for his handicap they sought legal advice to determine whether the fetal distress might have been the cause for his handicap. During the preparation of the case the chromosome test was repeated and with better preparations it was found that there was extra chromosomal material attached to the end of chromosome 7. Parental blood samples were also analyzed and found to be normal. It therefore appeared that this extra material had arisen in the formation of either egg or sperm and that this, rather than the obstetric management, was clearly the cause of his handicap. The parents were satisfied by the explanation and did not pursue their action.

---

were normal'. It will not be practical or cost effective to apply all the probes and therefore it will be necessary initially to make the appropriate clinical diagnosis to guide the best use of tests.

Another recent development using FISH probes is to make probes to the telomeres or tips of all the chromosomes. Using this, Flint[2] has shown that a further 6 percent of all previously undiagnosed mental handicap may be attributed to telomeric rearrangements or deletions. If this is confirmed in wider clinical studies then it is likely that this should also be used routinely in the assessment of a child with severe learning difficulties.

5.3 GENE DIAGNOSIS

Testing for mutations in individual genes has now become routine for many conditions, but each disease has produced its own diagnostic difficulties. One major problem is the fact that most single gene disorders can be caused by more than one mutation in the gene. This makes testing difficult. Molecular genetic tests may be classified as follows.

1 Diagnostic tests: these will identify all the mutations in the gene and therefore can be used both for diagnosis and to give a negative result for exclusion. Good examples are neurological disorders such as Huntington's disease and fragile X, where there are trinucleotide repeats and the presence or absence of the disease may be predicted by the number of repeat sequences.

2 Partially diagnostic tests: in some disorders there are a very large number of mutations that can cause the disease and a diagnosis may be made by testing for some of the commoner mutations. However, the absence of these mutations will not fully exclude the disorder.

3 Research tests: for many conditions the gene sequence responsible has been identified only recently and no diagnostic laboratory will be able to provide testing. Confirming a diagnosis in such cases will involve the time-consuming process of fully sequencing the gene.

4 Linkage tests: in situations where the location of a gene is known but the gene itself has not been identified, it may be possible to look at closely linked gene markers and by tracking these through the family it may be possible to predict those who are likely to have inherited the disease.

It is likely that approaches to molecular diagnosis will improve with the application of new technology. At present semi-automated gene sequencers can be used to screen for multiple mutations in a gene and an experimental technique called a gene chip has the potential to run up to 2000 individual gene tests on a multilayered plate a few centimeters in diameter. Such techniques will considerably expand the range of genetic diagnosis in the future.

5.4   SYNDROME DIAGNOSIS

There are now well over 2000 malformation syndromes recognized and at least half of these are associated with mental retardation.[3] The recognition of these syndromes depends considerably on clinical expertise since it is necessary to recognize a pattern of associated clinical features, in many cases including a characteristic facial appearance. In the case of Down's syndrome most pediatricians would recognize the facial appearance and the diagnosis can be confirmed by chromosome analysis. With rarer syndromes the assessment needs the expertise of a dysmorphologist (a geneticist or pediatrician with a specific interest in malformation syndromes). To aid their assessment they will have access to syndrome databases such as the London Dysmorphology Database, which provides a method of searching using the combinations of different clinical features.

As Cases 5.2 and 5.3 indicate, the recognition of a malformation syndrome may alter the course of medical litigation.

5.5   DEVELOPMENT OF GENETIC SERVICES

Medical genetics is a relatively new specialty and it has developed differently in Europe and North America. In the UK it has developed in regional centers providing comprehensive clinical and laboratory services in the public sector to populations of around 3 million. A similar pattern has developed in some other European countries such as the Netherlands. In North America the laboratories have tended to develop in the private sector and separately from the clinical services, which are often university based.

Some aspects of the clinical practice are particularly important from the medicolegal point of view. The first is the advice that might be given for other family members and their potential to have children with handicap. Clinical geneticists have a wider responsibility to the extended family and would have a duty to inform their patient when there is a significant risk of handicap elsewhere in the family. However, in most countries they would

---

Case 5.2

Sophie was born by forceps delivery at term. The delivery was uncomplicated but had been carried out by a relatively inexperienced doctor. There was more bruising than would usually be expected from forceps delivery and later, when this bruising had settled down; it was noted that she had some scarring over the side of the head which appeared to resemble the imprint of the forceps blade. Legal action was initiated and in the process of preparing a case for the defense a clinical geneticist was asked for an opinion. The geneticist recognized that Sophie had Setlis syndrome, which comprises bitemporal scarring resembling forcep marks, lax wrinkly skin, abnormal eyelashes and nose.[4] The plaintiff's lawyer had not considered such a possibility; however, when expert opinion was sought, the conclusion was that the case could not be persued further.

Case 5.3

In the 1960s thalidomide was used as a sedative and was prescribed in pregnancy. Shortly afterwards it was recognized as a teratogen causing major limb abnormalities and a financial settlement was made to those born with limb abnormalities after maternal exposure to the drug. Now, some 40 years; later there is a better understanding of limb abnormalities and in some cases the affected individuals might be better classified as malformation syndromes such as the Holt-Oram syndrome which comprises unilateral limb defect, sloping shoulders and an atrial septal defect in the heart. Holt-Oram syndrome is an autosomal dominant condition and thus it would be an explanation for the fact that some of the children who were thought to have been damaged by thalidomide have gone on to have children affected in a similar manner. The gene for Holt-Oram has recently been identified on chromosome 12 and it may be possible to confirm the diagnosis using molecular techniques.[5]

Case 5.4

The clinical geneticist Dr Smith is seeing a couple, Mr and Mrs Brown, who have had a handicapped child. It is found that the child has an unbalanced chromosome translocation between chromosomes 9 and 4, which has led to the child having additional extra material from chromosome 9 and some material from chromosome 4 missing. This is undoubtedly the cause of the child's mental handicap. The next stage is to test the parents to find out if either of them carries the translocation in balanced form. This shows that Mr Brown has the balanced translocation and that Mrs Brown has a normal female chromosome pattern. Mr and Mrs Brown would have around a 10 percent chance of having a further handicapped child, and could be offered prenatal diagnosis using amniocentesis and chromosome analysis.

This information also means that Mr Brown's two brothers or his sister might also carry the translocation and if they did they would also be at risk of having a handicapped child. Dr Smith would be negligent if he failed to inform Mr Brown of this possibility and should also advise Mr Brown about the mechanism of having the further tests carried out on his relatives. In the UK, Dr Smith would usually make arrangements for this information to be passed on by his patient to the other family members and for them to be seen in their local genetic center.

---

not have the right to approach other family members directly to inform them of this risk. Case 5.4 illustrates this dilemma.

The second aspect of clinical practice that may cause problems is the documentation of genetic counselling. Medical notes will usually record details of medical examination and treatment fully, but when it comes to genetic advice and counselling this is often percieved as being rather like a social chat and as such is not recorded. Genetic counselling may contain the details of the advice that was given with regard to the recurrence of mental handicap. It is well recognized that patients may take in relatively little of the information if they are anxious and they may misunderstand it completely. This misunderstanding may come to light years later when the patient says they understood there was no risk of recurrence while the doctor believes he or she had said there was a small but significant risk of recurrence. Without contemporaneous notes it would be difficult for the doctor to establish what was actually said. In such cases the patient's memory is generally much better since he or she will have only received genetic counselling on the one occasion, whereas the doctor may have counselled many patients in similar situations over the years. Thus clear documentation of counselling is essential in reducing the risk of litigation.

5.6   THE GENETICS OF CEREBRAL PALSY

There have been various definitions of cerebral palsy, but most definitions would include the fact that it is a persistent disorder of movement and posture, and that the motor development is deviant rather than immature and that it is non-progressive in its nature. It is better to consider cerebral palsy as a heterogeneous group of conditions. The clinical presentation depends on the pattern of motor involvement and whether there is an associated disorder of movement and coordination. Such a classification recognizes that there is no single cause but rather there are many different causes.

Most of the causes of cerebral palsy are acquired and hence the overall recurrence figures are small. The early studies indicated this. In 1950 Asher and Schonell[6] conducted a study of cerebral palsy in Birmingham, UK, and found only one affected sibling in 349 families. Similarly Gustavson et al.[7] in a study of 3150 families in Sweden only found 30 families in which there was a recurrence in siblings with normal parents. Where recurrence was found the pattern of handicap was similar. From these relatively large studies the empiric recurrence risk overall would be 1 percent or less.

Another approach to studying the genetic contribution to a disorder is to compare the rate in monozygous and dizygous twins. This is not particularly helpful in cerebral palsy. Virtually all studies have shown a three- to four-fold increase in twins or multiple births in cerebral palsy (e.g Griffiths[8], Goodman and Alberman[9]). The reasons for this increase are largely because multiple births are usually premature and this is one of the main non-genetic factors predisposing to cerebral palsy. Another factor will be the increased obstetric difficulty in delivering multiple births. From this it might be suggested that the second twin would be at greater risk as this twin will have longer *in utero* and potentially a greater risk of asphyxia. Most studies show a greater risk of death in the second-born twin but the data on cerebral palsy are conflicting. In the study by Griffiths[8] it was the first-born twin who had the greater risk of cerebral palsy. She suggests that this might be due not to anoxia but to a greater risk of cerebral compression in the birth canal. The twin studies do not show a greater concordance in monozygous compared with dizygous twins and it appears the variance in cerebral palsy with twins is largely due to perinatal or obstetric factors.

A better approach to understanding the genetic factors in cerebral palsy is to look at the recurrence in specific types of cerebral palsy and to dissect out the genetic factors. One of the best studies using this approach is that by Bundey and Griffiths published in 1977.[10] They undertook a complete ascertainment of all cases of cerebral palsy children in the West Midlands, UK, between 1952 and 1972. Of the 669 children with cerebral palsy they found only 3.6 percent had symmetrical spastic quadriplegia and within this group there was an overall recurrence risk of 1 in 9. The recurrence was similar with or without microcephaly. When the group was further analyzed there appeared to be some different patterns of handicap. Two families had postnatal microcephaly, myoclonic epilepsy, and spastic quadraplegia and as there was consanguinity and a similar ethnic origin in both families it was suggested that this particular pattern was autosomal recessive. In another family with athetoid spasticity the inheritance pattern suggested an X-linked inheritance.

This approach to improved clinical definition has been taken further in Birmingham by Mitchell and Bundey.[11] They looked at the relatively high frequency of non-progressive spasticity in the local Pakistani population. This population has a high rate of consanguinity. The group of 45 affected children in 16 families was still heterogeneous, but undoubtedly within it there were some autosomal recessive disorders. In one large consanguineous pedigree they were able to map a syndrome with severe mental retardation, spastic quadriplegia, and tapeto-retinal degeneration to chromosome 15q25.[12]

It is likely that similar studies in other consanguineous populations will identify further autosomal recessive forms of spastic quadriplegia. A study of cerebral palsy from Saudi Arabia showed a higher frequency of cerebral palsy in families and the most significant risk factors identified were a history of cerebral palsy in siblings and parental consanguinity.[13] In the genetically isolated Amish population a form of cerebral palsy with albinism called the Cross syndrome is recognized.[14]

The most common form of cerebral palsy is the asymmetrical hemiplegic form. This pattern is less likely to have a genetic basis. Most studies would suggest a 1–2 percent recurrence risk. In the few cases where it has recurred, it may be that the underlying predisposition is not for brain damage *per se* but for a greater risk of prematurity or some other obstetric complication.[15] In very rare cases it needs to be distinguished from migranous hemiplegia which may have an onset in childhood and if not adequately treated may leave permanent neurological damage.

In the diplegic form of cerebral palsy, genetic factors need to be considered very carefully. Hereditary spastic paraplegia can be mistaken for cerebral palsy if it has an early onset although it would tend to be progressive and therefore not strictly defined as cerebral palsy. In the Bundey and Griffiths study[10] the recurrence in siblings with symmetrical spastic diplegia was 2 out of 15 (13 percent). When Foley[16] carried out a study on the offspring of those with cerebral palsy to determine if there was a genetic risk, he only found 2 out of the 122 offspring who had a similar pattern of spasticity. Both of these had spastic diplegia. In view of the difficulty in excluding inherited forms of spastic paraplegia the recurrence risk for diplegic cerebral palsy is usually given as 10 percent in the absence of any adverse perinatal factors.

Athetoid or dystonic cerebral palsy has been associated with neonatal jaundice but in the absence of any significant neonatal factors it is important to consider autosomal recessive inheritance or, in the case of boys, X-linked recessive inheritance. Two X-linked forms have distinctive features. In the Allan-Herndon syndrome there is associated hypotonia, learning difficulties, and protruding ears[17] and in the X-linked form described by Pettigrew[18] there is associated Dandy-Walker malformation, basal ganglia disease and seizures. In the absence of a specific diagnosis or of a perinatal problem, the best figure to use for recurrence of athetoid cerebral palsy in further siblings is around 10 percent.

Ataxic cerebral palsy may not present until the child begins to walk independently and at that stage the child is noted to be ataxic. In many cases the computed tomography (CT) scan will demonstrate the presence of cerebellar hypoplasia. In such cases the likely pattern of inheritance is autosomal recessive. One specific disorder to exclude in this situation is carbohydrate-deficient glycoprotein disease, which is an autosomal recessive metabolic disease. It may be diagnosed by looking for abnormalities in the electrophoretic pattern of transferrin.[19]

5.7 METABOLIC DISORDERS PRESENTING AS CEREBRAL PALSY

There are a number of metabolic disorders that may produce either spasticity or dystonic movements and should therefore be considered in the context of 'inherited cerebral palsy'. In most cases there will be a progressive or episodic disturbance and therefore usually a rather different natural history from cerebral palsy. It is important to consider these disorders not only because there is usually a high recurrence risk and the opportunity of accurate prenatal diagnosis, but also because in some cases (e.g. holocarboxylase synthetase deficiency) there may be very effective metabolic treatment. The disorders are listed in Table 5.1 together with the method of diagnosis and pattern of inheritance.

On some occasions a magnetic resonance imaging (MRI) brain scan can be very helpful, identifying whether there is a metabolic abnormality underlying the handicap. Hoon[20] has shown that hypoxic-ischemic encephalopathy leaves a characteristic

hyperintense signal in the caudate and thalamus whereas mitochondrial disease and organic acidurias produce a different pattern of signals in the basal ganglia.

5.8 HEREDITARY SPASTIC PARAPLEGIA

One of the hallmarks of cerebral palsy is the presence of spasticity, but there are also many forms of inherited spasticity. The largest group is the inherited spastic paraplegias with or without associated clinical features. The pattern of spasticity is usually rather different from cerebral palsy as it predominantly affects the legs and is symmetrical. In most cases hereditary spastic paraplegia has an onset either in later childhood or in adult life, but there may be a considerable variation in the age of onset and certainly in the early-onset cases without a family history it may be almost impossible to distinguish from the diplegic form of cerebral palsy (See Case 5.5, p.85).

Great advances have been made in the genetic mapping of this group of disorders and in some cases the actual genes have been identified. It is therefore appropriate to use the newer classification based on molecular diagnosis.

Table 5.1 Metabolic disorders that present as cerebral palsy

Disease	Genetics	Clinical features	Diagnosis
Medium-chain acyl CoA dehydrogenase	AR	Severe hypoglycemia, lethargy, coma, and seizures	Hyperammonemia, fatty liver, mutation at position 985 of dehydrogenase gene in most patients
Glutaric aciduria type 1	AR	Dystonia, dyskinesia, opisthotonus, may be episodic or static, macrocephaly	Urine organic acids. Deficient glutaryl CoA dehydrogenase in cultured fibroblasts
Arginase deficiency	AR	Progressive spastic quadriplegia, seizures, MR, hyperactivity	Hyperammonemia, diaminoaciduria, increased argininemia
Arginosuccinic acid synthetase deficiency	AR	Episode episodes of lactic acidosis leading to neurological damage	Hyperammonemia, increased plasma citrulline. Confirmed enzyme deficiency in fibroblasts
Holocarboxylase synthetase deficiency	AR	Hypotonia, feeding difficulties, seizures, spasticity, MR. Associated with scaly skin and alopecia	Typical pattern of urine organic acids. Defect of biotin synthetase corrected by biotin supplements
Lesch-Nyhan syndrome	XR	Progressive spasticity, MR, and self-destructive behavior	Hypoxanthine guanine ribosyl transferase deficiency
Sjögren-Larsson syndrome	AR	Ichthyosiform erthroderma leading to scaly skin, spastic quadriplegia, MR	Increased hexadecanol in fibroblasts. Aldehyde dehydrogenase deficiency
Mitochondrial disorders	Mitochondrial	Various phenotypes including MELAS which produces strokes and mtDNA8993 mutation producing encephalopathy	Increased lactate. Ragged red fibers on muscle biopsy. DNA mutations detectable
Dopa responsive dystonia	AD	Dystonia with diurnal fluctuation	Decreased CSF dihydrobiopterin. Defect in GTP-cyclohydrolase
Factor V Leiden Protein C deficiency	AD/AR	Homozygotes may have placental and neonatal thrombosis leading to 'strokes'	Coagulation screen. DNA analysis

AR, autosomal recessive; AD, autosomal dominant; XR, X-linked recessive; MR, mental retardation.

Case 5.5

Philip was the first child born to an unrelated couple. The delivery was prolonged but his Apgar score was satisfactory and he went straight to the postnatal ward after delivery. His early motor milestones were normal but he was found to be delayed in walking and at 18 months the pediatrician noticed some increased tone and brisk reflexes in the legs. The possibility of cerebral palsy was considered. The question of litigation was raised as the parents were obviously concerned that he might have suffered injury from the prolonged delivery. When a specialist opinion was sought from a pediatric neurologist, he noted that Philip's mother had a slightly awkward gait and some nystagmus. She had equivocally brisk reflexes. The neurologist postulated that Philip might have X-linked spastic paraplegia and that his mother might be a mildly manifesting carrier. At that time there was no specific genetic test with which to confirm the hypothesis, but the situation has changed and today some more specialized laboratories can undertake genetic analysis for X-linked spastic paraplegia.

5.8.1 Spastic paraplegia 1 (SPG1) (L1CAM mutations)

In some families with X-linked spastic paraplegia there are additional problems such as mental handicap, indicating a clinical overlap with the MASA syndrome (Mental retardation, Aphasia, Shuffling gait, and Adducted thumbs). This latter condition has been mapped to Xq28 by a chromosomal rearrangement[21] and in a number of patients hydrocephalus with agenesis of the corpus callosum has been reported. At the same time the gene for X-linked hydrocephalus, which may also be associated with agenesis of the corpus callosum, was mapped to the same region. Eventually it was found that a single gene was responsible for all three conditions: X-linked spastic paraplegia, MASA syndrome, and X-linked hydrocephalus.[22] The gene involved produces a neural cell adhesion molecule called L1CAM, a glycoprotein expressed in axons and involved in neuronal migration. At the present time there is insufficient information available to relate mutations to specific phenotypes or neuropathology, but mutation analysis is available in a few diagnostic laboratories.

5.8.2 Spastic paraplegia 2 (SPG2) (PLP mutations)

The second X-linked form of spastic paraplegia was described as 'pure' spastic paraplegia, although there were often other neurological features such as optic atrophy, cerebellar ataxia, dysarthria, or nystagmus but not developmental delay. The gene for this form of spastic paraplegia was found to map to Xq21[23] and from this it was hypothesized and later proven that it involved the same locus as the neurodegenerative Pelizaeus-Merzbacher disease.[24] The mutations produce abnormalities in proteolipid protein (PLP) but it appears that SPG2 mutations, unlike those producing Pelizaeus-Merzbacher disease, do not produce clinical features in the first year of life or demyelination in the early MRI scans. The reason for this appears to be that the PLP gene produces two different myelin components which differ by the alternative splicing of one of the exons. One form is expressed in the early brain formation and is responsible for the more severe Pelizaeus–Merzbacher form, while the other mature form of PLP is expressed later and is responsible for spastic paraplegia 2. There are a number of other genetic disorders in which different mutations can produce different phenotypes and which have led to the reclassification of diseases.

5.8.3 Spastic paraplegia 3 (SPG3) (Stumpell disease)

This is probably the commonest form of hereditary spastic paraplegia and was originally described by Stumpell in 1880. It is autosomal dominant and there are many very large pedigrees identified. In the early 1980s Harding[25] tried to classify autosomal dominant hereditary spastic paraplegia into two groups. She described one with an earlier onset but a milder clinical course, and a second with a later onset but a more severe progressive course. This classification has been of some assistance in giving clinical prognosis but has now been superseded by the molecular classification. The later-onset form has been mapped to chromosome 14[26] but as yet no specific gene has been identified.

5.8.4   Spastic paraplegia 4 (SPG4)

The autosomal dominant forms of hereditary spastic paraplegia were found to be heterogeneous and a further locus was found on the short arm of chromosome 2.[27,28] In this case the gene mutation may be associated with a trinucleotide repeat. It is possible to draw some general conclusions from this finding. Trinucleotide repeats tend to be found in disorders of the central nervous system and if the repeat size increases when the genetic material is copied in the formation of egg and sperm it may become unstable and undergo an increase in repeat size. In other neurological disorders where this happens there will tend to be an earlier age of onset in the next generation. This phenomenon is known as anticipation. It follows, therefore, that this disorder may have a variable age of onset and that the age of onset may be earlier in successive generations.

5.8.5   Spastic paraplegia 5 (SPG5)

This form is autosomal recessive. In some of the original studies on hereditary spasticity there were a high proportion of cases with autosomal recessive inheritance, but there may be differences between populations. Many of the autosomal recessive forms of spasticity are associated with other features and except in inbred populations pure recessive spasticity is probably rare. Pure autosomal recessive spastic paraplegia was mapped using genetic linkage in Tunisian families[29] to the short arm of chromosome 8. The gene has not yet been identified.

5.8.6   Spastic paraplegia 6 (SPG6)

A further form of autosomal dominant hereditary spastic paraplegia similar to the early-onset form described by Harding has been linked to the long arm of chromosome 15.[30]

In addition to the 'pure' forms of spastic paraplegia there have been numerous reports of syndromes that include spastic paraplegia. Most of these have been confined to isolated case reports and as a source for future reference they are listed in Table 5.2 with the relevant McKusick number.[31]

One striking form of spasticity predominantly involving the facial muscles is congenital suprabulbar paresis or Worster-Drought syndrome.[32] The condition leads to speech difficulties and dribbling. It has on occasions been associated with fits and developmental delay. In a few cases there may be recurrence in the family, suggesting an autosomal dominant disorder with impaired penetrance.

5.9   MENTAL HANDICAP WITHOUT FOCAL NEUROLOGY

One of the most difficult areas in both pediatric neurology and medical genetics is the investigation of moderate to severe developmental delay without any specific neurological signs or associated physical abnormalities. The clinician in this situation has to work through a process of exclusion involving both environmental and genetic causes. Even then there will be a significant number of children in whom there will be no specific cause for their delay. In many series this will be as high as 40 percent of children with non-specific developmental delay. It is frustrating both for the parents and the clinicians, but it is likely that new developments in scanning technology and genetic testing will reduce the proportion of undiagnosed cases in the future. Two advances that have often been used to identify specific causes in this group of children are MRI scanning, which may identify neuronal migration defects or minor structural abnormalities, and tests

Table 5.2 Syndromes that include spastic paraplegia

Disease	Genetics	McKusick no.[31]
Spastic paraplegia and peripheral retinal degeneration	AR	270700
Spastic paraplegia and presenile dementia (Cross syndrome)	??	248900
Spastic paraplegia and Kallmann syndrome	??	308750
Spastic paraplegia and precocious puberty and MR	?AD	182820
Spastic paraplegia and pigmentary abnormalities	uncertain	270750
Spastic paraplegia and hereditary sensory neuropathy	AR	256840
Spastic paraplegia and macrocephaly	AR	600302
Spastic paraplegia, neuropathy, poikiloderma	AD	182815
Spastic paraplegia, myoclonic epilepsy	AR	270805
Spastic paraplegia and brachydactyly E	?AR	270710
Spastic paraplegia, palmoplantar hyperkeratosis, mental retardation	?XR	309560

AR, autosomal recessive; AD, autosomal dominant; XR, X-linked recessive; MR, mental retardation for fragile X mental retardation, which is now the second commonest cause of mental handicap.

Fragile X mental retardation derives its name from the chromosomal finding in the original patients studied. It was found that around 5 percent of the X chromosomes would develop a fragile site or unwinding of the heterochromatin on the long arm of the chromosome when the cells were grown in a culture medium deficient in folic acid. The patients in whom this occurred were moderately to severely handicapped but, unlike many handicapped persons, they did not have a particularly dysmorphic appearance or other physical abnormalities. They tended to have large heads and, as they became older, long ears and long facies. In terms of their psychomotor development they were more delayed in speech development and sometimes displayed autistic behaviour. The pattern of inheritance superficially resembled X-linked recessive inheritance, but there were a considerable number of females affected, usually in a milder form than males, and it appeared that on rare occasions the condition could be passed on from unaffected males since an unaffected father could have two carrier daughters (See Case 5.6 and 5.7).

These rather unusual genetic patterns were finally resolved[33] when the gene called FMR1 was discovered. The gene is located at the same position as the fragile site (viz. Xq28) and the mutation is a $(CCG)_n$ trinucleotide repeat. The disease starts with a slight expansion in the number of CCG repeats (60–200 repeats) which produces no symptoms and is referred to as the premutation. This may occur in unaffected males. However the premutation can increase during meiosis and therefore the next generation might be females who carry the full mutation of >200 repeats and are asymptomatic or only mildly affected as they have a second X chromosome to compensate for the mutation. If the mutation is passed on again to a boy, he will be fully affected with developmental delay and there will be the usual 50 percent risk of further male siblings being affected. It is always

---

Case 5.6

A girl was born by a water bath delivery at home. There was little documentation of the delivery other than the fact that the mother was pleased to have exercised her own choice in the method of delivery. The girl was slightly delayed in motor milestones but concerns came when her speech was markedly delayed and her behavior was described as autistic by the pediatrician. The pediatrician believed that there may have been neonatal problems around the time of delivery, but as part of his routine investigations ordered a DNA test for fragile X even though the handicapped child was a girl. He was surprised to find that she was a carrier of a large mutation in FMR1 gene as there was no family history of handicap but he eventually attributed the handicap to this. In the genetic follow-up it was found that the mother was also a carrier of the mutation but with a smaller expansion in the FMR1 gene. Prenatal diagnosis was offered to her in further pregnancies.

Case 5.7

Mrs Davies had two mentally handicapped brothers and when she came to start a family she was concerned that she might have a handicapped child similar to her brothers. The obstetrician checked the routine chromosome karyotype in an amniocentesis and when this was reported normal he reassured her 'that everything would be all right'. Unfortunately she had a son and it soon became apparent that he too was handicapped like his uncles. When the family were finally investigated by the clinical geneticist it was found that Mrs Davies' son had fragile X mental retardation and she was a carrier.

While the obstetrician had responded sympathetically to his patient's concerns, he was not sufficiently up to date with his genetic knowledge to consider fragile X and arrange the most appropriate test. He would probably be judged as negligent as he failed to refer Mrs Davies to the appropriate specialist and therefore she was not offered the correct prenatal test which would have allowed her the option of a termination of pregnancy.

There are many different forms of X-linked mental handicap and a family history such as this should be investigated preconceptually.

Table 5.3 X-linked syndromes other than fragile X syndrome presenting with mental handicap

Disease	Description	McKusick no.
Coffin-Lowry syndrome	Severe mental retardation, coarse facies, kyphosis	30360
FG syndrome	Broad forehead, frontal upsweep of hair, constipation	30545
Simpson-Golabi-Behmel syndrome	Neonatal overgrowth, severe mental retardation, cleft palate, coarse 'bulldog' facies	31287
Borjeson-Forsseman syndrome	Obesity, microcephaly, hypotonia, mental retardation	30190
X-linked alpha thalassemia mental retardation	Flat nasal bridge, triangular mouth, hypogonadism, alpha thalassemia, mental retardation	

more difficult to predict the outcome in female carriers but around 30 percent will be symptomatic.

In addition to fragile X being caused by mutations in FMR1 there is a second, much rarer form of fragile X mental retardation known as FraxE.[34] This is caused by an expansion in a location distal to FMR1 and can be tested for using a molecular genetic test.

In all studies of mental retardation there has been an excess of males over females. The main explanation of this is that there are a large number of X-linked syndromes with mental handicap. Although fragile X mental retardation will account for a significant proportion of cases, it is important to recognize some of the others if accurate genetic counseling is to be given. There are several good reviews[35,36] and Table 5.3 lists the main disorders.

If, at the end of the day, no cause is found for non-specific mental handicap, the geneticist will resort to using empiric recurrence risks based on the likelihood of recurrence after all recognizable causes of handicap are excluded. These figures indicate a recurrence of 5–10 percent.[37] This figure could be interpreted as suggesting on balance of probability that the cause is either due to a *de novo* mutation or due to non-genetic factors.

5.10   GENETICS OF BRAIN MALFORMATIONS

It is essential to have good neuroradiology in determining the cause of mental handicap. When a brain malformation is found it will indicate that the cause of the handicap was probably not due to perinatal asphyxia but due to prenatal or genetic factors.

5.10.1   Hydrocephalus

Hydrocephalus can be caused by a variety of different factors including prenatal infection, intracranial hemorrhage, postnatal meningitis, and genetic factors. In consanguineous populations autosomal recessive genes may cause hydrocephalus but in outbred Western populations the majority of cases in girls are unlikely to be genetic. In boys more care should be taken in the assessment. There is a well-recognized X-linked form of hydrocephalus which is usually associated with aqueduct stenosis and adducted thumbs. It is due to mutations in the L1CAM gene which also causes X-linked spastic paraplegia (see above).

5.10.2   Agenesis of the corpus callosum

This condition has been increasingly diagnosed with better scanning techniques. It may occur in partial form in children with normal intelligence and where present is not always the cause of developmental delay. When present with mental handicap, it is frequently associated with fits and spasticity. It may be caused by chromosome abnormalities, biochemical abnormalities (especially organic acidurias) and single gene syndromes.[38]

5.10.3   Holoprosencephaly

In this abnormality of the brain, the primitive forebrain (the prosencephalon) fails completely or partially to divide into two cerebral hemispheres. This affects the embryonic development of the face and is associated with hypotelorism (closely spaced eyes) and abnormalities of the nose and upper lip. The commonest single cause of holoprosencephaly is chromosome abnormality, especially trisomy 13 and deletions of 7qter.[39] In the case of trisomy 13 there will be other life-threatening malformations.

An autosomal dominant form with variable expressivity is recognized in which the facial features may be as minimal as a single central incisor and lack of smell (anosmia) due to malformation of the olfactory nerve.[40]

In the absence of a chromosome abnormality or a family history there is still a recurrence risk of 5 percent, suggesting there are still autosomal recessive genes causing this malformation that have not yet been found.

5.10.4 Cerebellar hypoplasia

Many cases of ataxic cerebral palsy will be found on neuro-imaging to have cerebellar hypoplasia. The cerebellar vermis and hemispheres may be reduced in size. Postmortem examination has shown that there may be atrophy of the granular layer and some degeneration of the Purkinje cells. The inheritance is usually autosomal recessive.

5.10.5 Lissencephaly

The term lissencephaly refers to the lack of gyral folds on the surface of the cortex. There are a number of causes to consider.[2,41] Type 1 (classical) lissencephaly may be isolated or, in the Miller-Dieker syndrome associated with a dysmorphic facial appearance and congenital heart disease together with almost complete absence of gyri. Chromosome studies with specific FISH studies may show deletions of chromosome 17p13. In type II lissencephaly (cobblestone) the eye should be examined carefully as there are autosomal recessive forms such as HARD (Hydrocephalus, Agyria, Retinal Dysplasia) and muscle–eye–brain disease which need to be excluded. Intrauterine infection may also cause lissencephaly and may be associated with chorioretinopathy. A brain scan may help to define the pattern of lissencephaly and this may be helpful in determining the etiology. A cobblestone pattern in the absence of muscle or eye disease is found in one autosomal recessive form.[42]

5.10.6 Neuronal migration defects

The advent of MRI scanning has identified a wide range of newly discovered defects in neuronal migration. Most cases, especially where the defect is unilateral or focal, are not genetic but some, such as subcortical band heteropia (double cortex syndrome) have occurred excusively in girls and are X-linked dominant. Chromosomal abnormalities and metabolic abnormalities should also be excluded.

5.11 FUTURE TRENDS

The overview presented in this chapter shows that there have been considerable advances in our understanding of genetic causes of cerebral palsy and mental handicap. This is likely to be reflected in medicolegal cases. Historically it was customary to attribute handicap, excluding Down's syndrome, as being due to anoxic damage occurring at the time of birth and litigation reflected this, with most cases being directed to finding negligence on the part of the obstetrician. However, with a greater understanding of genetic conditions has come an increasing range and sophistication of tests which may be used in prenatal diagnosis. Litigation now is increasingly looking at failure to provide accurate prenatal diagnosis and such cases may be successful for the plaintiff if a reasonable level of expertise has not been applied. In the future we may be looking at cases due to failure to provide the correct genetic counseling before birth and a handicapped child being born as a result of this failure. Clinicians should be aware of this trend and refer to their colleagues in clinical genetics where appropriate, ideally before pregnancy. For the geneticist one of the problems with this trend is the rapid pace of development in the specialty. It is appropriate for the geneticist to preface any counseling with the statement 'based on the knowledge available at present' and to advise patients to seek up-to-date knowledge if they are planning to delay their plans to start their family. From the point of view of the courts it can be very difficult to look back and accurately gauge the level of genetic knowledge available at the time the counseling was given.

It may not simply be in the field of birth injury and cerebral palsy that genetics will be important in establishing causation. One interesting finding from the work on Alzheimer's disease is that certain individuals with a certain apolipoprotein E genotype (homozygous E4) are more likely to react to brain injury with amyloid deposition. At present this is not thought to be relevant in giving a predisposition to cerebral palsy, but it may be that there are genetic factors in the ability to recover from head injury. This might add a new dimension to trauma litigation, in which the client's genotype is as important as the nature of the injury!

In conclusion, one trend is certain – genetics will not only increase our knowledge of disease but will also be increasingly important in various aspects of medicolegal work.

5.12 REFERENCES

1 Kuwano A, Ledbetter SA, Dobyns WB *et al.* Detection of deletions and cryptic translocations in the Miller–Dieker syndrome by in situ hybridization. *American Journal of Human Genetics* 1991; **49**: 707–14.

2 Flint J, Wilkie AOM, Buckle VJ, Winter RM, Holland AJ, McDermid HE. The detection of subtelomeric chromosome rearrangements in idiopathic mental retardation. *Nature Genetics* 1995; **9**: 132–9.

3 Patton MA. A computerised approach to dysmorphology. *MD Computing* 1987; **4**: 33–9.

4 Marion RW, Chitayat D, Hutcheon RG, Goldberg R, Shprintzen RJ, Cohen MM. Autosomal recessive inheritance in the Setleis bitemporal 'forceps mark' syndrome. *American Journal of Diseases of Children* 1987; **141**: 895–7.

5 Newbury-Ecob RA, Leanage R, Raeburn JA, Young ID. Holt Oram syndrome: a clinical and genetic study. *Journal of Medical Genetics* 1996; **33**: 300–7.

6 Asher P, Schonell FE. A survey of 400 cases of cerebral palsy in childhood. *Archives of Disease in Childhood* 1950; **25**: 360–79.

7 Gustavson KH, Hagberg B, Sanner G. Identical syndromes of cerebral palsy in the same family. *Acta Paediatrica Scandinavica* 1969; **58**: 330–40.

8 Griffiths M. Cerebral palsy in multiple pregnancy. *Developmental Medicine and Child Neurology* 1967; **9**: 713–31.

9 Goodman R, Alberman E. A twin study of congenital hemiplegia. *Developmental Medicine and Child Neurology* 1996; **38**: 3–12.

10 Bundey S, Griffiths MI. Recurrence risks in families of children with symmetrical spasticity. *Developmental Medicine and Child Neurology* 1977; **19**: 179–91.

11 Mitchell S, Bundey S. Symmetry of neurological signs in Pakistani patients with probable inherited spastic cerebral palsy. *Clinical Genetics* 1997; **51**: 7–14.

12 Mitchell SJ, McHale DP, Campbell DA *et al.* A syndrome of severe mental retardation, spasticity and tapetoretinal degeneration maps to chromosome 15q25. *American Journal of Human Genetics* 1998; **62**: 1070–6.

13 Al-Rajeh S, Bademosi O, Awada A, Ismail H, al-Shammasi S, Dawodu A. Cerebral palsy in Saudi Arabia: a case control study of risk factors. *Developmental Medicine and Child Neurology* 1991; **33**: 1048–52.

14 Cross HE, McKusick VA, Breen W. A new oculocutaneous syndrome with hypopigmentation. *Journal of Pediatrics* 1967; **70**: 398–406.

15 Palmer L, Petterson B, Blair E, Burton P. Family patterns of gestational age at delivery and growth in utero in moderate and severe cerebral palsy. *Developmental Medicine and Child Neurology* 1994; **36**: 1108–19.

16 Foley J. The offspring of people with cerebral palsy. *Developmental Medicine and Child Neurology* 1992; **32**: 972–8.

17 Stevenson RE, Goodman HO, Schwartz CE, Simensen RJ, McLean WT, Herndon CN. Allan Herndon syndrome I: clinical studies. *American Journal of Medical Genetics* 1990; **47**: 446–53

18 Pettigrew AJ, Jackson LG, Ledbetter DH. New X linked mental retardation disorder with Dandy Walker malformation, basal ganglia disease and seizures. *American Journal of Medical Genetics* 1991; **38**: 200–7.

19 Horslen SP, Clayton PT, Harding BN *et al.* Olivopontocerebellar atrophy of neonatal onset and disialotransferrin development deficiency syndrome. *Archives of Disease in Childhood* 1991; **66**: 1027–32.

20 Hoon AH, Reinhardt EM, Kelley RI, *et al.* Brain magnetic resonance imaging in suspected extrapyramidal cerebral palsy: observations in distinquishing genetic-metabolic from acquired causes. *Journal of Pediatrics* 1997; **131**: 240–5.

21 Winter RM, Davies KE, Bell MV, Huson SM, Patterson MN. MASA syndrome: further clinical delineation and chromosomal localisation. *Human Genetics* 1989; **82**: 367–70.

22 Jouet M, Rosenthal A, Armstrong G *et al.* X-linked spastic paraplegia (SPG1), MASA syndrome and X-linked hydrocephalus result from mutations in the L1 gene. *Nature Genetics* 1994; **7**: 402–7.

23 Keppen LD, Leppert MF, O'Connell P *et al.* Etiological heterogeneity in X linked spastic paraplegia. *American Journal of Human Genetics* 1987; **41**: 933–43.

24 Saugier-Veber P, Munnich A, Bonneau D *et al.* X-linked spastic paraplegia and Pelizaeus Merzbacher disease are allelic disorders at the proteolipid protein locus. *Nature Genetics* 1994; **6**: 257–61.

25 Harding AE. Hereditary 'pure' spastic paraplegia: a clinical and genetic study in 22 families. *Journal of Neurology, Neurosurgery and Psychiatry* 1981; **44**: 871–83.

26 Hazan J, Lamy C, Melki J, Munnich A, Recondo J, Wissenbach J. Autosomal dominant familial spastic paraplegia is genetically heterogeneous and one locus maps to chromosome 14q. *Nature Genetics* 1993; **5**: 163–7

27 Hazan J, Fonknechten N, Mavel D *et al.* Spastin, a new AAA protein, is altered in the most frequent form of autosomal dominant spastic paraplegia. *Nature Genetics* 1999; **23**: 296–303.

28 Nielsen J, Koefoed P, Abell R *et al.* CAG repeat expansion in autosomal dominant pure spastic paraplegia linked to chromosome 2p21–24. *Human Molecular Genetics* 1997; **6**: 1811–16.

29 Hentati A, Pericak-Vance MA, Hung WY *et al.* Linkage of pure autosomal recessive familial spastic paraplegia to chromosome 8 markers and evidence of genetic locus heterogeneity. *Human Molecular Genetics* 1994; **3**: 1263–7.

30 Fink JK, Wu CB, Jones SM *et al.* Autosomal dominant familial spastic paraplegia: tight linkage to chromo-

some 15q. *American Journal of Human Genetics* 1995; **56**: 188–92.

31 McKusick VA. *Mendelian inheritance in man: Catalogs of autosomal dominant, autosomal recessive and X linked phenotypes*, 12th edn. Baltimore and London: The Johns Hopkins University Press, 1994.

32 Patton MA, Baraitser M, Brett EM. A family with congenital suprabulbar paresis (Worster-Drought syndrome). *Clinical Genetics* 1986; **29**: 147–50 .

33 Richards RI, Sutherland GR. Fragile X syndrome: the molecular picture comes into focus. *Trends in Genetics* 1992; **8**: 249–55.

34 Dennis NR, Curtis G, Macpherson JN, Jacobs PA. Two families with Xq27.3 fragility, no detectable insert in the FMR1 gene, mild mental retardation, and absence of Martin-Bell phenotype. *American Journal of Medical Genetics* 1992; **43**: 232–6.

35 Glass IA. X linked mental retardation. *Journal of Medical Genetics* 1991; **28**: 361–71.

36 Lubs HA, Chiurazzi P, Arena JF, Schwartz C, Tranebaerg L, Neri G. XLMR genes: an update.

American Journal of Medical Genetics 1996; **64**: 147–57.

37 Crow YJ, Tolmie JL. Recurrence risks in mental retardation. *Journal of Medical Genetics* 1998; **35**: 177–82.

38 Dobyns WB. Absence makes the search grow longer (editorial). *American Journal of Human Genetics* 1996; **58**: 7–16.

39 Nanni L, Ming JE, Bocian M *et al.* The mutational spectrum of the sonic hedgehog gene in holoprosencephaly: SHH mutations cause a significant proportion of autosomal dominant holoprosencephaly. *Human Molecular Genetics* 1999; **8**: 2479–88.

40 Siebert JR, Cohen MM, Sulik KK, Shaw C-M, Lemire RJ. *Holoprosencephaly: an overview and atlas of cases.* New York: John Wiley & Sons, 1990.

41 Pilz DT, Quarrell OWJ. Syndromes with lissencephaly. *Journal of Medical Genetics* 1996; **33**: 319–23.

42 Dobyns WB, Patton MA, Stratton RF, Mastrobattista JM, Blanton SH, Northrup H. Cobblestone lissencephaly with normal eyes and muscle. *Neuropediatrics* 1996; **27**: 70–5.

6 Differential diagnosis of cerebral palsy

Robert C Vannucci

Contrary to the original opinion of Little and to more recent popular belief, not all cerebral palsy is caused by perinatal hypoxia/ischemia (asphyxia). Indeed, intrapartum asphyxia accounts for no more than 8–12 percent of all cases of cerebral palsy existing in infants, children, and adults. Other causes of cerebral palsy, to be reviewed below, are listed in Table 6.1, and include congenital malformations and syndromes, complications of prematurity, infectious disease, and several inborn errors of metabolism and neurodegenerative disorders.

6.1 TYPES OF CEREBRAL PALSY

The term 'cerebral palsy' encompasses a group of disorders of movement and posture caused by a non-progressive lesion of the developing brain. The term implies neither neuropathologic nor etiologic entities, but rather a heterogeneous collection of syndromes that are classified according to the type and distribution of motor abnormality. The number of affected individuals provides a major contribution to the overall population of handicapped children, with a prevalence of approximately 2 per 1000. Recent epidemiologic studies suggest an increasing prevalence, due primarily to increasing numbers of surviving very low birthweight infants who develop cerebral palsy.

The various cerebral palsy syndromes are classified in Table 6.2. They include spastic, dyskinetic, and ataxic forms. In spastic cerebral palsy, there is evidence on neurologic examination of hypertonicity (stiffness) of the muscles of the involved extremities, with an associated paucity of movement, hyperactive deep tendon reflexes, extensor plantar responses, and clonus. In spastic paraparesis (paraplegia), only the lower extremities are affected, with preservation of upper extremity function. In spastic diparesis (diplegia), all extremities are involved, but arm and hand function is better than leg and foot function. In spastic hemiparesis, there is involvement of both the arm and leg only on one side. Finally, in spastic quadriparesis

Table 6.1 Causes of cerebral palsy

Cause	Incidence (%)
Congenital malformations/syndromes	20–25
Complications of prematurity	5–10
Term intrapartum asphyxia	8–12
Postpartum insults	3–5
Other perinatal insults	
Toxic, metabolic, infectious, etc.	10–15
Unknown	33–54

Table 6.2 Cerebral palsy syndromes

Spastic
      Diparesis (diplegia)
      Paraparesis (paraplegia)
      Hemiparesis (hemiplegia)
      Quadriparesis (quadriplegia)
Dyskinetic
      Athetotic
      Choreic
      Dystonic
Ataxic

(quadriplegia), all extremities are involved and to an equal degree, usually severely.

The other types of cerebral palsy include the dyskinetic and ataxic forms. In dyskinetic cerebral palsy, involuntary movements (movements not under willful control) are apparent in the form of athetosis, chorea, dystonia, or some combination. Athetotic movements are slow, smooth, and writhing, involving predominantly distal muscles. Choreiform movements are rapid, irregular, unpredictable contractions of muscle groups, typically affecting proximal parts of the extremities. In dystonia, twisting, maintained distortions of the trunk and limbs are seen. Tone is variable in the dyskinetic syndromes. Associated findings include normal to reduced deep tendon reflexes, with an absence of clonus and pathologic reflex responses. Combinations of spasticity and dyskinesia can be seen in the same patient.

Ataxia indicates an incoordination of movement and stability. Difficulty in walking and hand control occurs, often in association with abnormal eye movements and difficulty in speech pronunciation (dysarthria). Deep tendon reflexes typically are reduced, but pathologic reflexes are absent.

Knowledge of the type of cerebral palsy exhibited by an individual patient provides a clue as to which part of the brain has been damaged and its etiology. Because motor dysfunction of the upper extremities is spared in spastic paraparesis, frequently the cause of this disorder is spinal in origin, either a congenital malformation or neoplasm. A familial form of spastic paraparesis also exists. Spastic diparesis typically is seen in children who have been born prematurely and who suffer periventricular leukomalacia (see below). Spastic hemiparesis occurs as a consequence of destruction of cortical or subcortical white matter of the cerebral hemisphere contralateral to the weakness. Frequent causes of hemiparesis include trauma, occlusive vascular disease (stroke), and infection. Spastic quadriparesis, the most severe form of cerebral palsy, occurs as a con-

sequence of asphyxia, but is also seen following trauma, infectious disease, and certain hereditary metabolic and neurodegenerative disorders. Dyskinetic forms of cerebral palsy indicate dysfunction of the basal ganglia of the brain, for which there are multiple etiologies, including asphyxia, kernicterus (hyperbilirubinemia), infectious disease, and certain metabolic disorders. The ataxic forms of cerebral palsy typically are prenatal in origin, related either to a congenital malformation or to a specific, often identifiable syndrome.

Many children with cerebral palsy exhibit other neurologic disturbances, but certainly not all. Infants and children with spastic hemiparesis often develop normally other than the obvious unilateral weakness. Language and cognition are usually normal, although the individuals are at increased risk for seizures. Like spastic hemiparesis, individuals with spastic paraparesis typically exhibit normal intellectual and language development. Seizures typically are not a problem in this group. Children with spastic diparesis can exhibit normal intellectual function, although they are at increased risk for the occurrence of either learning disability or mental retardation, the latter usually mild. The risk of seizures is increased. Children with spastic quadriplegia typically are retarded, and often severely to profoundly so. Seizures are quite frequent in this group, as are also visual and hearing impairments. These children frequently are microcephalic. In the dyskinetic and ataxic forms of cerebral palsy, the extent of any intellectual and language dysfunction is dependent upon the underlying cause of the motor disorder. In the absence of spasticity, children with athetotic cerebral palsy of asphyxial or kernicteric origin often exhibit normal intellectual development and language acquisition, although pronunciation can be compromised (dysarthria).

6.2 CAUSES OF CEREBRAL PALSY

As mentioned previously, there are multiple etiologies of cerebral palsy, all of which cause brain dysfunction or destruction during either prenatal or postnatal development. Acute insults to the adult brain can produce identical motor syndromes, but such affected individuals are not labeled as suffering from cerebral palsy, since their brains have previously undergone complete maturation. Accordingly, the designation of the term 'cerebral palsy' to individuals who have suffered brain insults during their formative years is strictly an arbitrary one.

6.2.1 Hypoxia-ischemia (asphyxia)

Hypoxia-ischemia or asphyxia causing brain damage can occur at any time during either the latter part of fetal life or postnatally. The two terms are relatively synonymous, asphyxia implying the existence of hypoxia and acidosis in tissues and blood, including the brain. Ischemia is defined as a reduction in or cessation of blood flow to the tissue, including the brain, and occurs as a consequence of cardiovascular depression arising from asphyxia or from occlusive vascular disease (see below). Experimental studies suggest that for brain damage to occur, at least some degree of ischemia must be present.

In the fetus, asphyxia arises as a consequence of either placental or umbilical cord dysfunction. These organs are the sole supply of oxygen and nutrients to the fetus, and also provide for the removal of carbon dioxide and lactic acid. The most frequent cause of asphyxia in postnatal infants and children is lung dysfunction, as seen in the respiratory distress syndrome of premature infants, pneumonia, and drowning, among others. Other causes of asphyxia include cardiac failure of multiple etiologies as well as acute exsanguination.

The topography or distribution of brain damage caused by asphyxia is to a large extent determined by the age of the fetus or newborn infant at the time of the insult. In the premature fetus or newborn infant, the white matter surrounding the lateral ventricles is most vulnerable to injury, producing so-called 'periventricular leukomalacia'. With increasing fetal age, the brunt of injury shifts to gray matter structures, specifically the cerebral cortex and basal ganglia. With partial, prolonged asphyxia occurring over hours, the cerebral cortex receives the brunt of injury in term infants, occasionally with involvement of the subcortical white matter. If the asphyxia is acute and severe in a full-term infant, then the predominant injury is focused on the basal ganglia, often with associated brainstem involvement. Similar distributions occur in the postnatal infant who was born at term.

6.2.2 Occlusive vascular disease (stroke)

Arterial occlusive vascular disease producing cerebral infarction (stroke) occurs in both the fetus and newborn infant as well as in the older infant and child. Previously, cerebral infarction due to arterial occlusive vascular disease was assumed to be of hypoxic-ischemic (asphyxial) origin, with or with-

Table 6.3 Causes of occlusive vascular disease

Sepsis
Meningitis
Asphyxia
Disseminated intravascular coagulation (DIC)
Congenital heart disease
Polycythemia (hyperviscosity)
Physical birth trauma
Demise of twin fetus
Developmental anomaly of carotid, vertebral, or basilar arteries
Placental embolization
Hypercoagulable states (antiphospholipid antibodies, protein S or C deficiency)

out associated venous occlusion. However, more recent investigations suggest that either embolic or thrombotic occlusion of one or more arteries supplying the brain produces a distinct clinical and pathologic entity. Large, single infarcts predominate in full-term infants, whereas multiple, small infarcts are more frequent in premature infants. The lesions typically involve the cerebral cortex and subcortical white matter, primarily in the territory of the middle cerebral artery and rarely in the distribution of the basilar artery. The causes of arterial occlusive vascular disease in the fetus and postnatal infant are numerous, with infectious disease and asphyxia being the most frequent, when an etiology can be identified (Table 6.3).

6.2.3 Trauma

Trauma to the brain can occur during the birth process or at any time thereafter. A traumatic insult occurring at birth is typically the consequence of an inappropriately applied vacuum extractor or forceps. Epidural or subdural hemorrhages occur, leading to compression of the underlying brain substance, occasionally with associated permanent damage. Occlusion of the venous sinuses with secondary hemorrhagic infarction of the cerebral hemispheres occurs with vacuum extraction. Lastly, contusions of the brain can occur, especially with inappropriate forceps manipulation.

Traumatic injuries to the postnatal brain occur as a consequence of falls, missiles, blunt trauma, or lacerations, as seen in motor vehicle accidents or child abuse.

6.2.4 Infectious disease

Children of all ages, including fetuses, suffer infectious disease, certain forms of which produce permanent brain damage. Of the infectious processes affecting the newborn infant, bacterial meningitis is the most frequent cause of brain damage, leading to cerebral palsy. The group B *Streptococcus* (GBS) is the leading offending agent. Viral encephalitis also can cause brain damage in any age group, including the fetus. The eponym 'TORCH' encompasses a few of these organisms, including cytomegalovirus and herpes simplex. Cytomegalovirus can cause major destruction of the brain during early to mid-fetal life, whereas the herpesvirus typically produces a focal encephalitis in the newborn or older infant or child. Many other viruses also produce encephalitis, occasionally with permanent brain injury.

Another infectious cause of brain damage is bacterial sepsis. In the premature infant, sepsis typically is nosocomial in origin, whereas in the full-term infant sepsis occurs usually as a consequence of prolonged rupture of the amniotic membranes, which also is a cause of meningitis. Although sepsis *per se* probably does not cause brain damage severe enough to lead to cerebral palsy, complications of sepsis can produce permanent brain injury. Such complications include disseminated intravascular coagulation and severe systemic hypotension (septic shock). In the older infant and child, sepsis severe enough to cause brain damage is most often seen in the immunocompromised patient.

6.2.5   Intracranial hemorrhage

Aside from trauma, the most common cause of intracranial hemorrhage is periventricular/interventricular hemorrhage. This entity is seen almost exclusively in infants born prematurely at or prior to 32 weeks gestation. The germinal matrix, a region of actively dividing primitive neurons and glia, surrounds the lateral ventricles during fetal life and is especially prone to hemorrhage if the infant is born prematurely or is otherwise stressed during fetal life. Hemorrhage into the germinal matrix often extravasates into the lateral ventricles and also into the parenchyma of the brain, causing permanent brain damage. Other non-traumatic causes of intracranial hemorrhage include congenital vascular malformations and coagulation defects.

6.2.6   Congenital malformations (anomalies)

Congenital malformations are frequently associated with permanent brain dysfunction, and

account for approximately 20 percent of all cases of cerebral palsy. Anomalies typically are divided into the embryonic induction disorders and disorders of neuronal proliferation and migration. Such anomalies can lead to permanent motor dysfunction with or without associated mental retardation and epilepsy. Some of the malformations are familial in nature, whereas others occur sporadically. Environmental influences also contribute to the occurrence of congenital malformations, including specific vitamin deficiency (folate), irradiation, maternal alcoholism, and drug abuse.

Certain congenital malformations are seen as a component of a specific syndrome, which might or might not be hereditary. The neurocutaneous disorders are well-known examples. Tuberous sclerosis is a neurocutaneous disorder causing mental retardation, cerebral palsy, and epilepsy. Congenital malformations of the brain occur as a consequence of aberrant neuronal migration leading to 'tubers' and benign neoplasms. Other well-known syndromes causing cerebral palsy, usually with associated mental retardation, include chromosomal aberrations and a variety of disorders, all of which are characterized by visually apparent somatic abnormalities which allow the clinician to make at least a tentative diagnosis, often confirmed by appropriate diagnostic testing (see below).

6.2.7   Metabolic disorders

Certain metabolic derangements occur in isolation, whereas others result from a hereditary inborn error of metabolism. The most common metabolic derangement in the newborn infant is hypoglycemia, for which there are multiple causes, including intrauterine growth retardation, asphyxia, and diabetes in the mother. It is generally conceded that for brain damage to occur, the hypoglycemia must be severe, protracted, and lead to symptoms in the newborn infant. Hypocalcemia in the newborn infant is not thought to cause permanent brain damage.

A large number of inborn errors of metabolism exist, essentially all due to a hereditary deficiency in a specific enzyme which drives a cellular biochemical reaction (Table 6.4). Some, but certainly not all, of these disorders can present in the immediate newborn period. Such disorders include those of amino acid metabolism and transport, carbohydrate metabolism, lipid metabolism, metal metabolism, purine and pyrimidine metabolism, organic acidurias, and lysosomal and peroxisomal disorders. Some of these inborn errors of metabolism

Table 6.4 Inborn errors of metabolism

Disorders of amino acid metabolism or transport
Disorders of carbohydrate metabolism
Disorders of lipid metabolism
Mitochondrial disorders
Organic acidurias
Lysosomal storage disorders
Peroxisomal disorders
Lipidosis
Disorders of metal metabolism
Disorders of purine and pyrimidine metabolism

are amenable to treatment in the form of dietary manipulation or drug intervention; accordingly, their early identification is important from a therapeutic perspective. Untreated, the affected infants and children often show signs of neurologic deterioration, which precludes the diagnosis of cerebral palsy, which by definition is a 'static encephalopathy'. However, some children with these disorders, including those with mitochondrial abnormalities, do not exhibit a progression of their disease, but rather remain static or show very slow deterioration over many, many years. Accordingly, such children are often somewhat falsely labeled as having cerebral palsy of unexplained cause.

6.3 NEUROLOGIC ASSESSMENT

Having reviewed the causes of cerebral palsy, albeit superficially, a discussion of the neurologic assessment and diagnostic procedures to ascertain as precise an etiology as possible is in order. The neurologic evaluation of the premature and full-term newborn infant is derived from the 'classic' neurologic examination of the older infant, child, and adult, but with certain modifications. Given the relative lack of cooperative interaction between the examiner and infant, the assessment is largely observational, as is the case in infants of slightly older ages. However, the examination itself can provide valuable information regarding the nature and location of anatomic or functional deficits referable to the central or peripheral nervous system, thereby providing important clues regarding the underlying cause of any observed neurologic dysfunction, which might eventually manifest itself in the form of cerebral palsy with or without mental retardation, learning disability, or epilepsy.

As in any medical evaluation, the neurologic assessment of the newborn and older infant begins with a thorough historical review of maternal (and paternal) data relevant to the situation at hand (Table 6.5). For the newborn infant, most required information is available from the maternal pregnancy and delivery records, supplemented by interviews with one or both parents. More detailed historical accounts of maternal exposure to infectious disease or elicit drugs, family history of neurologic abnormalities or death in early life, and the mother's own perception of fetal well-being might provide important causal information regarding a neurologically compromised newborn infant. Knowledge of the delivery process and the status of the infant at and shortly following birth completes the historical survey.

Table 6.5 Pregnancy and birth history

Age, gravidity, parity
Pre-pregnancy health status
    Nutrition
    Chronic disease:
        Diabetes, hypertension, heart disease, anemia, cancer, rheumatic disease
    Infectious disease:
        Syphilis, tuberculosis, AIDS, other venereal disease
Pregnancy health status
    Nutrition/vitamins
    Exposure to infection:
        Respiratory illness, rash, adenopathy
    Glucose intolerance
    Hypertension
    Blood type/Rh
    Tobacco, alcohol, drug exposure
Obstetrical conditions
    Pelvic anatomy
    Placental position and size
    Vaginal/urinary infection
Fetal status
    Growth
    Activity
    Multiple fetuses
    Ultrasonic abnormalities
    Biophysical profile
Family history
    Cerebral palsy, mental retardation, epilepsy, metabolic disease
    Death or disability in early life
Birth
    Route of delivery
    Anesthesia/analgesia
    Fetal heart rate monitoring
    Scalp or umbilical cord pH
    Gestational age (average, small, large for)
    Instrumentation
    Apgar scores
    Need for resuscitation
    Early postnatal status

Table 6.6 The neurologic evaluation

General appearance and physiognomy
Level of consciousness
Mechanical signs: head, spine, extremities
Cranial nerves
Motor: strength, tone, movements
Sensation: light touch, pain
Deep tendon reflexes
Primitive reflexes: Moro, grasp, suck, root, etc.
Autonomic: heart rate pattern, respiratory pattern, bladder and bowel function

Having obtained as adequate a maternal and fetal-newborn history as possible, the physician proceeds with the medical evaluation of the infant, derived from elements of the classic neurologic examination combined with a developmental assessment of gestational age (Table 6.6). The physical component of the neurologic examination includes visualization and palpation of the head, spine, and extremities. The entire body is observed for visibly apparent congenital anomalies, birthmarks, or bruises. The head and spine are palpated to ascertain the presence of deformities, the position of the sutures, and the size and shape of the fontanels. The presence of excessive head molding (caput) or cephalohematoma is determined. The circumference of the head is measured and plotted on a standardized growth chart, taking gestational age into account. Finally, each side of the head is gently tapped with a finger to ascertain its resonance (presence or absence of a 'cracked-pot' sound), which might provide a clue as to the underlying presence of hydrocephalus or an epidural or subdural fluid collection. The size and shape of the head provide important information regarding the occurrence of a remote or chronic insult to the fetal brain. When fetal brain growth has been compromised, head size will be decreased relative especially to body or crown–rump length, and the sutures might overlap. In contrast, a large head with split sutures denotes an underlying large brain, usually the consequence of congenital obstructive hydrocephalus or, less likely, a mass lesion. Postnatally, a rapidly expanding head with split sutures indicates the occurrence of cerebral edema or acquired, progressive hydrocephalus, as results from intraventricular hemorrhage in a premature infant.

Following the general physical examination, neurologic function is ascertained as described in Table 6.7. The gestational age of the newborn infant at the time of birth must be taken into account, since the more premature the infant at birth, the more primitive the neurologic findings. Specifically, reflex activity is less well developed and reduced muscular tone (hypotonia) is a characteristic finding. Premature infants are more difficult to arouse, as they sleep for more extended intervals than do full-term infants. The Dubowitz and Ballard scoring systems are scales used by physicians to ascertain the degree of prematurity in a newborn infant.

The neurologic assessment of the older infant and child is similar to that obtained in the newborn infant, and includes both historical and physical components. As the child grows older, interaction between the examiner and patient becomes feasible. After the age of 3 years, the infant under optimal circumstances is fully cooperative and interactive.

Premature or full-term newborn infants who become neurologically ill in the early postnatal period as a result of a central nervous system disturbance typically exhibit one of the following clinical presentations: (A) normal at birth with neurologic compromise thereafter; (B) ill at birth with evolving (deteriorating or improving)

Table 6.7 Neurologic presentations classified according to etiology in newborn infants

A	B	C
IVH (premature)	Intrapartum hypoxia-ischemia (asphyxia)	Congenital malformations
Hypoxia-ischemia	Cerebral birth trauma	Prenatal infections
Hypoglycemia	Intrapartum hemorrhage	Prenatal hypoxia-ischemia
Kernicterus	Certain metabolic and degenerative diseases	Certain metabolic and degenerative diseases
Sepsis/meningitis		
Alcohol or narcotic addiction		
Certain metabolic and degenerative diseases		

A = Normal at birth; sick thereafter.
B = Ill at birth; improvement or deterioration thereafter.
C = Ill at birth; unchanged thereafter.

Table 6.8 Conditions that mimic perinatal asphyxia

Sepsis or meningitis (bacterial)
Viral encephalitis
Congenital malformations
Sedation or analgesia
Metabolic encephalopathy
Neuromuscular disease
Birth trauma

neurologic deficits thereafter; and (C) ill at birth with fixed neurologic deficits. The most frequent and specific causes of these three clinical presentations are shown in Table 6.7. A fourth category also exists, in which a newborn infant appears well at or following birth only to exhibit evidence of developmental delay or other neurologic disturbance (i.e. cerebral palsy) months or even years later. Diagnostic investigation then uncovers an abnormality of brain structure or function typically of prenatal origin. Possible causes in this situation include congenital malformations, intrauterine infection, prepartum hypoxia-ischemia or hemorrhage, and certain metabolic and degenerative diseases (see above).

Fetuses who have suffered an insult severe enough to produce brain damage immediately prior to birth exhibit a spectrum of abnormalities within the newborn period. Acute brain damage is manifest by an immediate acute encephalopathy which will evolve over several days to a week or more (see above). Fetuses who are asphyxiated shortly prior to or at the time of delivery will be depressed at birth with low Apgar scores and a need for major resuscitation. Thereafter, they usually exhibit evidence of 'multi-organ injury' in addition to an encephalopathy. Blood obtained from the umbilical cord vessels at delivery or from an artery shortly after birth will show evidence of a metabolic or mixed acidosis. Newborn infants who suffer physical birth trauma might exhibit a lucid interval of several hours, followed by neurologic compromise thereafter. Periventricular/intraventricular hemorrhage severe enough to cause brain damage also is characterized by the occurrence of an acute encephalopathy.

A tentative diagnosis of acute hypoxic-ischemic encephalopathy in the newborn infant dictates that other insults to the brain that mimic the condition have been considered and effectively excluded by appropriate diagnostic procedures (see below and Table 6.8). Thus, a continuum of systemic and neurologic deficits is required for a diagnosis of acute hypoxic-ischemic encephalopathy, without which causation and prognosis for the occurrence of cerebral palsy become speculative at best.

6.4   DIAGNOSTIC PROCEDURES

Recommended specific diagnostic procedures to be accomplished in newborn and older infants and children exhibiting neurologic compromise are dependent upon the differential localization of the deficits and the differential diagnosis of presumed causes. The neuro-imaging procedure of choice is ultrasound (US), computed tomography (CT), or magnetic resonance imaging (MRI). An electroencephalogram (EEG) is usually reserved for those patients with seizures, although such a study can also be useful as a screening test to ascertain cerebral involvement by a toxic, metabolic, or infectious process. The EEG, when conducted in a newborn infant, also provides prognostic information regarding long-term neurologic function. Hematologic, microbiologic, and metabolic studies are indicated in many infants, and their conduct is dependent upon the tentative differential diagnosis. Lumbar puncture is indicated in those patients suspected of suffering acute central nervous system infection (meningitis, encephalitis) or hemorrhage not obvious on US or CT. Genetic testing and chromosomal karyotyping are indicated in infants and children exhibiting somatic dysmorphism or one or more anomalies of organs including the brain.

Radiographic procedures have become invaluable in assessing the nature and extent of damage to the brain of an infant or child who has recently or remotely sustained an insult severe enough to produce tissue injury. In addition, the evolution of the brain lesions can be ascertained by sequentially scanning any individual infant; and, to some extent, the interval between the initial radiographic study and the antecedent stress can be documented. This allows the clinician to determine more accurately whether brain damage has occurred before or during parturition.

MRI has become a valuable radiographic tool, not only for elucidating the presence, distribution, and severity of acute lesions, especially those arising from perinatal cerebral hypoxia-ischemia, but also for characterizing the presence and extent of the ultimate brain damage. Chronic, end-stage lesions consist of T2-weighted hyperintensities, with or without cyst formation of periventricular or subcortical white matter, representing prior white matter necrosis (periventricular leukomalacia), gliosis, or delayed myelination, especially in premature infants. Prior cerebral cortical, basal ganglia, and thalamic or brainstem damage is seen as structural abnormalities consisting of atrophy, cystic degeneration, and persistently abnormal signals on either T1- or T2-weighted images. Ventricular dilatation or distortion might accompany the gray or white matter lesions. Certain metabolic, especially mitochondrial, disorders also exhibit characteristic MRI findings.

For the infant or child suspected of suffering a metabolic disorder, blood and urine are collected for biochemical analyses. Routine laboratory screening includes the complete blood count, glucose, blood urea nitrogen, calcium, phosphorus, magnesium, electrolytes, liver function studies, and selected enzymes. Blood and urine amino and organic acid analysis should be accomplished as well as blood lactate and pyruvate. Other biochemical studies are conducted upon clinical indication.

6.5 MEDICOLEGAL IMPLICATIONS

The neurologic assessment of a newborn or older infant or child is designed to answer many questions about the immature brain, including the following: (1) is an affliction of the brain present; (2) if an ailment exists, what is its underlying cause and when did it begin; (3) what management strategies are available to influence favorably the ultimate outcome, if available; and (4) what is the ultimate neurologic prognosis? These four questions are intimately related, the answers to which require the following: (1) a thorough knowledge of the antecedent prenatal, intrapartum, and postpartum history; (2) a detailed systemic and neurologic examination; (3) the selection and proper interpretation of appropriate diagnostic studies; and (4) sequential follow-up evaluations.

The use of the neurologic assessment for the prognostic identification of newborns at risk for later abnormal development, including cerebral palsy, must be interpreted with some degree of caution, except in situations where multiple, unequivocal clinical signs or a laboratory investigation indicate severe damage to the brain. To some extent, the developing nervous system has the capacity for reorganization following at least some types of injury (neuronal plasticity). Neuronal plasticity and biological variations among human infants probably account for our inability to prognosticate with a high degree of accuracy the ultimate neurologic outcome of any single newborn. However, with these limitations in mind, certain generalizations can be made regarding the association between abnormal neonatal neurologic signs and the later development of cerebral palsy, mental retardation, learning disability, or epilepsy. These generalizations include the following:

1 The full-term newborn infant with a negative family history, negative prenatal, intrapartum, and neonatal history, and a normal physical and neurologic examination has a negligible chance of subsequent abnormal neurologic development related to perinatal causes. The incidence of cerebral palsy, mental retardation, learning disability, or epilepsy in such an infant is no greater than that of the general population.
2 Signs of neurologic dysfunction should be apparent in a newborn whose brain has been acutely damaged by an immediate prepartum or intrapartum insult. In contrast, a newborn who suffered a remote injury to the brain earlier in fetal life might not show signs of neurologic dysfunction in the immediate newborn period.
3 Certain neurologic symptoms and signs, even though infrequent in their occurrence, have considerable predictive power for later abnormal neurologic function. These symptoms and signs include altered consciousness or hypotonia lasting more than 1 week, a weak cry for more than 2 days, or an inability to suck, requiring gavage feedings.
4 Combinations of symptoms and signs are more significant than a single abnormality.
5 The total duration of the existence of abnormal neurologic signs does not necessarily add to or detract from their significance. In general, the longer one or more abnormal neurologic signs persist, the worse the ultimate neurologic outcome.
6 Signs of neurologic dysfunction occurring in the presence of neuropathologic lesions, identifiable on neuro-imaging, are more predictive of subsequent neurologic abnormality than are signs with no demonstrable brain lesion.

6.6   SELECTED REFERENCES

1 Barkovich AJ. *Pediatric neuroimaging.* New York: Raven Press, 1990.

2 Barkovich AJ, Truwit CL. Brain damage from perinatal asphyxia: correlation of MR findings with gestational age. *American Journal of Neuroradiology* 1990; **11:** 1087–96.

3 Barmada MA, Moossy J, Shuman RM. Cerebral infarction with arterial occlusion in neonates. *Annals of Neurology* 1979; **6:** 495–502.

4 Calvert SA, Hoskins EM, Fong KW, Forsyth SC. Periventricular leukomalacia: ultrasonic diagnosis and neurological outcome. *Acta Paediatrica Scandinavica* 1986; **75:** 489–96.

5 Finer NN, Robertson CM, Richards RT, Pinnell LE, Petters KL. Hypoxic-ischemic encephalopathy in term neonates: perinatal factors and outcome. *Journal of Pediatrics* 1981; **98:** 112–17.

6 Freeman JM, Nelson KB. Intrapartum asphyxia and cerebral palsy. *Pediatrics* 1988; **82:** 240–9.

7 Graziani LJ, Pasto M, Stanley C *et al.* Neonatal neurosonographic correlates of cerebral palsy in preterm infants. *Pediatrics* 1986; **78:** 88–95.

8 Gutberlet RL, Cornblath M. Neonatal hypoglycemia revisited. *Pediatrics* 1976; **58:** 10–17.

9 Menkes JH. Metabolic diseases of the nervous system: heredodegenerative diseases. In: Menkes JH ed. *Textbook of child neurology.* Baltimore: Williams and Wilkins, 1990: 29–212.

10 Miller G. Cerebral palsies. In: Miller G, Ramer JC eds. *Static encephalopathies of infancy and childhood.* New York: Raven Press, 1992: 11–26.

11 Nelson KB, Ellenberg JH. Neonatal signs as predictors of cerebral palsy. *Pediatrics* 1979; **64:** 225–32.

12 Papile L-A. Intracranial hemorrhage. In: Fanaroff AA, Martin RJ eds. *Neonatal-perinatal medicine VI.* St Louis: Mosby, 1997: 891–9.

13 Sarnat HB. Embryology and malformations of the CNS. In: Fanaroff AA, Martin RJ eds. *Neonatal-perinatal medicine VI.* St. Louis: Mosby, 1997: 826–56.

14 Sarnat HB, Sarnat MS. Neonatal encephalopathy following fetal distress – a clinical and electroencephalographic study. *Archives of Neurology* 1976; **33:** 695–706.

15 Vannucci RC. Acute perinatal brain injury: intracranial hemorrhage. In: Cohen WR, Acker DB, Friedman EA eds. *Management of labor II.* Rockville, MD: Aspen Publishers, 1989: 245–82.

16 Vannucci RC. Hypoxia-ischemia: clinical aspects. In: Fanaroff AA, Martin RJ eds. *Neonatal-perinatal medicine VI.* St Louis: Mosby, 1997: 877–91.

17 Vannucci RC, Yager JY. Newborn neurologic assessment. In: Fanaroff AA, Martin RJ eds. *Neonatal-perinatal medicine VI.* St Louis: Mosby, 1997: 812–26.

18 Volpe JJ. *Neurology of the newborn III.* Philadelphia: WB Saunders, 1995.

7 Brain development: normal and abnormal

Waney Squier

The brain is a very complicated organ consisting of the nerve cells or neurons and a variety of supporting cells or glia. The function of the glial cells is to provide protection and nutrition for nerve cells, to insulate nerve processes and so increase the speed and efficiency of impulse transmission, and to react to injury and produce scar tissue. Other cells cover the surfaces of the brain, forming a barrier and creating a highly protected environment.

The nerve cells are arranged in groups or nuclei forming specialized interconnected structures within the brain which subserve individual functions. These structures develop in a well-defined temporal sequence. This is an extremely complex series of processes which begins at conception and continues well into the third decade of life.

Disturbance of early brain development results in malformation. Disruption of the development of a particular structure will result in its malformation only during the period of formation of the structure. Damaging events occurring after a structure has formed will lead not to malformation but to destruction. In this way insults occurring during brain development may be precisely timed according to the pattern of malformation of the individual structures.

The *causes* of injury and disturbance of brain development are multiple and are described in more detail in Chapters 3 and 8. Injurious agents may leave specific hallmarks allowing their identification in later life but this is only seen in the minority of cases.

Timing of injury can be much more precise. This is especially true in the early part of gestation when major developmental processes are under way, and, as noted above, timing of injury is reflected in specific malformations. In later development, when the main structures of the brain have formed, timing of an insult is less precise and depends upon recognition of general patterns of injury which reflect specific vulnerability of the already formed structures. These patterns are described in detail in Chapter 8.

In order to understand the timing of disruptions of brain development some knowledge of normal brain development is helpful.

For the purposes of this review brain development is subdivided into six major processes:

1 Formation of main structures of the brain
2 Cell proliferation and brain growth
3 Neuronal migration

4   Differentiation
5   Programmed cell death
6   Myelination.

Our knowledge and understanding of these processes and their genetic control have been gained from observations of specific malformations in human disease and from experimental studies on transgenic animal models. The impact of brain damage on clinical disease varies at each stage; while severe disruptions of early development are likely to be lethal in intrauterine life, disruptions of neuronal migration are now commonly recognized as a cause of neurological disease. More subtle alterations of later brain development and maturation are less likely to be recognized due to the absence of a macroscopically or radiologically visible malformation, milder and less readily defined clinical manifestations and association with a normal lifespan.

7.1   FORMATION OF MAJOR BRAIN STRUCTURES: 0–20 WEEKS

The major structures of the brain are formed in the first 20 weeks of gestation. The brain and spinal cord are determined in the first days after conception as a plate of cells running in a longitudinal streak in the very early embryo. This plate rolls up to form a tube which is the precursor of the primitive nervous system (Fig. 7.1). The tube fuses in a zip-like fashion, beginning in the cervical region at 22 days. Fusion is complete at the posterior end by 28 days. Induction of the neural streak, its rolling up and fusion (neurulation) are controlled by a number of secreted molecular signals under genetic control.[1]

From 30 days the anterior part of the neural tube differentiates into three regions: the fore, mid and hindbrain (Fig. 7.2). The forebrain develops lateral pouches which become the cerebral hemispheres. The midbrain is formed by thickening of the tissues around the central canal which persists as the narrow aqueduct of Sylvius, while in the hindbrain the central canal dilates to form the fourth ventricle and cells migrate from germinal centers in its margins to form the brainstem nuclei and the cerebellum (see Plate 1). The brainstem nuclei develop very early, by 5 weeks.

Groups of cells in the inferior parts of the cerebral vesicles form the basal ganglia and thalamus. Bundles of fibers, the projections of neurons in the developing cerebral cortex and deep nuclei, form the dense white matter tracts connecting the various parts of the nervous system. Motor projection fibers from the cerebral cortex grow down between the developing basal ganglia and thalamus to form the internal capsule and then extend into the brainstem as the corticospinal tract, carrying motor projections to the spinal cord and ultimately supplying the muscles. Other large bundles of fibers cross the midline connecting the two cerebral hemispheres. Of these, the largest and most important is the corpus callosum which forms a thick band of fibers crossing dorsal to the lateral ventricles. This structure begins to form in the lamina terminalis, the most anterior part of the neural tube, at 11 weeks. It grows from front to back and growth is complete by 17 weeks of gestation.

7.1.1   Disorders of brain formation: 0–20 weeks

7.1.1.1   Neural tube defects

Failure of fusion of the neural tube results in a range of malformations which may also involve

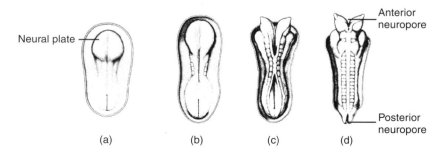

Figure 7.1 Dorsal views of the embryo showing the earliest stages of the nervous system. (a,b) The neural plate with a central groove. At 18 days (b) the plate is beginning to roll up. (c) Fusion beginning in the cervical region. By 23 days most of the tube has fused but anterior and posterior ends remain open (d).

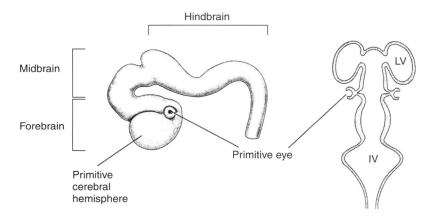

Figure 7.2 Lateral view of the human embryonic brain at 6 weeks and dorsal view representing development of the ventricular system (LV, lateral ventricle, IV, fourth ventricle).

the adjacent coverings of the nervous system, bones, and skin. These all arise on or before 28 days of development. The most severe outcome of failure of fusion is anencephaly, where most of the forebrain and cranium is absent. This malformation is incompatible with life for more than a few days after birth. Less serious defects include encephaloceles, where brain tissue protrudes through a defect in the overlying skull, or myeloceles, which are due to similar defects in the spinal cord and its coverings. The most familiar clinical presentation of these spinal defects is spina bifida. Both genetic and environmental factors appear to have a role in causing neural tube defects. This has been manifest by the marked geographical and racial variations in the incidence of spina bifida and the profound effects of folate administration in reducing its incidence.[2]

7.2.1.2   *Holoprosencephaly*

Failure of normal growth and separation of the anterior brain into the paired cerebral hemispheres result in holoprosencephaly. In this condition there is a single cerebral 'holosphere' with a single ventricle. Midline structures do not develop. The anomaly is not rare, occurring in up to 1.2 per 10 000 live births.[3] Twelve sites on 11 chromosomes have been implicated in this malformation. Holoprosencephaly is associated with midline facial defects involving the nose and eyes. The nose may be small or absent and the eyes too closely placed; in the most severe forms only a single central eye is present (cyclopia). Only infants with the mildest forms of holoprosencephaly survive for more than a few days after birth.

7.2.1.3   *Agenesis of the corpus callosum*

Agenesis of the corpus callosum is not uncommon and may occur alone or as part of a large number of brain malformation syndromes.[4] Isolated agenesis of the corpus callosum is occasionally found incidentally at post mortem without any apparent clinical manifestations. Partial agenesis of the corpus callosum almost always involves the later-forming posterior part. Complete failure of development of the corpus callosum has a secondary effect on the gyral pattern of the adjacent medial surface of the cerebral hemispheres. The cingulate gyrus, which normally curves in an anteroposterior direction immediately above the corpus callosum, fails to form and instead the medial surfaces of the hemispheres have radially disposed gyri (Plate 2).

Defects in the anterior or middle part of the corpus callosum imply an origin after completion of its development. An example of such a defect, due to amniocentesis injury at 16 weeks, is illustrated in Chapter 8 (Plate 18).

Septo-optic dysplasia is another developmental anomaly of midline structures associated with hypoplasia of the corpus callosum. In this syndrome the anterior septum is absent, there is optic nerve hypoplasia and hypothalamic and pituitary dysfunction. The cause of this malformation is unknown but early intrauterine destructive lesions have been described.[5]

7.2   CELL PROLIFERATION AND BRAIN GROWTH: CONCEPTION TO 12 YEARS

The early neural tube consists of a thin layer of cells surrounding the central canal. The cell layers rapidly increase in number and differentiate into ventricular, intermediate, and marginal zones. The ventricular zone, which lies immediately beneath the ependymal lining of the central canal, becomes the germinal matrix zone where active cell proliferation occurs producing neurons and later the supporting glial cells (Plate 3). Cell proliferation is most active between 8 and 16 weeks of gestation. As the brain grows the germinal matrix recedes, and instead of lining the entire ventricular system, remains as several well-defined masses in the anterior and posterior horns of the lateral ventricles. This tissue is composed of densely packed, immature, dividing, nerve cell precursors and is amply supplied with blood through a network of thin-walled capillaries. These small blood vessels have little structural support and are a potential source of bleeding in adverse conditions. After 36 weeks of gestation the germinal matrix is resorbed and the risk of periventricular hemorrhage is dramatically reduced.

Brain growth is very rapid between 20 and 40 weeks when a six-fold increase in weight occurs. The cerebral surface is smooth at 20 weeks but as it increases in size it undergoes folding in order to accommodate the enormous expansion in cortical volume and so the familiar gyral pattern is formed (Fig. 7.3, Plate 4). Further brain growth continues after birth and by 2 years the brain weight is over three times that at birth, due largely to an increase in myelin. Growth continues at a slower rate until about 12 years when adult weight is attained.

7.2.1 Disorders of brain growth

Rare syndromes are recognized when the brain is normally structured but either too large or too small due to over- or underproduction of cells. Failure of adequate cell production is also part of a number of rare and serious malformation syndromes.

Microcephaly means a small head and *microcephaly vera* is a genetic form with depletion of neurons. However, a small head is more commonly due to reduced brain volume secondary to an early destructive event, which may be identified by brain scans or pathological examination. The distinction of the different etiologies of microcephaly is important for counseling for future pregnancies.

7.3 NEURONAL MIGRATION: 6–20 WEEKS

Neurons are generated in the germinal zone close to the ventricular lining and they all have to migrate in

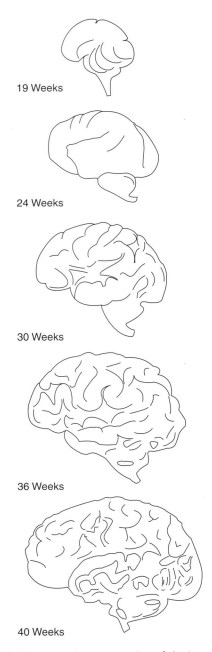

19 Weeks

24 Weeks

30 Weeks

36 Weeks

40 Weeks

Figure 7.3 Diagrammatic representation of the increase in size and complexity of the brain between 19 and 40 weeks of gestation (courtesy of Maria Dambska and Kristyna Wisniewski).

order to reach their final position in the mature brain. Neuronal migration has been the subject of considerable interest in the last two decades, particularly since the widespread use of high-resolution magnetic resonance imaging (MRI) scans has allowed recognition of neuronal migration disorders, which are an underlying cause of many human neurological symptoms, notably epilepsy.

Several major migrational pathways are known, contributing to formation of the cerebral cortex, the deep cerebral nuclei, the brainstem nuclei, and the cerebellum (Plate 1). The pathways involved in neuronal migration to the cerebral cortex have been particularly well described and recently reviewed.[6,7]

Neurons destined to form part of the cerebral cortex leave the germinal matrix after their final mitotic division and migrate to the developing cortical plate with the assistance of radial glial fibers. These are the processes of primitive astrocytes which align themselves radially with their processes extending between the ventricular zone and the brain surface. The migrating neurons attach themselves to these glial fibers and migrate along them to the presumptive cortical plate (Plate 5). Some neurons also migrate horizontally in the cortical plate.[8] Migration depends on the relationship between primitive neurons and radial glial cells and also on interaction with the extracellular matrix. Studies of human migration disorders and their counterparts in animal models have demonstrated the importance of the intraneuronal cytoskeletal systems, including actin and microtubules, which are closely involved in developing cell processes, axon outgrowth, and cell motility.[3]

Neuronal migration to the developing cerebral cortex occurs in successive waves between 6 and 21 weeks of gestation. There is no good evidence for continuing migration to the cortex after this time in the human brain.[9]

The first arriving cells form a primitive cortical band known as the preplate. This is split into a superficial marginal zone and a subplate zone by subsequently migrating cells. The marginal zone contains a population of cells known as Cajal–Retzius cells which have an important role in guiding subsequently arriving neurons to their correct location in the cortex and thus ordering proper cortical lamination.[10] Cajal–Retzius cells express a protein called reelin under the control of growth factors.[11] Further control of migration is exercised by extracellular matrix proteins and the integrity of the pial membrane on the surface of the brain.

All newly arriving cells migrate first to the marginal zone and contact Cajal–Retzius cells before moving to their final position in the cortex. The earliest arriving cells form the deepest layers and the later arriving the more superficial layers and so the cortex is formed in an 'inside-out' fashion.

The deep layer of the preplate, the subplate, appears to function as a relay station guiding axons growing into the cortex to their correct targets.[12] Cells of the marginal and subplate zones are not readily identified after the first weeks of postnatal life. They may be lost by programmed cell death, by dilution in the rapidly growing brain, or by conversion into other neuronal types.

7.3.1 Failed or inadequate migration

Failed or inadequate migration may be focal or diffuse. When widespread it is usually genetically determined while focal anomalies of migration tend to be due to damage such as trauma, infection, or ischemia.

Failure of migration is associated with a spectrum of pathological changes from heterotopia, where neurons have been arrested in the course of migration, to more complex and widespread disorders of cortical structure.

7.3.1.1 Type 1 lissencephaly

In type 1 (classical) lissencephaly, the brain is smooth and the cortex contains reduced numbers of neurons (Plate 6). There is an ill-defined inferior cortical border and neurons are seen straggling throughout the underlying white matter. It is associated with mutations at chromosome 17p13.[13]

Children with this disorder are profoundly neurologically impaired with severe seizures. The pathogenesis of type 1 lissencephaly probably involves failed proliferation as well as failed migration of cells.

7.3.1.2 X-Linked lissencephaly

Another well-described and genetically determined form of failure of neuronal migration is X-linked lissencephaly. This is associated with a locus at Xq22.[14] Females with this mutation have a 'double cortex' (Fig. 7.4, Plate 7). Beneath an apparently normally formed and folded cortex there is a second, less regular, band of neurons separated from the normal cortex by a thin, irregular strip of white matter. The mechanism of this malformation is thought to be related to 'X inactivation'. Every female cell carries two X chromosomes, only one of which is functional, the other is normally inactivated. In this condition it is thought that those cells with the active normal X chromosome are able to migrate and form a cortex while the cells bearing an active mutant X chromosome migrate incompletely and form the straggling 'double layer' of the cortex. Those few males

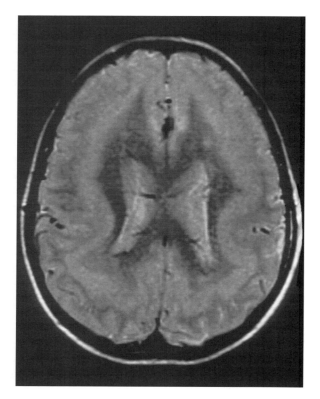

Figure 7.4 Horizontal MRI scan of 'double-cortex' syndrome showing a thick band of gray matter lying beneath an apparently normal cortex.

who survive with this mutation have a completely smooth brain[15] and die in early life. Females may survive into adult life but are often of low intelligence and suffer from epilepsy.

7.3.1.3 Neuronal heterotopia

Focal failure of neuronal migration leaves clusters of neurons stranded as heterotopia *en route* for the cortex (see Plate 8). They may be close to the ventricular wall, when migration fails completely, within the white matter or immediately beneath the cortex. The non-migrated neurons may show evidence of immaturity[16] and the cortex overlying heterotopia is usually malformed. This form of focal periventricular or white matter heterotopia is not uncommon clinically. It is usually sporadic but has been described in early fetal traumatic injury[17] (see Case 8.2, Plate 18).

Heterotopia may also be genetically determined. In X-linked periventricular heterotopia, which is linked to a locus at Xq28,[18] multiple masses of unmigrated neurons form nodules in the lining of the ventricles. Females survive, are often of normal intelligence but have seizures. Males have a higher rate of associated malformations and tend to die young.

Interruption of the hindbrain migration pathways results in abnormal clusters of incompletely migrated neurons in the meninges of the brainstem. This usually follows insult before 20 weeks of gestation.

7.3.2 Excessive migration

Lesions in the pial limiting membrane of the brain surface are associated with heterotopic neuronal clusters in the leptomeninges on the brain surface. These appear to result from overmigration of neurons onto the brain surface through defects in the glial/pial limiting membrane. Focal surface heterotopias are seen following focal traumatic lesions[19] and in experimental models with defects in the glial limiting membrane and altered extracellular proteins[20] (Plate 9) and in other disorders such as the fetal alcohol syndrome.[21]

7.3.2.1 Type 2 lissencephaly

Severe and generalized overmigration causes almost the entire brain surface to be effaced by massive migration of neuroblasts through the pial membrane onto the brain surface, inhibiting normal cortical folding[22] (Plate 10). Several different syndromes share this malformation; in the most severe of them there is also malformation of the eye together with a form of congenital muscular dystrophy. These syndromes include Fukuyama muscular dystrophy, an autosomal recessive condition most commonly seen in Japan, muscle–eye–brain disease which is most frequent in Finland, and the Walker-Warburg syndrome which is seen throughout the world.

In Fukuyama muscular dystrophy a mutation has been identified in a gene on chromosome 9 which codes for a secreted protein, fukutin, which is normally present in the extracellular matrix. The association of this brain malformation with congenital muscular dystrophy is consistent with a deficiency of a component of the extracellular matrix common to both muscle and brain.

The gene for muscle–eye–brain disease has not yet been identified but it is thought to reside on chromosome 1, while no linkage has been described for Walker-Warburg syndrome.[3]

Patients with lissencephaly are developmentally delayed and may have dysmorphic features and arthrogryposis (congenital fixation of joints).

7.4 CORTICAL DIFFERENTIATION

Once neurons have reached the cortical plate further stages of development and differentiation take place before the mature, laminated cortical structure is achieved.

Simple lamination of the cortex is first identified by 16 weeks of gestation. By term all of the neurons will have acquired their characteristic phenotypic appearance and the characteristic six layers of the adult cortex are identified.[23] Neuronal differentiation is partly determined at a very early stage, in the germinal matrix, before migration has even begun, but there are other later further influences, including establishment of functional connections with other neurons.

Between 20 and 40 weeks of gestation the brain weight increases six-fold and there is an enormous increase in the size of the cerebral cortex. In order to accommodate the huge cortex within the cranial cavity the cortex becomes folded. At 20 weeks only a few primitive indentations are seen but by term the adult pattern of gyri and sulci is virtually complete (see Plate 4).

7.4.1 Cortical dysplasia

This is a cortical malformation with a wide spectrum of pathologies of varying severity. Cortical dysplasias may be small focal malformations or they may be widespread. Their histological features range from very minor alterations in cortical lamination to areas of completely disordered cortical formation including the presence of bizarrely formed giant neurons and glial cells, and the persistence of embryonic cells and structures (Plate 11).

Their time of origin in development is uncertain but a classification has been proposed which bases timing on the presence or absence of specific histological features.[24] The presence of underlying neuronal heterotopias indicates an origin before 20 weeks of gestation, but some forms of cortical dysplasia may be acquired later. While the development of bizarre giant cells has been ascribed to an early genetic aberration with nuclear heteroploidy,[25,26] Marin-Padilla has shown that increase in neuronal size and complexity of the dendritic tree can occur following injury in postnatal life.[27] The clinical significance of cortical dysplasias is that they are related to intractable epilepsy and are frequently recognized in MRI scans.

The mildest form of cortical dysplasia is *microdysgenesis*, which is recognized only by microscopy and consists of minor disorganization in the arrangement of neurons in the cortex, the presence of single or small groups of neurons scattered in the white matter and increased cellularity of the most superficial cortical layer, the molecular layer. This may be due to altered migration or to failure of involution of the Cajal–Retzius cells. In some cases abnormal myelinated fibers are also seen in the molecular layer[28] (Plate 12). Micro-dygenesis appears to be more common in patients with epilepsy.[29,30]

7.4.2 Polymicrogyria

The macroscopic appearance of polymicrogyria is of areas of the brain surface with many small, irregular and crowded gyri (Plate 8). The histological features are variable; essentially, there is abnormal fusion of the superficial layers of adjacent gyri with large blood vessels denoting the seam lines. Beneath this the cortical architecture is disturbed, there may be fewer laminae than normal with the cortex forming an undulating band beneath the fused superficial layers. In some cases the neurons are even more disorganized and form irregular nodules. The overlying meninges may be thickened or contain ectopic groups of neurons and glial cells.

The pathogenesis of polymicrogyria remains uncertain. It is frequently classified as a neuronal migration disorder but probably represents disruption of later cortical maturation and folding in the postmigrational period. It is not unusual to identify focal clusters of neuronal heterotopia in the zone beneath a focus of polymicrogyria, suggesting that a degree of migration failure may be associated with this malformation. Neuronal death or damage to the pial surface may cause the abnormal fusion of the superficial cortical layers. Polymicrogyria has been shown to arise before but not after 28 weeks of gestation.[31,32]

Several causes have been proposed. Sporadic polymicrogyria is generalized or patchy and often occurs on the edge of a destructive lesion (see Case 8.4, Plate 20) or in watershed areas, suggesting that ischemia plays a part in some cases. Polymicrogyria also occurs in infants with congenital cytomegalovirus infection, when the virus may be directly toxic to neurons or destroy endothelial cells and impair capillary blood flow producing cortical ischemia. Some forms of polymicrogyria are clearly inherited; in these cases the malformation is bilateral and symmetric.[33,34]

Patients with polymicrogyria present with epilepsy; some also have neurological symptoms and developmental delay.

7.5 PROGRAMMED CELL DEATH

Up to 50 percent of the cells produced in the fetal brain will die by programmed cell death before the brain reaches maturity. This mechanism allows for removal of cells which do not establish viable contacts with others and is responsible for involution of those transient structures which only function during fetal life, for example the subplate and Cajal–Retzius cells. Programmed cell death is a form of suicide in which a cascade of intracellular enzymes is activated, some dependent on gene transcription, which ultimately leads to breakdown of the nuclear DNA (see Chapter 8). The morphological appearance of cells undergoing programmed cell death is that of apoptosis, the nucleus becomes shrunken and deeply basophilic, ultimately breaking up into rounded masses.[35] This appearance has long been recognized as one of the characteristic forms of cell death in the immature brain.[36]

7.5.1 Disorders of programmed cell death

The role of disorders of programmed cell death in malformation is uncertain but they have been implicated in a number of disorders of brain growth, including microcephaly and macrocephaly. The excess cells in the white matter and cortical molecular layer in microdysgenesis may result from failure of programmed cell death and this mechanism was proposed for minor structural anomalies described in schizophrenia.[37]

7.6 MYELINATION

Defective myelination can have a profound effect on neurological development. A number of well-recognized inherited diseases (the leukodystrophies) result in failure of normal myelin production.

In a proportion of cases of cerebral palsy neuropathological examination reveals only reduced myelin volume in the absence of marked scarring or gliosis or cortical and basal ganglia damage.[38] This may result from injury to oligodendrocytes (the cells responsible for myelination) or their pre-cursors due to chronic intrauterine oxygen or nutritional deprivation at a sensitive time in their development.

Ischemia in the last trimester of gestation and the neonatal period damages myelin, causing a spectrum of damage from severe cystic leukomalacia to milder widespread reduction in volume of myelin with diffuse gliosis (see Chapter 8).

In assessing the child with reduced myelin volume it is important to distinguish between delayed and defective myelination and repeated MRI studies may be needed to establish the diagnosis.

7.7 REFERENCES

1 Scotting PJ, Rex M. Transcription factors in early development of the central nervous system. *Neuropathology and Applied Neurobiology* 1996; **22**: 469–81.

2 Copp AJ. Prevention of neural tube defects: vitamins, enzymes and genes. *Current Opinion in Neurology* 1998; **11**: 97–102.

3 Walsh CA. Genetic malformations of the human cerebral cortex. *Neuron* 1999; **23**: 19–29.

4 Norman MG, McGillivray MG, Lakousek DK, Hill A, Poskitt KJ. Crossing the midline. In: *Anonymous congenital malformations of the brain*. Oxford: Oxford University Press, 2000: 309–31.

5 Roessmann U, Velasco ME, Small EJ, Hori A. Neuropathology of 'septo-optic dysplasia' (de Morsier syndrome) with immunohistochemical studies of the hypothalamus and pituitary gland. *Journal of Neuropathology and Experimental Neurology* 1987; **46**: 597–608.

6 Uher BF, Golden JA. Neuronal migration defects of the cerebral cortex: a destination debacle. *Clinical Genetics* 2000; **58**: 16–24.

7 Parnavelas JG. The origin and migration of cortical neurones: new vistas. *Trends in Neuroscience* 2000; **23**: 126–31.

8 Rakic P. Specification of cerebral cortical areas. *Science* 1988; **241**: 170–6

9 Evrard P, Marret S, Gressens P. Environmental and genetic determinants of neural migration and post-migratory survival. *Acta Paediatrica Supplement* 1997; **422**: 20–6.

10 Flint AC, Kriegstein AR. Mechanisms underlying neuronal migration disorders and epilepsy. *Current Opinion in Neurology* 1997; **10**: 92–7.

11 Ringstedt T, Linnarsson S, Wagner J *et al*. BDNF regulates reelin expression and Cajal-Retzius cell development in the cerebral cortex. *Neuron* 1998; **21**: 305–15.

12 Molnar Z, Blakemore C. How do thalamic axons find their way to the cortex? *Trends in Neuroscience* 1995; **18**: 389–97.

13 Lo NC, Chong CS, Smith AC, Dobyns WB, Carrozzo R, Ledbetter DH. Point mutations and an intragenic deletion in LIS1, the lissencephaly causative gene in isolated lissencephaly sequence and Miller-Dieker syndrome. *Human Molecular Genetics* 1997; **6**: 157–64.

14 Gleeson JG, Allen KM, Fox JW *et al.* Doublecortin, a brain-specific gene mutated in human X-linked lissencephaly and double cortex syndrome, encodes a putative signaling protein. *Cell* 1998; **92**: 63–72.

15 Pinard JM, Motte J, Chiron C, Brian R, Andermann E, Dulac O. Subcortical laminar heterotopia and lissencephaly in two families: a single X linked dominant gene. *Journal of Neurology, Neurosurgery and Psychiatry* 1994; **57**: 914–20.

16 Hannan AJ, Servotte S, Katsnelson A *et al.* Characterization of nodular neuronal heterotopia in children. *Brain* 1999; **122**: 219–38.

17 Squier M, Chamberlain P, Zaiwalla Z *et al.* Five cases of brain injury following amniocentesis in mid-term pregnancy. *Developmental Medicine and Child Neurology* 2000; **42**: 554–60.

18 Eksioglu YZ, Scheffer IE, Cardenas P *et al.* Periventricular heterotopia: an X-linked dominant epilepsy locus causing aberrant cerebral cortical development. *Neuron* 1996; **16**: 77–87.

19 Choi BH, Matthias SC. Cortical dysplasia associated with massive ectopia of neurons and glial cells within the subarachnoid space. *Acta Neuropathologica Berlin* 1987; **73**: 105–9.

20 Blackshear PJ, Silver J, Nairn AC *et al.* Widespread neuronal ectopia associated with secondary defects in cerebrocortical chondroitin sulfate proteoglycans and basal lamina in MARCKS-deficient mice. *Experimental Neurology* 1997; **145**: 46–61.

21 Clarren SK, Alvord-EC J, Sumi SM, Streissguth AP, Smith DW. Brain malformations related to prenatal exposure to ethanol. *Journal of Pediatrics* 1978; **92**: 64–7.

22 Squier MV. Development of the cortical dysplasia of type II lissencephaly. *Neuropathology and Applied Neurobiology* 1993; **19**: 209–13.

23 Marin-Padilla M. Review of perinatal brain damage, repair and neurological sequelae in the premature born infant. *International Pediatrics* 1995; **10** Suppl 1: 26–33.

24 Mischel PS, Nguyen LP, Vinters HV. Cerebral cortical dysplasia associated with pediatric epilepsy. Review of neuropathologic features and proposal for a grading system. *Journal of Neuropathology and Experimental Neurology* 1995; **54**: 137–53.

25 Farrell MA, DeRosa MJ, Curran JG *et al.* Neuropathologic findings in cortical resections (including hemispherectomies) performed for the treatment of intractable childhood epilepsy. *Acta Neuropathologica Berlin* 1992; **83**: 246–59.

26 Manz HJ, Phillips TM, Rowden G, McCullough DC. Unilateral megalencephaly, cerebral cortical dysplasia, neuronal hypertrophy, and heterotopia: cytomorphometric, fluorometric cytochemical, and biochemical analyses. *Acta Neuropathologica Berlin* 1979; **45**: 97–103.

27 Marin-Padilla M. Developmental neuropathology and impact of perinatal brain damage. II: white matter lesions of the neocortex. *Journal of Neuropathology and Experimental Neurology* 1997; **56**: 219–35.

28 Thom M, Holton JL, D'Arrigo C *et al.* Microdysgenesis with abnormal cortical myelinated fibres in temporal lobe epilepsy: a histopathological study with calbindin D-28-K immunohistochemistry. *Neuropathology and Applied Neurobiology* 2000; **26**: 251–7.

29 Hardiman O, Burke T, Phillips J *et al.* Microdysgenesis in resected temporal neocortex: incidence and clinical significance in focal epilepsy. *Neurology* 1988; **38**: 1041–7.

30 Meencke HJ. The density of dystopic neurons in the white matter of the gyrus frontalis inferior in epilepsies. *Journal of Neurology* 1983; **230**: 171–81.

31 Barth PG. Disorders of neuronal migration. *Canadian Journal of Neurological Sciences* 1987; **14**: 1–16.

32 Ferrer I, Xumetra A, Santamaria J. Cerebral malformation induced by prenatal X-irradiation: an autoradiographic and Golgi study. *Journal of Anatomy* 1984; **138**: 81–93.

33 Dobyns WB, Truwit CL. Lissencephaly and other malformations of cortical development: 1995 update. *Neuropediatrics* 1995; **26**: 132–47.

34 Guerrini R, Dubeau F, Dulac O *et al.* Bilateral parasagittal parietooccipital polymicrogyria and epilepsy. *Annals of Neurology* 1997; **41** :65–73.

35 Kerr JF, Wyllie AH, Currie AR. Apoptosis: a basic biological phenomenon with wide-ranging implications in tissue kinetics. *British Journal of Cancer* 1972; **26**: 239–57.

36 Larroche JC. Symposium: recent advances in fetal and neonatal neuropathology. Concluding remarks. *Neuropathology and Applied Neurobiology* 1996; **22**: 502–3.

37 Akbarian S, Vinuela A, Kim JJ, Potkin SG, Bunney-WE Jr, Jones EG. Distorted distribution of nicotinamide-adenine dinucleotide phosphate-diaphorase neurons in temporal lobe of schizophrenics implies anomalous cortical development. *Archives of General Psychiatry* 1993; **50**: 178–87.

38 Chattha AS, Richardson EPJ. Cerebral white-matter hypoplasia. *Archives of Neurology* 1977; **34**: 137–41.

8 Pathology of fetal and neonatal brain damage: identifying the timing

Waney Squier

The developing brain may be damaged by a considerable number of insults. The resulting pattern of brain damage depends on the nature of the insult, its severity, and particularly on the period in development when the insult occurs. This is, of course, independent of birth and a significant proportion of injuries occur during intrauterine life.[1]

The purpose of this chapter is to review the histopathology of these patterns of damage. Their identification on magnetic resonance imaging (MRI) scans is potentially a powerful source of information regarding causation and timing of injuries in the brain-damaged child.

8.1 SPECIFIC INSULTS CAPABLE OF DAMAGING THE FETAL BRAIN

A number of insults are known to disrupt normal brain development although the mechanisms of their action are not fully understood. They are listed in Tables 8.1–8.4 and include drugs and toxins, metabolic disorders, infections (both fetal and maternal), irradiation and most important of all reduced blood flow and oxygen supply.

8.1.1 Hypoxia-ischemia: asphyxia (Table 8.1)

Hypoxia (lack of oxygen), ischemia (lack of blood supply), and asphyxia (a combination of reduced oxygen and blood flow with a build-up of toxic metabolic by-products causing acidosis) are perhaps the most important causes of damage to the developing human brain. In human fetuses the exact nature of the insult and the contribution of each of these elements cannot be determined and the general term hypoxic-ischemic injury (HII) will be used.

Some 6 per 1000 newborn infants suffer from asphyxia around the time of birth, half of these have

Table 8.1 Hypoxia-ischemia: asphyxia. Factors that modify pattern of brain damage

Insult	Fetal
Severity	Developmental age
Duration	Temperature
Pattern (single, repeated)	Growth retardation
	Metabolic state

severe and permanent neurological handicaps and 1 infant per 1000 dies of the resulting brain damage. Many more infants suffer permanent neurological damage as a result of hypoxia or ischemia *in utero*. The precise number affected by HII *in utero* is difficult to determine. These insults are often clinically undetected and the resulting brain damage indistinguishable from that resulting from other less common insults such as metabolic disease or materno-fetal infections. For this reason care must be taken to exclude specific diseases, particularly those that may have implications for future pregnancies, before a diagnosis of hypoxic-ischemic injury is made. Chapter 4 describes in detail the effects of asphyxia on the developing brain.

8.1.2   Toxins (Table 8.2)

Exposure to cigarette smoke (in which there are multiple toxins including nicotine), alcohol, and recreational drugs may all damage the fetal brain.[2] All result in microcephaly and disorders of cognition in later life. Fetal alcohol exposure also leads to disruption of brain development.[3]

Several malformation syndromes have been described in children of women with epilepsy treated with anticonvulsants.[4] Epidemiological studies have shown an association between cerebral palsy and maternal iodine deficiency in pregnancy.[5] The effects may be mediated by astrocyte damage: these cells are the targets of thyroid hormone during development.[6]

Table 8.2 Toxins that are known to damage the developing brain

Cigarette smoke
Alcohol
Cocaine
Anticonvulsants
Anticoagulants
Iodine deficiency
Lead
Mercury
Irradiation

Lead toxicity impairs cognitive function by disruption of normal neurotransmission.[7] Mercury poisoning *in utero* causes altered neurological development.[8] It is widespread in fish-eating populations around the world.

The adverse effects of irradiation on the developing brain were seen in survivors of Hiroshima. In animal models irradiation impairs neuronal migration and stimulates apoptotic cell death.[9]

8.1.3   Metabolic diseases (Table 8.3)

There is an increasing list of metabolic diseases which can influence brain development. Some have their effects in early intrauterine life, interfering with brain formation and resulting in malformations, e.g. pyruvate dehydrogenase deficiency, Zellweger's syndrome[10] and non-ketotic hyperglycinemia.[11] Others appear to act later and result in defective myelination or cerebral atrophy, for example glutaric aciduria type 1.[12]

In hyperbilirubinemia bilirubin is deposited in the neurons of the cerebral gray matter causing yellow discoloration of the nuclei or *kernicterus*. The deposited pigment is toxic to neurons. This syndrome is now seen infrequently due to prompt treatment of neonatal jaundice and prevention of Rhesus incompatibility disease. Bilirubin discoloration of the brain is more frequently seen in severe cerebral edema with breakdown of the blood–brain barrier allowing bilirubin to be deposited widely throughout the brain in the presence of only low serum levels of the pigment.

Blood-clotting disorders such as alloimmune thrombocytopenia and factor V Leiden mutation are increasingly recognized as potential causes of

Table 8.3 Metabolic causes of damage to the developing brain

Zellweger's syndrome
Neonatal adrenoleukodystrophy
Glutaric aciduria type II
Non-ketotic hyperglycinemia
Menkes disease
GM2 gangliosidosis
Ornithine carbamyl transferase deficiency
Hyperbilirubinemia
Lesch-Nyhan syndrome
Dopa-responsive dystonia
Hypoglycemia
Mitochondrial diseases: including pyruvate dehydrogenase deficiency
Blood-clotting disorders

fetal and neonatal brain damage[13,14] due to intrauterine cerebral hemorrhage.

8.1.3.1 Hypoglycemia

Little is known of the effects of increased or reduced blood sugar on the fetal brain or the effects of severe uncontrolled maternal diabetes in pregnancy. However, a pattern of brain damage has been observed in newborn infants who have suffered severe hypoglycemia in the neonatal period. Cases with pure hypoglycemia and without associated asphyxia or seizures are very uncommon and neuropathological descriptions of resulting brain injury are few. In these few, neuropathological studies the distribution of damage differed from that seen in HII with most severe involvement of the occipital cortex and no evidence of watershed distribution or ulegyria.[15,16] Further, the selective neuronal damage tended to involve the more superficial cortical layers, a pattern also seen in a rat model.[17]

Recently, imaging studies have added further evidence for this specific pattern of brain involvement in neonatal hypoglycemia.[18–20] In all of these studies, the predominant involvement of the parieto-occipital cerebral cortex and underlying white matter has been stressed.

The metabolic factors underlying this specific distribution of damage are unknown but magnetic resonance spectroscopy of neonatal brains has shown relatively high lactate levels in the parieto-occipital regions in the immature brain which may reflect persistent glycolytic metabolism and thus vulnerability to hypoglycemia in this region of the immature brain.

While severe hypoglycemia may alone produce brain damage, lesser degrees may act together with other insults such as HII or seizures and contribute to final damage. It has been shown that hypoglycemia accentuates hypoxic brain damage in the immature brain – the reverse of the situation in the adult.[21]

8.1.3.2 Mitochondrial diseases

Mitochondrial diseases are now recognized to cause malformation and tissue destruction in fetal and neonatal life. Mitochondrial defects occur in a variety of diseases which have in common failure of energy metabolism. The most common pathology is necrotizing encephalomyelopathy with patchy tissue loss, capillary proliferation and widespread astrocytic gliosis. In pyruvate dehydrogenase deficiency there is extensive loss of white matter as well as cortical malformation and neuronal heterotopias.[22] Cystic cerebral damage and calcification have also been described in mitochondrial disease in intrauterine life.[23]

8.1.4 Infections (Table 8.4)

8.1.4.1 Fetal infections

The most important specific infections of the fetal brain are listed in Table 8.4. Viruses most commonly cause fetal brain damage by crossing the placenta, while bacterial infections in intrauterine life are extremely rare.

Each of the organisms mentioned has specific pathological features, but they all cause damage and death of neurons with resultant tissue loss and glial scarring. The hallmark of viral infections in the fetal brain is widespread and intense mineralization which is readily identified on computed tomography (CT) scans. In the case of cytomegalovirus (CMV), the mineral is often seen as a thick periventricular band (Plate 13). The pattern of mineralization is distinct from that seen after HII.

Fetal viral infections rarely involve the brain in isolation and additional damage may be found in other organs, including the eyes, liver, and skin.

8.1.4.2 Materno-fetal infections

During the last few years an association has been recognized between ascending maternal infections (involving the placenta and amniotic membranes) and fetal brain damage, in particular white matter lesions and cortical malformation.[24] This association was made initially by epidemiological studies[25] and has been supported by subsequent work demonstrating the presence of markers of inflammatory diseases in the brains and amniotic fluid of infants with white matter lesions.[26] The inflammatory markers include cytokines, interleukins 1 and 6 and tumor necrosis factor.[27] The cytokines are a

Table 8.4 Infections that may damage the fetal brain

Direct fetal infections, including:
Toxoplasma
Rubella
Cytomegalovirus
Herpes
Varicella
HIV
Materno-fetal intrauterine infection and inflammation

group of polypeptides which have multiple functions, including both enhancing and suppressing inflammation, and which also act as growth factors. They may be developmentally regulated and their levels elevated by a number of insults including infection and HII. They may cross the placenta but are also produced within areas of brain damage.[28]

8.2 GENERAL RESPONSES OF THE BRAIN TO INJURY

Following an insult to the brain a series of cellular reactions is set in progress. These have the effect of limiting damage by increasing vascular supply, removing dead tissue, and repairing damage by forming glial scar tissue in and around the damaged area. Nerve cells that have died are not regenerated, although it is now apparent that some compensatory growth and increase in size of neurons may take place in adjacent tissues.[29,30]

The clinical significance of these changes is that they take place in a defined temporal sequence and their identification on scans or in pathological specimens allows timing of an insult.

8.2.1 Edema

Edema (brain swelling) occurs very soon, within 1 hour of injury and usually subsides by 7 days. It results from damage to the walls of small blood vessels allowing fluid to escape into the interstitial spaces between cells and from swelling of the astrocytic glial cells.

Edema may be localized to a damaged area or be generalized throughout the brain. The white matter, particularly where fiber bundles are tightly packed, often shows the most severe edema. This is exemplified by abnormal signal intensity in the posterior limb of the internal capsule on MRI scans. This sign has been identified in infants with hypoxic-ischemic encephalopathy and is an accurate predictor of poor neurodevelopmental outcome.[31]

The brain may also show generalized swelling which is seen on ultrasound, CT, and MRI scans. The ventricles may be compressed and cortical sulci narrowed by swelling; and the distinction between gray and white matter is lost. Clinically, edema is identified by fullness of the fontanel, separation of cranial sutures, and increased head circumference. Compression and damage to the cerebral tissues and coning (that is, herniation of

hindbrain structures out of the foramen magnum at the base of the skull) are rare in neonates as there is considerable space around the infant brain for swelling and the cranial sutures may widen to further accommodate the swollen brain.

8.2.2 Cell death

Several processes of cell death are described, the best characterized are necrosis and apoptosis. Their precise definition and identification remain the subject of debate but necrosis is generally regarded as passive cell death (or murder) while apoptosis is an energy-dependent process (suicide) requiring activation of a series of enzymes resulting in degradation of nuclear DNA.[32] Apoptosis resembles the form of death seen as part of normal brain development (programmed cell death) and occurs more frequently after insults in the immature than the adult brain.

In cells undergoing *necrosis*, hematoxylin and eosin-stained sections show cytoplasmic swelling with bright pink cytoplasm (eosinophilia) at about 5–6 hours after injury (Plate 14). The nuclear membrane breaks down and the nuclear chromatin disintegrates into an irregular web (nucleolysis). Necrosis often provokes an inflammatory response.

When a cell undergoes *apoptosis* it shrinks and the nucleus rounds up, becoming uniformly dense, and stains deep blue (basophilia) (Plate 14). The nucleus then breaks up into a number of rounded basophilic masses (apoptotic bodies). The entire process takes about 12 hours.

Both forms of cell death may be seen in the same part of the brain following an insult. The factors determining which route a cell takes to die are not known but are related to cell maturity and the severity of insult.[33]

8.2.3 Microglial response

Microglial cells are the brain's intrinsic population of phagocytic cells or macrophages. They initially respond within hours of an insult, and within 2–3 days develop into large cells with ample cytoplasm in which ingested tissue debris may be identified. These cells remove dead tissue and their activity contributes to the formation of cysts in areas of necrosis. In the days following hemorrhage red cells may be seen within macrophages, later they are broken down but hemosiderin (iron pigment) may remain for months or years, serving as a useful marker of previous hemorrhage both in histological preparations and on MRI scans.

Microglial cells at the inner margin of the hippocampal dentate gyrus are a reliable indication of previous episodes of HII in infants below 9 months of age[34] (Plate 15).

8.2.4 Reactive gliosis

The astrocytic glial-supporting cells of the brain respond to injury by enlarging, proliferating, and later developing fibrillary processes. They express a specific protein, glial fibrillary acidic protein (GFAP), which can be demonstrated by special staining methods. A glial response is seen from 17 weeks of gestation.[35,36] Large areas of gliosis may be identified on MRI scans by altered signal intensity.

8.2.5 Capillary response

Capillaries are the smallest vessels bringing blood to the tissues of the brain and have thin walls formed by a single cell layer, the endothelium. The endothelium is metabolically highly active, transporting substances between blood and brain cells, and as such is also very sensitive to HII. Following injury, capillaries in tissues adjacent to the damaged area undergo a series of changes, endothelial nuclei become larger, the cells become thicker and at 5–8 days after injury the capillaries branch and proliferate. This response appears to limit the extent of damage as inhibition of capillary response results in larger areas of brain damage.[37] Prolonged hypoxia in the fetal sheep results in proliferation of blood vessels[38] but other insults may also influence capillary response, for example chronic metabolic insufficiency in Leigh's disease, a mitochondrial disorder, results in widespread and prominent increase in capillaries.[22]

Increased vascularity is readily identified on MRI scans and is the explanation for 'cortical highlighting', a characteristic increase in signal seen about 1 week after severe HII in term infants (see Case 8.10, Plate 33).

8.2.6 Cyst formation

Following death of areas of brain tissue macrophages enter and ingest debris, removing it via the bloodstream. Small areas of damage collapse and are replaced by glial scar tissue but larger areas become cystic. In the fetal and neonatal brain cyst formation takes a minimum of 7–10 days.

Evolving damage is identifiable on ultrasound scans which initially show 'flares'; later, cysts are identified, which are also identified on CT and MRI scans.

8.2.7 Mineralization

Minerals, particularly calcium, are readily laid down in areas of damaged tissue in the fetal brain. Mineral accumulates within macrophages and nerve cells and their processes and stains intense blue in hematoxylin and eosin-stained preparations. The petrified outlines of nerve cells damaged by HII may persist for many years surrounded by dense reactive gliosis (Plate 16). Mineralization is well demonstrated in CT scans and may indicate the etiology of injury. In viral infection calcification is often dense and widespread or may form a dense periventricular band (see Plate 13). Following HII, calcification is less frequent and the distribution is in the pattern characteristic of the injury. The thalamus, basal ganglia, and brainstem are most frequently involved.

8.3 PATTERNS OF DAMAGE RELATED TO DEVELOPMENTAL AGE

8.3.1 Early: less than 28 weeks

8.3.1.1 Major malformations

Damage in the early months of gestation is characterized by disruption of specific developmental processes leading to malformations. The stages of brain development and brain malformations are described in more detail in Chapter 7. While much has been learned from experimental animal models, the timing in these models cannot be accurately related to timing of injury in the human brain due to the very different rates of brain maturation between species. Examples cited here are derived from well-documented human cases.

Damage in the first trimester of pregnancy leads to severe and gross malformations such as anencephaly or holoprosencephaly which are lethal in fetal or early neonatal life.

Less severe or very focal damage in the second trimester can cause malformation by interfering with development of specific structures. Several examples from individual cases are described below.

8.3.1.2 The corpus callosum

The corpus callosum is the major commissure carrying fibers interconnecting the two cerebral hemispheres. It first appears as a rudimentary structure at 11 weeks of gestation and over the next 6 weeks grows in a predominantly rostro-caudal direction.

Partial agenesis or interference with the development of the corpus callosum will lead to absence of its posterior part as this is the last part to form.

8.3.1.3   The inferior olives

These nuclei have a specific developmental timetable and disturbance in their development may allow the timing of brain damage to be pinpointed (see Case 8.1).

The inferior olivary nuclei are collections of nerve cells forming bilateral crenelated structures in the brainstem. They are a relay station in the pathway between cerebral hemispheres, cerebellum, and spinal cord and are part of the circuit controlling balance, power, and coordination of movements.

Neurons migrate into the brainstem to form the inferior olives in the first 12 weeks of gestation. They migrate both around the surface and across the brainstem to reach their destination (see Plate 1). Interruption of this migration results in ectopic neurons either on the surface of the brainstem or within the parenchyma in an abnormal position. When the olives are first formed they are simple 'C'-shaped structures, but as they grow and acquire new connections they increase in size and complexity and develop their characteristic folded appearance. This takes place between 7 and 22 weeks.

8.3.1.4   Neuronal heterotopias

As detailed in Chapter 7, all neurons migrate from the site where they are formed in the germinal matrix to their final position in the mature brain. In the human cerebral hemispheres this is complete by 21 weeks.[39,40] Migration around the brainstem is complete by 20 weeks.[41] If migration is interrupted then neurons are stranded in ectopic sites, as clusters or bands in the white matter or in the brainstem leptomeninges. The cortex overlying neuronal heterotopias is also usually malformed due to disturbance of the normal neuronal complement. Many syndromes of neuronal heterotopia are genetically determined[42] and these tend to have widespread and symmetrical masses of heterotopic neurons. Sporadic cases may result from trauma, hemorrhage, ischemia, or infection.[24,43]

Two cases are illustrated in which a well-documented injury in the second trimester resulted in neuronal heterotopias (Cases 8.2 and 8.3). Case 8.2, as well as having damage to the corpus callosum, had cortical damage and heterotopic neurons (see Plate 18c,d,e).

8.3.1.5   Cortical malformations and polymicrogyria

Cortical malformations encompass a variety of disturbances of cortical structure which may arise at various times in development.[44] Some of the more subtle alterations of cortical structure may also be due to secondary rearrangements of cell position following acquired damage in later life.[30] Polymicrogyria is the term used to describe a cortex in which the gyri are too small and too numerous when viewed with the naked eye. Histological

---

Case 8.1 (Plate 17)

Traumatic amniocentesis at 16 weeks. The baby had a scar in the scalp over the occiput. CT scan showed cerebellar hypoplasia and a small brain. The infant had a single seizure and died at $2^{1}/_{2}$ years. Plate 17 illustrates the brainstem with a normal control. The olivary malformation suggests that the nucleus developed normally until at least 12 weeks of age. However, further maturation (between 17 and 22 weeks) was impaired, the olives being simple and immature.

Case 8.2 (Plate 18)

Traumatic amniocentesis at 16 weeks gestation. The baby had a scar on the scalp, developed hemiplegia and intractable epilepsy. MRI scans showed atrophy of the left cerebral hemisphere, a defect in the anterior corpus callosum and cortical thickening in the left Sylvian fissure with underlying neuronal heterotopia. Hemispherectomy was performed to relieve epilepsy.

Case 8.3 (Plate 19)

This infant was born at 37 weeks with Apgar scores of 8 at 1 and 5 minutes. She suffered severe motor impairment, seizures and developmental delay and died at 7^1/$_2$ months.

Post-mortem examination showed an atrophic brain with widespread cortical malformation and an old cystic infarction in the territory of the middle cerebral artery. Histology of the brain showed a polymicrogyric cortex with underlying heterotopic neurons. Further enquiry into the clinical history revealed that at 19 weeks of pregnancy the mother was the subject of a physical attack and required hospital admission when severe abdominal bruising was noted. The nature of the brain damage shows interference with neuronal migration and is consistent with injury before 21 weeks of gestation.

Case 8.4 (Plate 20)

The mother attempted suicide while 22 weeks pregnant and suffered hypovolemic shock, requiring blood transfusion. Fetal arthrogryposis and cerebral ventriculomegaly were identified on ultrasound scans.

The pregnancy continued and the baby was born at 36 weeks and died at 9 hours of age. Examination of the brain revealed massive destruction, with much of the cerebral hemispheres being replaced by a thin-walled cyst (hydranencephaly). At the edge of the cyst the cortex was disturbed and the neuronal layers thrown into a series of folds. This represents the ischemic 'penumbra', a zone which suffered sublethal damage on the border of the totally infarcted area of brain.
(Case courtesy of Dr Helen Porter)

---

examination of polymicrogyria reveals a number of different architectural patterns, a consistent feature being fusion of the superficial layers of adjacent gyri.[41] Several patterns of clustered or festooned bands of neurons have been described. Histologically verified cases of polymicrogyria have been described following injuries before 28 weeks of gestation[45–47] but not after this time.

8.3.2   Mid-gestation: 28–36 weeks

8.3.2.1   White matter damage

During this period of mid-gestation the developing white matter bears the brunt of injury following generalized HII. Although neuropathologic study shows little cortical damage in preterm infants with white matter damage there is evidence that cortical, as well as white matter, growth is reduced at term.[48] The reason for the vulnerability of the immature white matter is not entirely understood. For many years it has been believed that the anatomy of the vascular supply to the white matter at this stage is an important factor, with the deep white matter representing a watershed territory, the end field between main areas of supply.[49] However, Kuban and Gilles[50] in a detailed anatomic study failed to demonstrate a watershed zone. Studies of blood flow to the white matter show it to be low at this developmental stage[51] and blood vessel density in the white matter is lower between 28 and 36 weeks than in earlier or later periods of development.[52]

An additional, and probably very important, factor may be the intrinsic vulnerability of the developing oligodendroglial cells to HII. This is a stage of active migration and proliferation of oligodendrocytes and the onset of myelination. *In vitro* studies have shown them to be susceptible to glutamate toxicity. Glutamate is released in excessive amounts when nerve cells or their processes are damaged by HII. Oligodendroglia have glutamate receptors and may thus be damaged by excess glutamate in much the same way as nerve cells.[53, 54]

Three patterns of white matter damage, periventricular leukomalacia, telencephalic leukoencephalopathy, and multicystic leukoencephalopathy, are described below. The pathology is not distinct but rather represents a spectrum of severity of damage. It must not be assumed that white matter damage is always the result of HII. Materno-fetal infections and metabolic disease can cause damage to the white matter indistinguishable from that resulting from HII. Both hypoxia-ischemia and infection cause elevation of proinflammatory cytokines which may mediate white matter damage.[27]

Although deep white matter damage is most commonly observed between 28 and 36 weeks it has also been documented to occur at and after term. Damage to the white matter in the parietal region underlying primary motor cortex is well recognized in term neonates who have suffered neonatal encephalopathy.[55,56] This pattern of damage with ulegyria in the motor cortex, subjacent white matter damage and status marmoratus of the basal nuclei has been recognized pathologically for some years.[57]

A considerable proportion of white matter damage occurs during intrauterine life.[1,58] Obstetric antecedents associated with white matter lesions include materno-fetal infections,[25] intrauterine growth retardation, and oligohydramnios,[59] hemorrhage in the first trimester, maternal urinary tract infection, and neonatal acidosis at birth.[60] These associations suggest that chronic fetal hypoxia and placental insufficiency may be a cause of white matter damage, as has been shown in the experimental sheep model.[37] As these factors are difficult to observe clinically they may go undocumented. Relatively few cases have histories of identified adverse obstetric events.

8.3.2.1.1 Periventricular leukomalacia

The macroscopic appearance of periventricular leukomalacia is of small areas of necrosis, several millimeters in diameter, in the deep white matter, most commonly in the frontal and occipital regions. The lesions appear yellow due to calcium deposition and may become centrally cavitated and cystic. The surrounding white matter is often congested and light brown in color (Plate 21).

Microscopy shows widespread glial proliferation and capillary reactive changes. The infarcts may contain macrophages and are surrounded by glial cells and mineralized cells and processes. There is often axonal damage adjacent to areas of infarction. Damaged axons may be swollen or show rounded 'axon retraction balls' (see Plate 23).

The evolution of periventricular leukomalacia may be to cyst formation (see below) while smaller areas of damage may be replaced by glial tissue. This almost invariably leads to tissue loss and reduced volume of myelinated white matter with compensatory dilatation of the lateral ventricles. The periventricular white matter is firm, gray, and gliosed; the altered structure of the tissue is reflected in altered signal on MRI scans.

Case 8.5 (Plate 22)

This infant was born at 28 weeks gestation just 1 week after his mother had had emergency surgery for a bleeding renal vascular malformation. During this emergency the maternal blood pressure had fallen to very low levels. The baby was born spontaneously but died 1 hour after birth.

Case 8.6 (Plate 23)

This infant was born very prematurely at 24 weeks gestation and survived a stormy course for 6 weeks during which time he suffered a germinal matrix hemorrhage. He finally collapsed with bowel perforation and died 6 hours later. MRI scan showed altered signal in the white matter and a stained section of a horizontal slice through the brain shows the earliest changes of white matter damage. These changes are consistent with damage a few hours before death. (MRI courtesy of Dr Mary Rutherford)

Case 8.7 (Plate 24)

The baby was born at 30 weeks with Apgar scores of 8 at 1 minute and 9 at 5 minutes. There was no birth asphyxia. Hyaline membrane disease developed and on day 1 ultrasound scans showed bilateral echodensities. By day 12 there were bilateral cysts in the periventricular white matter. At 4 months CT scan showed cerebral atrophy but no cysts were seen. The infant developed spastic quadriplegia and died at 11 months of age.

Case 8.8 (Plate 25)

The infant died 1 day after term delivery. The fetus was in a breech position until 35 weeks when he underwent spontaneous version. After that the fetal movements were reduced. During version the fetus may have compressed the umbilical cord, reducing blood supply. The intervening 5 weeks before death was sufficient time for the damaged white matter to undergo cystic change.

8.3.2.1.2 *Telencephalic leukoencephalopathy*

This term was coined by Gilles and co-workers[61] and describes diffuse reactive changes throughout the white matter of the cerebral hemispheres without focal infarction or cyst formation. The cellular changes are similar to those seen in periventricular leukomalacia and include gliosis, reactive capillary proliferation, and macrophage infiltration.

8.3.2.1.3 *Multicystic leukoencephalopathy*

In this condition the white matter contains many large cysts which may almost completely replace it, leaving a thin rim of gliotic cortex over the surface. Deep gray structures are usually firm and gliotic. Cysts may be predominantly periventricular or subcortical; in the latter case the neurodevelopmental prognosis is much worse.[62]

Most cases described in the literature have occurred between 30 and 44 weeks of gestation and almost all are associated with a sudden interference in fetal blood supply due to maternal hypotension. A number of cases have been recorded, with causes including maternal hypotension in anaphylactic shock, road traffic accident, or butane intoxication.[63,64]

8.3.2.1.4 *Posterior limb of the internal capsule*

Recent MRI studies of neonates have shown frequent involvement of the posterior limb of the internal capsule in hypoxic-ischemic damage.[31] Babies with this kind of damage have a poor prognosis and always develop some form of cerebral palsy.

The histological correlate of the altered signal is edema. Many of these infants also have severe damage in the adjacent deep gray nuclei, ventrolateral nucleus of the thalamus, and posterior putamen. This constellation of changes is illustrated in.Case 8.12, Plate 38.

8.3.2.2 **Germinal matrix hemorrhage**

Germinal matrix hemorrhage is the second major pathology in midterm and characteristically occurs in infants under 36 weeks of age (Plate 26). At this age the matrix is not fully involuted and its delicate blood vessels are liable to rupture. Germinal matrix hemorrhage is common in very low birthweight infants less than 24 weeks of age.[65] It tends to occur between 12 and 72 hours after birth in sick neonates in whom autoregulation of cerebral blood flow is disturbed.[66,67] It may also occur during intrauterine life.[1,58]

Other patterns of fetal intracranial hemorrhage may result from clotting disorders, of which alloimmune thrombocytopenia is the most common. An association of intraventricular hemorrhage with amniotic sac inflammation has been noted.[13,68]

The complications of germinal matrix hemorrhage include rupture into the ventricular system (intraventricular hemorrhage) and venous infarction of adjacent cerebral parenchyma (parenchymal hemorrhagic infarction).

Both have serious implications for future neurological development, while hemorrhages confined to the germinal matrix and without involvement of adjacent parenchyma have a good prognosis.[69]

Rupture of the hemorrhage through the ependyma into the ventricular system is associated with a poor prognosis due to the damaging effects of blood in the ventricular system. These effects are multiple. Blood clots may block narrow pathways of cerebrospinal fluid (CSF) flow and cause acute obstruction and hydrocephalus (Plate 27). Blood also acts as an irritant on the ependymal lining of the ventricular system causing the ependyma to be shed and replaced by gliosis. This prolific glial growth may itself block CSF flow and cause hydrocephalus of more chronic onset. Histological evidence of old blood pigment and iron in the damaged lining confirms a hemorrhagic etiology (Plate 28).

Blood may also obstruct the arachnoid villi where CSF drains back into the venous system and cause enlargement of CSF spaces both within the ventricles and the surface of the brain, a condition known as 'communicating hydrocephalus'.

Case 8.9 (Plate 29)

This twin was born prematurely at 23 weeks gestation. At 2 days of age bilateral germinal matrix and intraventricular hemorrhages were identified on MRI scan. He died at 14 days of age. (MRI courtesy of Dr Mary Rutherford)

8.3.2.3   Parenchymal hemorrhagic infarction

A sinister complication of germinal matrix hemorrhage is infarction of the adjacent white matter which greatly worsens the prognosis[69] (Plate 30).

About 15 percent of cases develop this complication,[70] which is usually unilateral and leads to asymmetrical ventricular dilatation. Originally, the damage to the white matter was thought to result from direct extension of hemorrhage into the tissues but histological studies show perivascular hemorrhage around draining veins indicating raised venous pressure and failure of venous drainage with stasis of blood flow as a cause of infarction. This is thought to result from mechanical obstruction of the draining veins by blood clot.

The long-term sequelae are severe, as damage to the white matter causes destruction of motor fibers resulting in the spastic diplegic form of cerebral palsy.

8.3.3   Late gestation: term

As the brain approaches maturity it is the gray matter which is mainly, but not exclusively, vulnerable to HII. The pattern of gray matter damage is partly due to distribution of blood flow and vascular supply: the 'watershed zones' between main arterial supplies are especially vulnerable. Columnar necrosis of the cortex and ulegyria are also characteristic of the term brain.

The deep gray nuclei, especially the putamen and the thalamus, are also frequently involved in term HII but damage to these nuclei is also seen at other gestational ages if the injury is sufficiently severe and acute.

The reasons for vulnerability of specific cell types are unknown but are probably related to maturity, acquisition of specific neurotransmitters, and calcium-binding proteins, and the ability to produce anti-apoptotic factors. These factors are discussed in more detail in Chapter 4.

Distinctive patterns of damage following severe HII in the term infant are well recognized.[56,71,72] Typically the deep gray matter of the posterior putamen, ventrolateral nucleus of the thalamus, midbrain, and lateral geniculate bodies are involved, together with the peri-rolandic cortex and its underlying white matter as well as white matter elsewhere (Case 8.12, Plate 38).

8.3.3.1   Cortex: watershed zones

Watershed zones are the areas of the brain at the peripheries of fields of supply of the main cerebral vessels, and have the most tenuous blood supply (Plate 31). The main cortical watershed zones in the neonatal brain are in the parasagittal region between the areas of supply of middle, anterior, and posterior cerebral arteries and in the lateral aspect of the cortex in the parieto-occipital region between middle and posterior cerebral arteries.

8.3.3.2   Cortex: columnar necrosis

The capillary supply to the cortex is still not completely mature at term. It consists of delicate capillaries which enter the cortex at right-angles from the leptomeninges, and which have few lateral anastomoses. Reduction of flow leads to necrosis of cells furthest away from these vessels and survival only of those cells close to them.[73] This results in a pattern of columnar necrosis which is seen at any gestational age until term, although it is uncommon in human cases. It is well described in the rat model of cerebral ischemia.[74] As the cortex which has been damaged in this way matures, bands of glial cells grow into the necrotic zones and surviving perivascular cells form rounded masses (Plate 32).

8.3.3.3   Cortex: ulegyria

This pattern of damage is seen characteristically in the term brain after the gyral pattern has been established but is rarely seen in the adult brain. In

Case 8.10 (Plate 33)

This infant of 12 weeks survived 9 days after severe HII following trauma.

Case 8.11 (Plate 34)

Term delivery by cesarean section for antepartum hemorrhage. There was severe birth asphyxia. The child developed spastic quadriplegia, seizures and cortical blindness and died at 5 years of age.

this condition the cortex at the depths of sulci is more severely damaged than the gyral crests. It has been suggested that vulnerability of the depths of sulci results from reduced vascular supply consequent upon cortical folding. Cerebral swelling with compression of surface vessels within sulci may also contribute. The accentuation of damage in sulcal depths is seen in Case 8.10, Plate 33.

In long-term survivors, the cortex of the depths of sulci becomes gliosed, thin, and atrophic, in contrast to the normal thick cortex in the crests of gyri. This has led to the description of the remaining gyri as 'mushrooms'.

Other patterns of cortical damage include selective neuronal death. This may be laminar, in which cortical layers III–V are most vulnerable. Laminar destruction of neurons is seen in the adult brain. Plate 35 shows an extremely unusual example in an early fetal brain at 20 weeks of gestation. Selective neuronal death is also well recognized in the hippocampus. Here specific groups of cells such as the CA1 and CA3 regions of Ammon's horn or the internal layer of cells of the hippocampal dentate gyrus are particularly vulnerable.

8.3.3.4 Deep gray nuclei

The deep gray nuclei are vulnerable in severe term HII,[75] but damage to these nuclei is also described in much younger fetuses.[76,77] The thalamus and posterior part of the putamen are frequently involved at term.[55,56] There may be necrosis and cystic change, but in babies who survive there is usually more subtle damage and the basal nuclei become atrophic, causing dilatation of the third ventricle. Dead neurons may be identified as mineralized ghosts surrounded by dense gliosis (see Plate 16b).

8.3.3.5 Status marmoratus

At about 6 months of age the deep gray nuclei are myelinated. It is at this stage that status marmoratus is first seen: an abnormal marbled appearance visible with the naked eye and on scans. It is due to myelination of aberrant glial bundles which have formed as a scarring reaction to earlier HII (Plate 36).

8.3.3.6 Cerebellum

The cerebellar cortex may be damaged by HII as any other part of the cortex but selective cerebellar damage by HII is extremely uncommon. I have seen one case with a clear history of severe birth asphyxia at term who subsequently developed a spastic quadriplegia cerebral palsy with epilepsy. Scans showed cerebellar atrophy. Subsequent histological examination revealed typical hypoxic-ischemic damage in the cerebellar cortex with mild atrophy of the hippocampus and the cerebral white matter. An exhaustive search for neurodegenerative diseases or other causes of cerebellar atrophy was negative. There was no evidence of primary cerebellar hypoplasia or a malformation syndrome.

8.4 INFLUENCE OF THE NATURE OF INSULT ON PATTERNS OF DAMAGE

The final pattern of brain damage following HII is the result of complex interactions of a number of factors which are incompletely understood in the human fetus but include the age at the time of insult, metabolic state of the fetus, and the nature and severity of the insult itself.

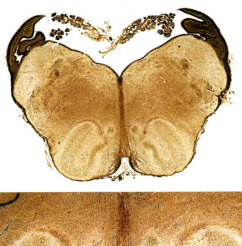

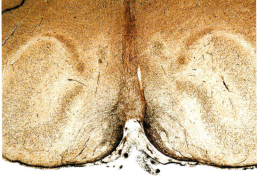

Plate 1 Section through the brainstem of a 10-week fetus showing migration of neurons (stained black) from the lateral margins of the fourth ventricle. Cells migrate dorsally to form the cerebellum and ventrally to form the brainstem nuclei. There are cells migrating over the surface and streaming into the ventral part of the medulla to populate the immature olivary nuclei (lower picture).

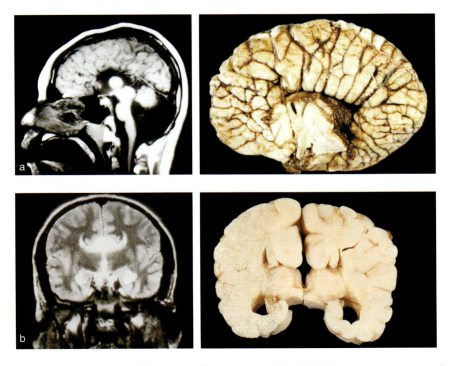

Plate 2 (a) Sagittal MRI scan (left) of agenesis of the corpus callosum. Note radial gyri. Similar appearances are seen in the medial aspect of a fixed cerebral hemisphere (right). (b) Coronal MRI showing laterally displaced ventricles in a 'Viking's horn' brain slice appearance.

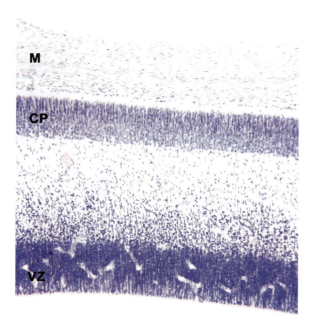

Plate 3 Developing brain wall at about 10 weeks of gestation. The thick ventricular zone (VZ) lines the ventricle and is the site of cell proliferation. Cells are migrating out through the future white matter to the cortical plate (CP) the precursor of the cerebral cortex. Above are the thick, well vascularized meninges (M).

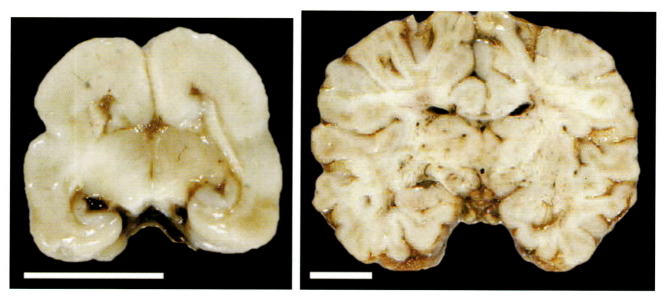

Plate 4 Coronal slices of fixed brains at 20 weeks gestation (a) and at term (b). Scale bar = 2 cm.

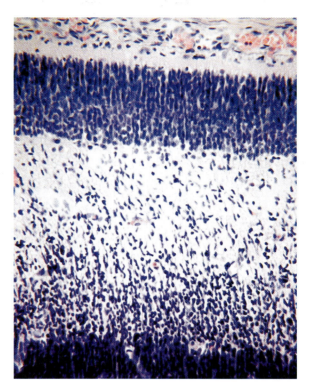

Plate 5 Radial migration at 10 weeks. Migrating cells are elongated along very delicate glial processes. Cells arriving in the cortical plate are aligned in regular columns along glial fiber guides.

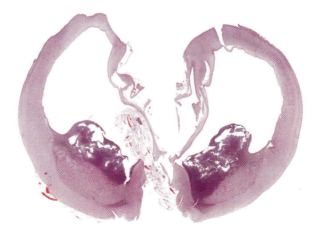

Plate 6 Stained section of lissencephalic brain at term. Note the smooth and thin brain wall with very large lateral ventricles and big residual masses of germinal matrix.

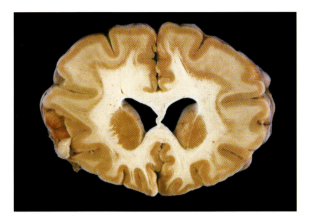

Plate 7 Coronal fixed brain slice showing a thick band of nerve cells underlying a well-formed cortex. Note the inferior part of the cortex is normal.

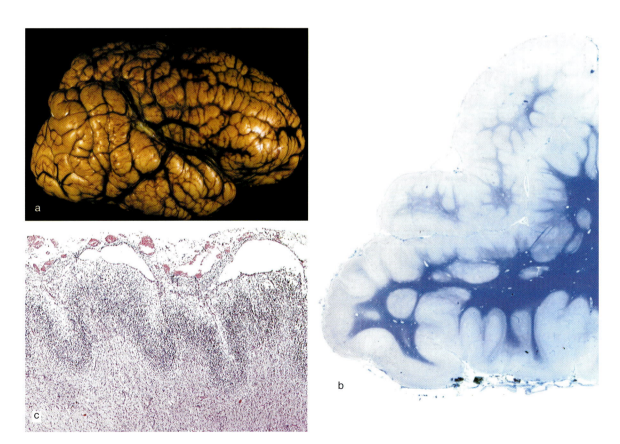

Plate 8 (a) Surface of a brain showing polymicrogyria. Many gyri appear coarse and thickened but they have a fine nodularity due to fusion of many small underlying gyri. (b) Stained section of the brain in (a). Note the multiply folded gyri and heterotopic groups of neurons in the underlying white matter. (c) Polymicrogyria in a fetal brain. The cortex is represented by an undulating band of neurons (stained blue). The overlying meninges are partly adherent to the brain surface and large vessels can be seen dipping into the cortex between folds in the band of neurons.

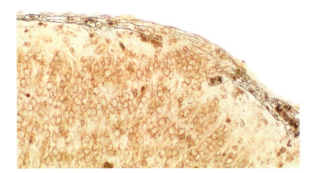

Plate 9 Section of a mouse brain stained with reticulin to show the delicate fibers of the pial membrane, the innermost layer of the leptomeninges which cover the brain surface. Neurons are migrating through the superficial cortex and out onto the brain surface though gaps in the pial membrane. Photo courtesy of Perry Blackshear.

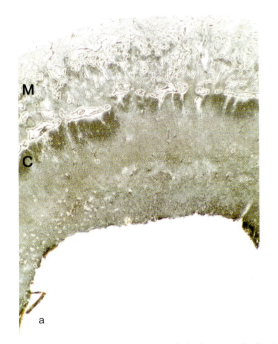

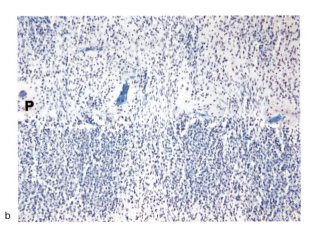

Plate 10 (a) Low-power image of the brain wall of a 20-week fetus with type II lissencephaly. A few clusters of cells (stained black) remain in the position of the normal cortical plate (C) but many more have migrated out into the leptomeninges (M) through gaps in the pial membrane. Overmigrated cells form small groups interspersed with thick, densely vascular leptomeninges. (b) A high-power picture of type II lissencephaly at 20 weeks showing three abnormal breaks in the pial membrane (P) where cells are streaming from the cortical plate (below) into the leptomeninges.

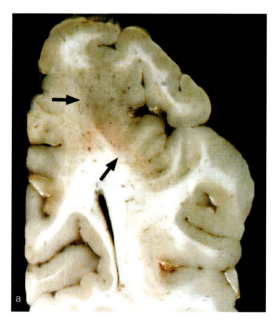
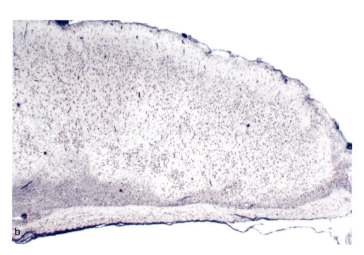

Plate 11 (a) Coronal slice of fixed brain. This specimen was resected from an infant for severe epilepsy. There is a focus of dysplastic cortex (arrows) but cortex elsewhere is macroscopically normal. Small groups of unmigrated, heterotopic neurons are seen close to the ventricular wall at the tail of the lower arrow. (b) Stained section of dysplastic cortex which is thickened with an irregular deep border. Neurons are not arranged in regular laminae but form clusters, particularly in the deeper layers.

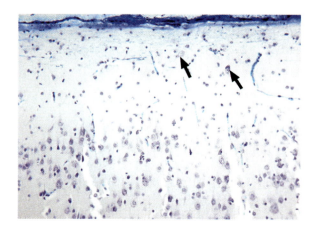

Plate 12 Stained section of the cortex in microdysgenesis. Neurons are frequent in the superficial layer (two are marked with arrows). This layer should be relatively free of neurons. The upper margin of the second layer is ragged. There are a number of myelinated fibers running horizontally in the upper layers of the cortex just below the surface of the brain.

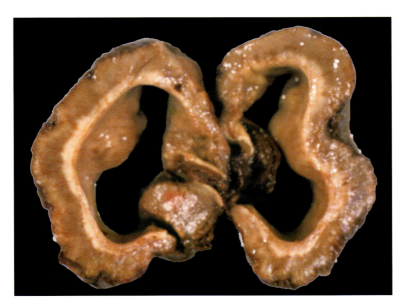

Plate 13 Cytomegalovirus infection. Coronal slice of fixed brain of a neonate with cytomegalovirus. Note the dense white periventricular band of mineralization.

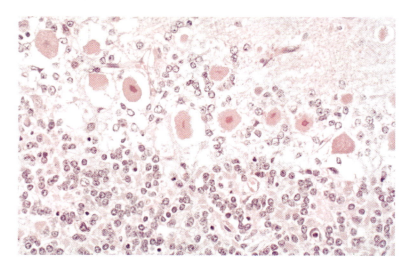

Plate 14 Apoptosis and necrosis. Section of cerebellar cortex 48 hours after severe hypoxic-ischemic injury, stained with hematoxylin and eosin. The large Purkinje cells are necrotic. They have bright pink (eosinophilic) cytoplasm and their nuclei are small and poorly defined as they disintegrate (nucleolysis). In contrast, many cells in the deeper granule cell layer are undergoing apoptosis. Their nuclei are shrunken and rounded and stain dark blue.

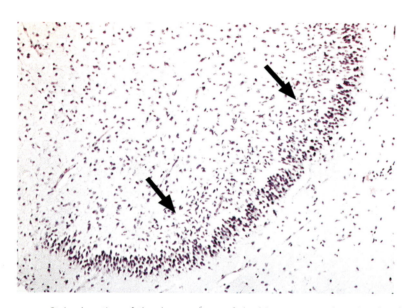

Plate 15 Microglial response. Stained section of the dentate gyrus of the hippocampus. There is a band of small elongated cells (arrows) close to the inner margin of the dentate gyrus. These are reactive microglial cells, an indication of previous hypoxic-ischemic injury in the infant.

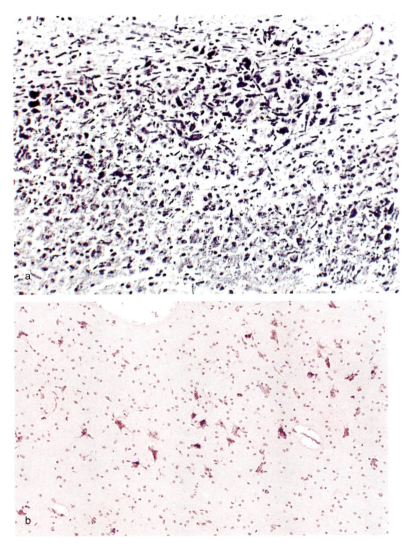

Plate 16 Mineralization. (a) Section of fetal brain 12 days after injury stained with luxol fast blue and cresyl violet. Many cell bodies and fibers in the upper part of the picture stain intense blue due to deposition of mineral within them. The tissues in the lower part of the picture appear granular due to necrosis. (b) Section of the thalamus stained with hematoxylin and eosin. This child died 7 years after severe birth asphyxia. The ghosts of damaged nerve cells containing deposits of mineral appear dark purple; many small round nuclei of glial cells are seen between them. No remaining normal neurons are identified.

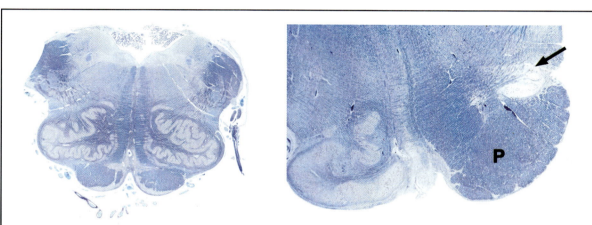

Plate 17 Intrauterine trauma at 16 weeks. Slices through the brainstem of a normal control (left) and Case 8.1 (right). The right olivary nucleus (arrow) is very small and immature and the left is not normally folded. The left pyramidal tract (P), which carries motor fibers to the spinal cord, is absent.

Case 8.1

Traumatic amniocentesis at 16 weeks. The baby had a scar in the scalp over the occiput. CT scan showed cerebellar hypoplasia and a small brain. The infant had a single seizure and died at 2$\frac{1}{2}$ years. Plate 17 illustrates the brainstem with a normal control. The olivary malformation suggests that the nucleus developed normally until at least 12 weeks of age. However, further maturation (between 17 and 22 weeks) was impaired, the olives being simple and immature.

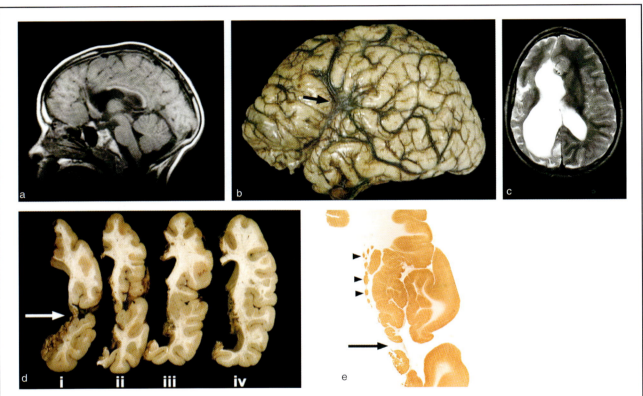

Plate 18 Intrauterine trauma at 16 weeks. (a) Sagittal MRI showing a defect in the anterior corpus callosum. Note the presence of the cingulate gyrus posteriorly, evidence that the corpus callosum had formed normally prior to damage. (b) Surface of the hemisphere following fixation. The arrow indicates a cortical scar. (c) Horizontal MRI scan showing atrophy of the left cerebral hemisphere and a focal cortical abnormality. (d) Coronal slices through the fixed hemisphere show thin and damaged anterior corpus callosum (i, ii). A cortical defect is obvious in i (arrow) and thickened, irregular adjacent cortex is seen in ii–iv. (e) Section of part of the hemisphere stained to show nerve cells brown clearly demonstrates the cortical defect (arrow), the thickened dysplastic adjacent cortex and many nodules of heterotopic neurons (arrowheads) which have failed to complete migration underlying the abnormal cortex.

Case 8.2

Traumatic amniocentesis at 16 weeks gestation. The baby had a scar on the scalp, developed hemiplegia and intractable epilepsy. MRI scans showed atrophy of the left cerebral hemisphere, a defect in the anterior corpus callosum and cortical thickening in the left Sylvian fissure with underlying neuronal heterotopia. Hemispherectomy was performed to relieve epilepsy.

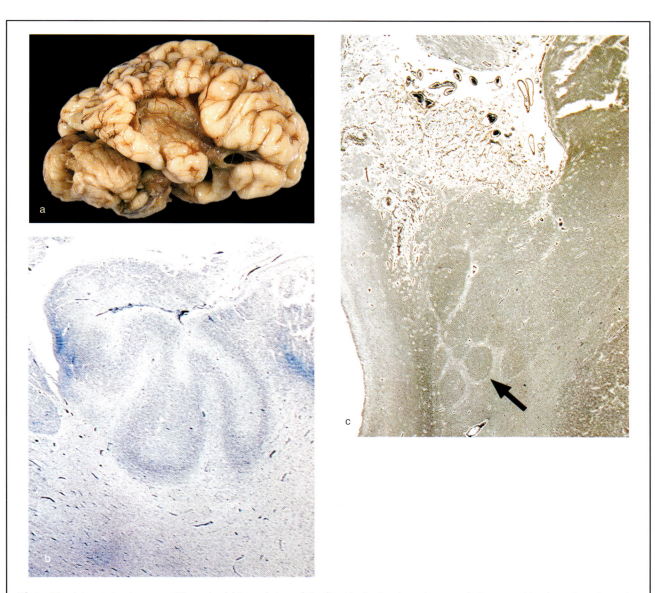

Plate 19 Intrauterine trauma at 19 weeks. (a) Lateral view of the fixed brain showing a large cortical cyst resulting from tissue loss. The adjacent gyri are irregular. (b) Part of the abnormal cortex showing an undulating band of neurons (stained blue) characteristic of polymicrogyria. (c) Reticulin-stained section shows deep heterotopic neurons (arrow) and thickened meninges in the overlying damaged cortex.

Case 8.3

This infant was born at 37 weeks with Apgar scores of 8 at 1 and 5 minutes. She suffered severe motor impairment, seizures and developmental delay and died at $7^1/_2$ months.

Post-mortem examination showed an atrophic brain with widespread cortical malformation and an old cystic infarction in the territory of the middle cerebral artery. Histology of the brain showed a polymicrogyric cortex with underlying heterotopic neurons. Further enquiry into the clinical history revealed that at 19 weeks of pregnancy the mother was the subject of a physical attack and required hospital admission when severe abdominal bruising was noted. The nature of the brain damage shows interference with neuronal migration and is consistent with injury before 21 weeks of gestation.

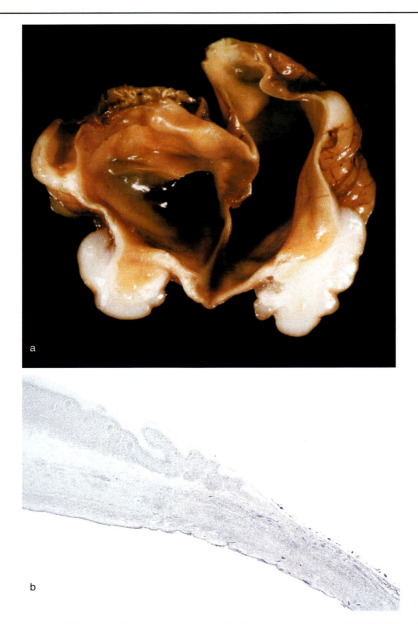

Plate 20 Intrauterine ischemia at 22 weeks. (a) Coronal slice of the fixed brain shows preservation of only small areas of cortex in the inferior parts of the brain. Elsewhere the entire brain is virtually a cyst with a thin membranous wall. The ventricles are dilated and their lining bloodstained. (b) Section of the cortex adjacent to the cystic brain wall shows irregular cortical folding.

Case 8.4

The mother attempted suicide while 22 weeks pregnant and suffered hypovolemic shock, requiring blood transfusion. Fetal arthrogryposis and cerebral ventriculomegaly were identified on ultrasound scans.

The pregnancy continued and the baby was born at 36 weeks and died at 9 hours of age. Examination of the brain revealed massive destruction, with much of the cerebral hemispheres being replaced by a thin-walled cyst (hydranencephaly). At the edge of the cyst the cortex was disturbed and the neuronal layers thrown into a series of folds. This represents the ischemic 'penumbra', a zone which suffered sublethal damage on the border of the totally infarcted area of brain. (Case Courtesy of Dr Helen Porter)

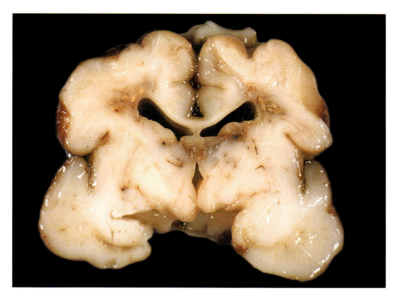

Plate 21 Periventricular leukomalacia. Coronal slice of a fixed brain showing multiple small cystic lesions with yellow walls in the deep white matter close to the lateral ventricles.

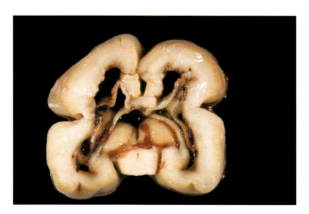

Plate 22 Intrauterine ischemia at 27 weeks. Hemorrhagic necrosis of the entire deep periventricular white matter. There was associated damage to deep gray nuclei and the brainstem.

Case 8.5

This infant was born at 28 weeks gestation just 1 week after his mother had emergency surgery for a bleeding renal vascular malformation. During this emergency the maternal blood pressure had fallen to very low levels. The baby was born spontaneously but died 1 hour after birth.

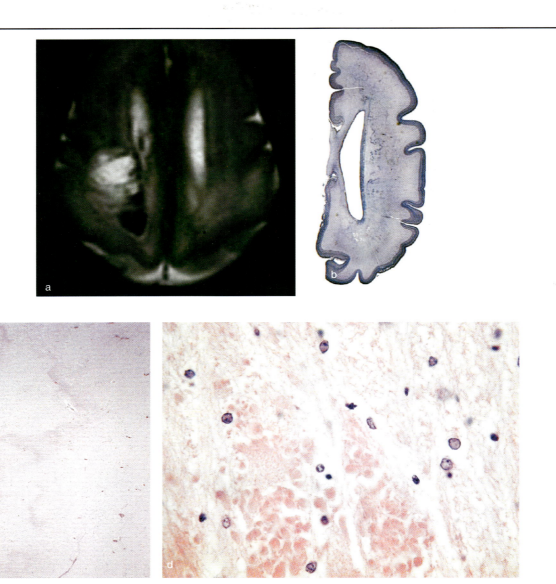

Plate 23 Acute periventricular infarction. (a) Horizontal MRI scan shows a large hemorrhage in the left hemisphere. There is patchy altered signal in the right hemisphere. (b) A horizontal section of the right hemisphere shows an irregular, serpignious band in the white matter close to the ventricular wall. (c) Low-power histology shows the serpignious deep pink band of early 'coagulative necrosis' with hematoxylin and eosin staining. (d) Higher power histology shows the pink color to result from clusters of swollen disrupted axons – 'axon retraction balls'. Many cells in this area are shrunken and deep blue in color as they undergo apoptosis.

Case 8.6

This infant was born very prematurely at 24 weeks gestation and survived a stormy course for 6 weeks during which tine he suffered a germinal matrix hemorrhage. He finally collapsed with bowel perforation and died 6 hours later. MRI scan showed altered signal in the white matter and a stained section of a horizontal slice through the brain shows the earliest changes of white matter damage. These changes are consistent with damage a few hours before death. (MRI Courtesy of Dr Mary Rutherford)

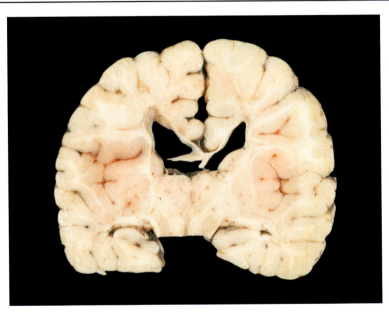

Plate 24 Old periventricular leukomalacia. Coronal slice through the fixed brain shows dilatation of the lateral ventricles (more marked on the left) and a thin corpus callosum due to reduction in volume of white matter. The periventricular tissues show little macroscopic change but microscopic examination revealed extensive gliosis in which the remnants of a cyst were found. The cysts had collapsed and were replaced by glial scar tissue.

Case 8.7

The baby was born at 30 weeks with Apgar scores of 8 at 1 minute and 9 at 5 minutes. There was no birth asphyxia. Hyaline membrane disease developed and on day 1 ultrasound scans showed bilateral echodensities. By day 12 there were bilateral cysts in the periventricular white matter. At 4 months CT scan showed cerebral atrophy but no cysts were seen. The infant developed spastic quadriplegia and died at 11 months of age.

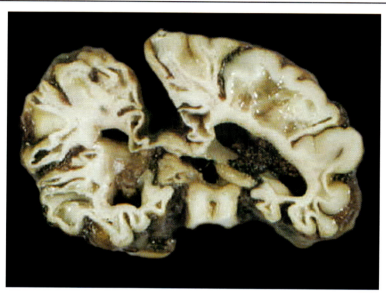

Plate 25 Multicystic leukomalacia. Coronal slice of a fixed brain which is severely atrophic. There are multiple large cysts in the white matter. Cortex over these cysts tends to be thin but in other areas it is well preserved.

Case 8.8

The infant died 1 day after term delivery. The fetus was in breech position until 35 weeks when he underwent spontaneous version. After that the fetal movements were reduced. During version the fetus may have compressed the umbilical cord, reducing blood supply. The intervening 5 weeks before death was sufficient time for the damaged white matter to undergo cystic change.

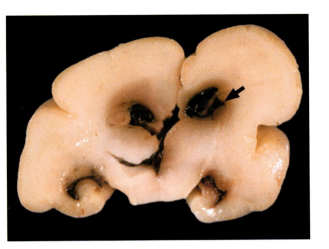

Plate 26 Germinal matrix hemorrhage. Coronal slice of a fixed brain showing a germinal matrix hemorrhage close to the wall of the right lateral ventricle (arrow). Blood has ruptured into both lateral ventricles.

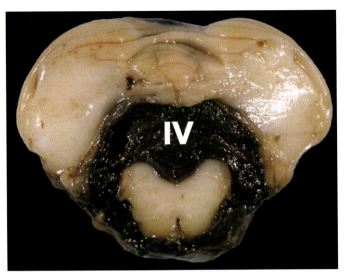

Plate 27 Intraventricular hemorrhage. Fixed brain slice showing the inferior aspect of the cerebellum and the brainstem. Blood clot is distending the fourth ventricle (IV), has tracked out through the lateral exit foramen, and forms a thick clot all around the brainstem.

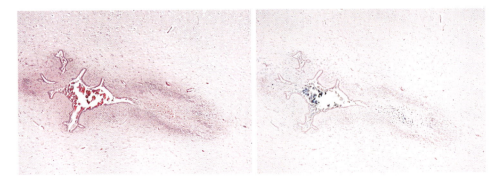

Plate 28 Aqueduct stenosis. Sections through the midbrain of a child with hydrocephalus due to aqueduct stenosis following intraventricular hemorrhage. The section on the left (a) is stained with hematoxylin and eosin. The site of the original aqueduct is marked by a band of deep purple cells. Much of the lumen has been occluded by reactive glial cells. Only a narrow, forked channel remains. Several smaller channels or ependymal rosettes are seen close to the walls of the stenosed aqueduct. (b) This section has been stained to show iron, which is deep blue. Iron remaining from destruction of red blood cells due to old hemorrhage is seen in the lumen of the stenosed aqueduct and in the glial tissue occluding the lumen.

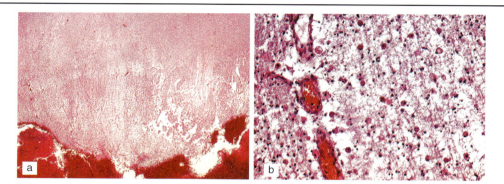

Plate 29 Early parenchymal hemorrhagic infarction. (a) Low-power section of the brain wall adjacent to a large germinal matrix hemorrhage. The deep white matter is pale and edematous close to the blood clot. (b) High-power picture of the tissue shown in (a). The tissue is very edematous and blood vessels are congested. Many large round cells are seen. These are macrophages with small nuclei and a large mass of cytoplasm in which intact red cells may occasionally be seen. The macrophages take up red cells in the damaged tissues and transport the debris away through the vascular system. Due to the slowed venous blood flow they cannot escape by this means and so remain in the infarcted tissue.

Case 8.9

This twin was born prematurely at 23 weeks gestation. At 2 days of age bilateral germinal matrix and intraventricular hemorrhages were identified on MRI scan. He died at 14 days of age. (MRI courtesy of Dr Mary Rutherford)

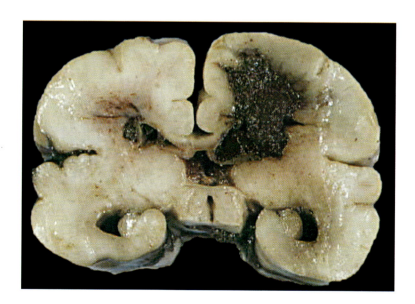

Plate 30 Parenchymal hemorrhagic infarction. Coronal slice of fixed brain. On the right side blood clot is seen in the lateral ventricle with a large wedge of parenchymal hemorrhagic infarction fanning out into adjacent white matter. A smaller germinal matrix hemorrhage is present in the left hemisphere, where large congested veins are seen in the adjacent parenchyma.

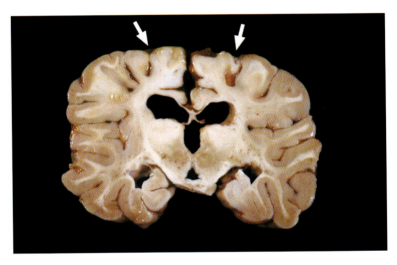

Plate 31 Coronal slice of fixed brain of a child with cerebral palsy. The cortex is deficient in the depths of parasagittal sulci (arrows), one of the cortical watershed areas. Elsewhere the cortex is well preserved. The deep gray nuclei are atrophic, as is the white matter, and the corpus callosum is extremely thin. The ventricular system is dilated.

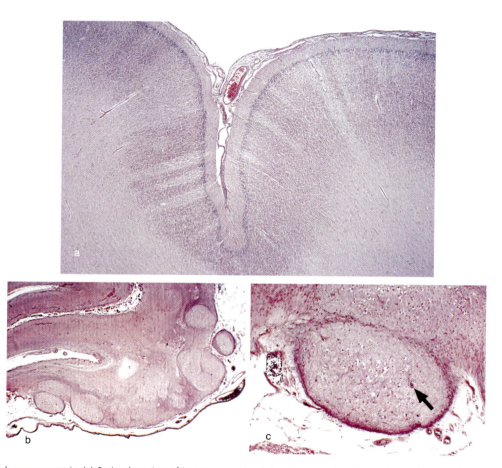

Plate 32 Columnar necrosis. (a) Stained section of immature cortex following hypoxic-ischemic injury showing the pattern of columnar necrosis. Viable cells remain around vessels which enter the brain at right angles to the surface. (b) Edge of an old area of cortical infarction. The neurons are found in rounded masses separated by bands of glial cells (stained purple). (c) At higher power the nodules of neurons have a central blood vessel (arrow). This is the result of sparing of cells around blood vessels; more distant neurons have died and been replaced by glial cells.

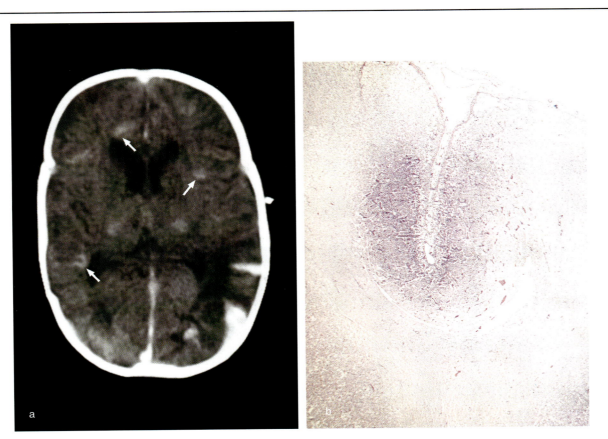

Plate 33 (a) MRI scan shows increased cortical signal (cortical highlighting) at the bases of sulci (arrows). (b) Histology shows the reactive capillary proliferation which is more intense in the sulcal depths.

Case 8.10

This infant of 12 weeks survived 9 days after severe hypoxic-ischemic injury following trauma.

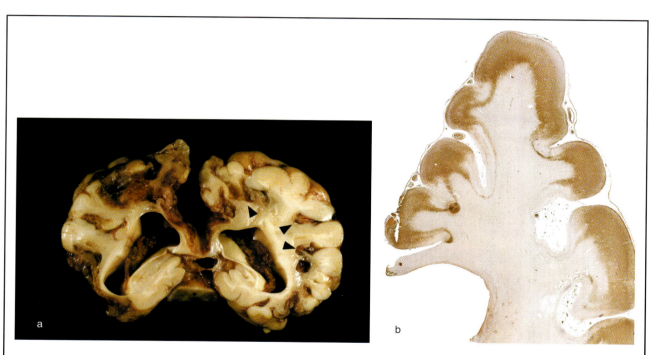

Plate 34 Old hypoxic-ischemic injury (HII) with ulegyria. (a) A coronal slice of fixed brain shows dilated ventricles due to reduced volume of brain tissue. There has been extensive cortical loss most marked in depths of sulci (arrowheads). Sparing of superficial cortex gives some gyri the appearance of mushrooms. (b) Section of brain with old HII showing ulegyria. The nerve cells are stained brown. Note the selective loss of nerve cells from the depths of sulci.

Case 8.11

Term delivery by cesarean section for antepartum hemorrhage. There was severe birth asphyxia. The child developed spastic quadriplegia, seizures and cortical blindness and died at 5 years of age.

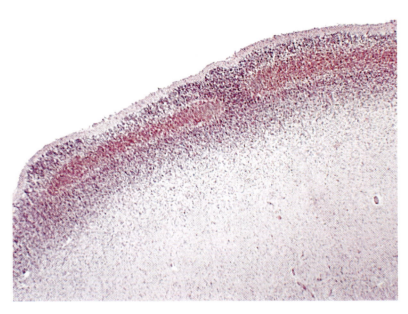

Plate 35   Laminar necrosis. Stained section of fetal brain showing large zones of laminar necrosis (stained pink) within the cortex.

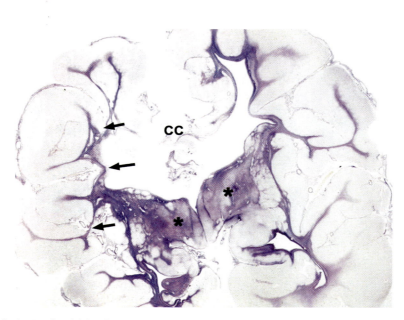

Plate 36 Section of the brain of a child with cerebral palsy who died aged 6 following severe birth asphyxia due to uterine rupture. The section is stained to show glial tissue purple. There is intense and abnormal gliosis of the thalamus (status marmoratus, asterisks). There is also ulegyria (arrows). The white matter is atrophied and gliotic and the corpus callosum (CC) reduced to a thin membrane.

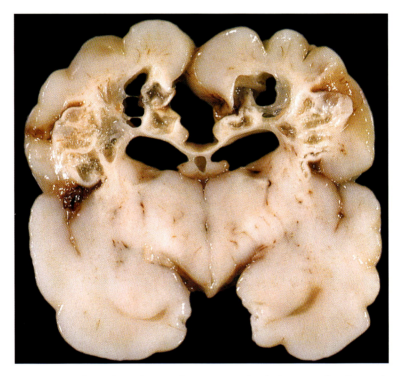

Plate 37 Coronal slice of fixed brain of an infant of 27 weeks gestation who died at 7 weeks of age. She was growth retarded and died with necrotizing enteroclitis. There is bilateral cystic damage to the white matter in the territory of the middle cerebral arteries. Elsewhere the cortex is well preserved and normally developed.

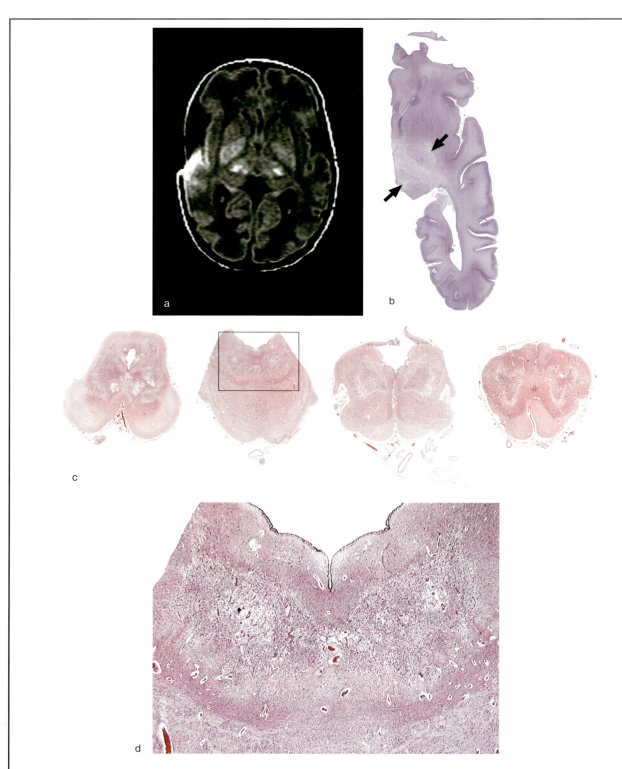

Plate 38 (a) Horizontal MRI scan showing high signal in the deep gray nuclei. Comparison with (b), a stained section of the right hemisphere, shows necrosis of thalamus and putamen (arrows). The posterior limb of the internal capsule, which runs between them, is pale due to edema. (c) Sections of the brainstem show bilateral necrosis extending through its entire length. The boxed area is shown in high power in (d) where congested and proliferating capillaries are seen with pale areas of tissue loss between them.

Case 8.12

This baby was born at 28 weeks of gestation; at 4 weeks of age he suffered with necrotizing entero-colitis and collapsed with intestinal perforation. One week after this, MRI scan demonstrated high signal in the thalamus and putamen with edema of the posterior limb of the internal capsule. The baby died at 8 weeks.

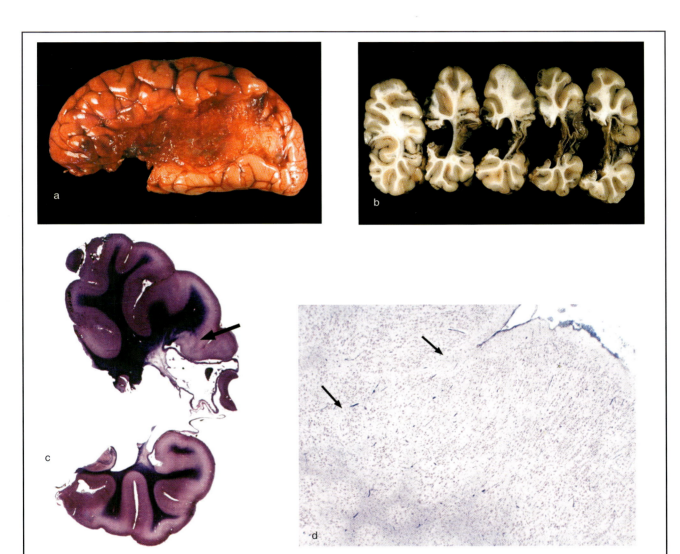

Plate 39 Old infarction. (a) The lateral aspect of a fresh hemispherectomy specimen showing a large, old cystic infarction where the cortex has been replaced by a thin glial membrane. (b) Coronal slices through the fixed hemisphere demonstrate the extent of the cystic replacement of cortex. (c) A coronal section through the old cyst shows the tissue defect covered by a thin membrane (white matter is stained deep blue). The cortex on the border of the cyst is irregular (arrow). (d) High-power image of the bordering cortex shows marked dysplasia. Neurons are not arranged in regular horizontal laminae but form clusters or columns. There are groups of incompletely migrated neurons deep to the deep cortical border. Arrows mark a seam line where the most superficial layers of adjacent gyri have fused.

Case 8.13

Pregnancy and delivery were normal. The baby had an apneic attack 1 hour after birth and seizures from day 1. Severe epilepsy was treated by hemispherectomy at 11 years of age.

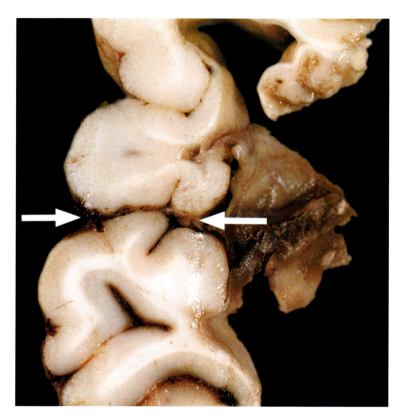

Plate 40　Schizencephaly. Fixed brain slice showing a cleft extending through the entire brain wall (arrows). The old blood clot close to the ventricular end of the cyst suggests earlier hemorrhage. The adjacent cortex is dysplastic if damage occurs before 28 weeks of gestation.

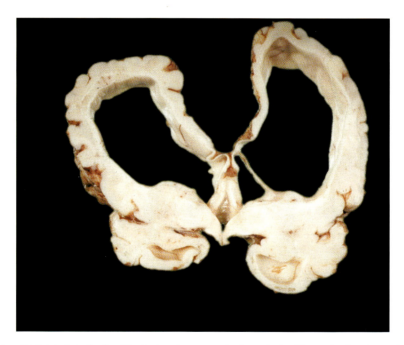

Plate 41 Hydrocephalus. Coronal slice of a fixed brain showing severe hydrocephalus. The cortex has formed normally but is stretched by the ventricular expansion. The white matter is very attenuated and thin.

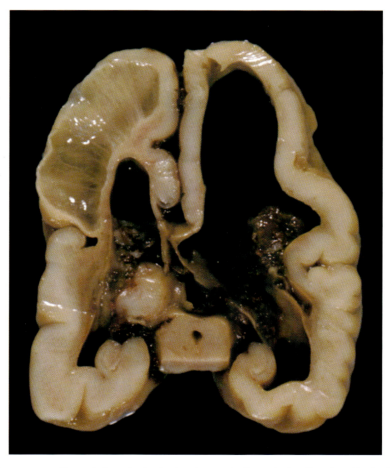

Plate 42   Hydrocephalus *ex vacuo*. Coronal slice of a brain showing marked ventricular dilatation. The brain wall is thin. There is an old cystic cavity involving white matter and cortex on the left side. Blood clot is seen in the ventricles.

8.4.1 Chronic partial asphyxia

Chronic partial asphyxia in the human fetus probably occurs in conditions of placental insufficiency and may be associated with placental infarctions, retroplacental hemorrhage, and intrauterine growth retardation. Individual cases are not frequently identified but there is an association between white matter damage in humans and intrauterine growth retardation and acidosis at birth.[59,60] Chronic partial asphyxia of the fetus causes redistribution of blood to the brain, heart, and adrenals while within the brain blood flow is diverted from the cerebral hemispheres in favor of the vital centers in the brainstem.[78]

The sheep model of placental insufficiency shows increase in capillary size and gliosis of the white matter as well as cerebellar damage,[37] and in the rat chronic hypoxemia results in reduced growth of white matter and cortex.[79]

In the human fetus chronic partial asphyxia alone may cause white matter damage including periventricular leukomalacia, telencephalic leukomalacia, diffuse white matter gliosis, or generalized reduction in volume of the white matter.

Redistribution of blood flow to the brainstem in these infants makes the cerebral hemispheres particularly vulnerable to HII. Infarction of frontal and parietal regions is a common pattern of damage as is bilateral infarction in the territory of the middle cerebral arteries (Plate 37). Infants compromised by chronic partial asphyxia *in utero* may be unable to tolerate even normal delivery which may prove hazardous and precipitate catastrophic hemispheric damage. Over 100 years ago Freud first proposed the concept that difficulties at birth may be the result of brain injury rather than its cause.[80]

8.4.2 Repeated brief ischemia

Brief repeated episodes of ischemia in term lambs lead to damage in the cortex, basal ganglia, and white matter (see Chapter 4). The equivalent pattern of injury involving predominantly cortex and deep nuclei is seen in term human infants suffering severe asphyxia at birth.[55,56] During difficult delivery repeated episodes of asphyxia are caused by strong uterine contractions and reflected in abnormal CTG tracings.

In these infants there may be sufficient time for some redistribution of blood flow and the characteristic pattern of damage involves the cerebral hemispheres.[78,81] Multi-organ involvement with cardiac or renal damage is usually also present.

8.4.3 Acute near-total asphyxia

A pattern of brain damage involving extensive brainstem and basal ganglia necrosis with relative cortical sparing is seen in acute near-total asphyxia[75,77,81] or following cardiac arrest.[82] Although occasionally seen in adults it is much more common in infants and has been described as early as 24 weeks of intrauterine life.[35] The brainstem nuclei develop very early in intrauterine life and are not uncommonly damaged in vascular accidents in the earliest months of gestation.[83,84]

Pathological findings are distinctive with symmetrical bilateral necrosis of brainstem nuclei extending uniformly from the lowest levels of the medulla through the midbrain to the thalamus and basal ganglia of the brain. The cortex shows only minimal damage.

8.5 ARTERIAL INFARCTION

Arterial infarction describes death of the tissue supplied by a single large artery, and may also sometimes be described as a 'stroke'.

The middle cerebral arteries are most commonly involved; the left more frequently than the right, possibly due to its straighter course allowing easier access of emboli to the small brain vessels. The posterior cerebral arteries are involved next in order of frequency followed by the anterior cerebral, carotid, and vertebro-basilar systems.[85]

Most arterial infarctions occur in prenatal life, although premature infants are at high risk in the pre- and perinatal periods.[86] There is usually no identified predisposing cause, Apgar scores are high

---

Case 8.12 (Plate 38)

This baby was born at 28 weeks of gestation; at 4 weeks of age he suffered from necrotizing enterocolitis and collapsed with intestinal perforation. One week after this, MRI scan demonstrated high signal in the thalamus and putamen with edema of the posterior limb of the internal capsule. The baby died at 8 weeks.

Case 8.13 (Plate 39)

Pregnancy and delivery were normal. The baby had an apneic attack 1 hour after birth and seizures from day 1. Severe epilepsy was treated by hemispherectomy at 11 years of age.

---

and there is no encephalopathy or asphyxia. The usual presenting feature is neonatal seizures. Early histological examination may show thrombus within the artery but in most cases the arteries are normal.[87]

The damaged area is initially edematous, but as necrotic tissue is resorbed the infarcted area becomes cystic. Examination of the edges of the cyst may give pathological clues to the timing of the initial infarction; malformations in the borders of the cyst indicate an early intrauterine origin before cortex formation is complete.[47]

These histological features indicate that the cortex was damaged in early development, before 21 weeks of gestation.

8.6   PORENCEPHALY

This, by definition, implies a hole in the cerebral tissues and is most appropriately used to describe a well-circumscribed cystic lesion in the brain which most commonly results from arterial infarction, but hemorrhage may cause similar appearances. The term is often used more widely in practice, particularly among neuroradiologists who have extended the term to include unilateral enlargement of the lateral ventricles, assuming direct communication with a pre-existing porencephalic cyst.

8.7   SCHIZENCEPHALY

This term describes a cleft in the brain wall extending from the ventricle to the meningeal surface. The cleft may be lined by cortex which is often dysplastic. The initial description by Yakovlev and Wadsworth[88] considered that these were malformations rather than destructive lesions, and demonstration of mutations in the homeobox gene *EM X 2* in some patients with schizencephaly lent some support to this hypothesis.[42] However, there is also an argument that these lesions are probably due to tissue loss from infarction. The cyst resulting from a full thickness brain wall infarction may collapse to give a linear cleft-like appearance both

on scans and on naked eye examination of the brain (Plate 40). Barkovich and Kjos showed multiple areas of cortical damage in patients with schizencephaly, further supporting a vascular or ischemic etiology.[89]

8.8   HYDRANENCEPHALY

This term denotes destruction of major parts of both cerebral hemispheres, usually the bilateral territories of supply of the middle cerebral arteries.

The infarction does not necessarily result from bilateral obstruction of the middle cerebral arteries but may result from profound hypotension or reduction of flow in the anterior circulation (from the internal carotid arteries) with the posterior circulation providing sufficient supply to spare limited areas of the cerebral hemispheres in the frontal poles, parasagittal areas, and occipital poles.

A precipitating event is rarely identified and babies with this catastrophic form of brain damage may have normal deliveries and early life, presenting with neurological symptoms weeks or months later.[90] It is likely that many of these infants may have been predisposed to their damage by chronic placental insufficiency with redistribution of blood away from the anterior part of the brain.[78]

8.9   HYDROCEPHALUS

Hydrocephalus is the dilatation of the fluid-filled spaces within or over the surface of the brain due to increase in volume or pressure of CSF in the cranial cavity (Plate 41). CSF is formed within the ventricles from fronds of vascular tissue called the choroid plexus. It flows through the ventricles to bathe the surface of the brain and is resorbed into the venous system at the arachnoid granulations, specialized structures in the sagittal venous sinus which runs in the membranes over the surface of the midline of the brain.

Hydrocephalus may be caused by excessive production of CSF, failure of drainage of CSF or obstruction to its flow. Excess CSF production is the result of overgrowth of the choroid plexus and is rare. Failure of drainage occurs when the arachnoid granulations fail to develop, which is also extremely rare, or more frequently when they are damaged by blood or inflammatory debris in the CSF. This form of hydrocephalus, in which CSF flow is preserved between the ventricles and the brain surface, is termed 'communicating hydrocephalus'. Obstruction to CSF flow commonly occurs in the narrow parts of the ventricular system, the foramina of Monro which drain the lateral ventricles, the aqueduct of Sylvius, a long narrow channel through the brainstem, or at the exit foramina of the fourth ventricle. When these pathways are blocked the proximal part of the ventricular system will enlarge, causing 'obstructive hydrocephalus'.

Compensatory ventricular dilatation 'hydrocephalus ex vacuo' results from loss of brain tissue or its failure to grow.

8.9.1 Causes of hydrocephalus

The causes of hydrocephalus are multiple and vary with developmental stage at onset. Thus hydrocephalus is associated with malformations in many early fetal cases; in later intrauterine life destructive lesions and hemorrhage are more common while cases developing in postnatal life are more likely to be associated with infections such as meningitis or brain tumors.

8.9.2 Fetal ventriculomegaly

This may be identified on routine anomaly scans by 17–20 weeks of gestation and needs to be verified by careful measurement on repeated scans as ventricular size normally undergoes considerable change at this developmental stage.

About one-quarter of cases so identified have isolated ventriculomegaly and most will have a good prognosis and develop normally. Review of published series shows that cognitive or motor delay is usually mild and occurs in about 9 percent of isolated mild ventriculomegaly. With increasing ventricular size (>12 mm) the likelihood of abnormal postnatal neurodevelopment increases to 23 percent.[91] The majority of cases of fetal ventriculomegaly have other associated malformations, either in the central nervous system or elsewhere, and chromosome anomalies are identified in 30 percent of these.[92]

Only 10 percent of fetal ventriculomegaly is due to hemorrhage or infection,[93] the majority are malformative or idiopathic.

8.9.3 Obstructive hydrocephalus

Obstructure hydrocephalus is due to obstruction to the normal flow of CSF and the clinical and imaging manifestations depend on the site of obstruction.

8.9.3.1 Obstruction of the foramina of Monro

The foramina of Monro are narrow channels that drain CSF from the lateral ventricles into the midline third ventricle. Obstruction in fetal and neonatal life is uncommon but may occur acutely in intraventricular hemorrhage. In later life colloid cysts are more frequent causes of acute hydrocephalus due to obstruction of the foramina of Monro.

8.9.3.2 Obstruction of the aqueduct of Sylvius

The aqueduct of Sylvius is a long narrow channel running through the brainstem connecting the third and fourth ventricles. It originates as the central canal of the primitive neural tube in the midbrain and brainstem.

'Aqueduct stenosis' is responsible for one-third of cases of hydrocephalus diagnosed in the neonatal period,[94] but hydrocephalus due to aqueduct stenosis may not present until months or even years later. Obstruction of the aqueduct causes dilatation of the lateral and third ventricles; the fourth ventricle is unaffected. The causes of aqueduct stenosis are many and are not readily identified on brain scans.

Primary aqueduct stenosis is thought to be an early malformation in which the aqueduct is represented by multiple, narrow, or branching channels. The absence of reactive gliosis or damage to the ependyma suggests that this is a genuine malformation but does not preclude very early inflammation. In animal models viral infection and vitamin deficiency can produce similar changes.[95]

Lateral compression may produce aqueduct narrowing with the aqueduct forming a thin slit running in a dorsoventral direction. This may be secondary to hydrocephalus when the dilated ventricles cause enlargement of the hemispheres which then compress the aqueduct.[96] External compression of the aqueduct may also result from an intrinsic brainstem tumor or from a mass such as an aneurysm of the vein of Galen overlying the brainstem.

Much more commonly in pathological practice aqueduct obstruction results from inflammation of the ependymal lining of the aqueduct. Blood, infection, and tissue debris in the CSF cause inflammation of the delicate ependymal lining of the CSF pathways. The damaged ependyma is shed and replaced by proliferating glial cells which may bulge into and narrow the lumen. Regenerative attempts by the ependyma are seen as rosettes or strips of ependyma buried in the exuberant glial tissue. When hemorrhage is the initial cause of the inflammation, iron or hemosiderin pigment may be detected in the gliotic tissues and persist for many months or years (see Plate 28).

8.9.3.3 *Obstruction of the exit foramina of the fourth ventricle*

The lateral foramina (foramina of Lushka) or midline foramen (foramen of Magendie) draining the fourth ventricle may also be obstructed by inflammation or blood clot (see Plate 27). Obstruction here causes dilatation of the fourth, third, and lateral ventricles and the aqueduct of Sylvius is patent or enlarged.

8.9.3.4 *'Encysted' fourth ventricle*

Occasionally the fourth ventricle is the primary site of infection or hemorrhage. The outflow foramina may be blocked in addition to the distal part of the aqueduct, thus closing off all outflow from the ventricle and producing a cyst. Continued CSF production from choroid plexus in the fourth ventricle leads to its enlargement. The large fourth ventricle may produce secondary compression of the midbrain.

8.9.4 Communicating hydrocephalus

In communicating hydrocephalus the CSF spaces both within the brain but also over its surface are enlarged. Very rarely arachnoid granulations are congenitally absent and CSF cannot drain into the venous system. More frequently blood clot or inflammation following infection in the meninges may obstruct the arachnoid granulations. CSF drainage is also impaired in sinus thrombosis.

8.9.5 Hydrocephalus ex vacuo

Parenchymal tissue loss from infarction or hemorrhage will result in increased ventricular volume (Plate 42). This may be symmetrical as in diffuse periventricular leukomalacia or asymmetrical as following unilateral germinal matrix hemorrhage associated with parenchymal venous infarction.

Ventricular dilatation is seen in a number of brain malformation syndromes without obstruction of CSF flow and it may be assumed that the large CSF spaces result from failure of normal brain growth.

8.10 REFERENCES

1 de-Vries LS, Eken P, Groenendaal F, Rademaker KJ, Hoogervorst B, Bruinse HW. Antenatal onset of haemorrhagic and/or ischaemic lesions in preterm infants: prevalence and associated obstetric variables. *Archives of Disease in Childhood Fetal and Neonatal Edition* 1998; **78**: F51–56.

2 Ferriero DM, Dempsey DA. Impact of addictive and harmful substances on fetal brain development. *Current Opinion in Neurology* 1999; **12**: 161–6.

3 Clarren SK, Alvord-EC J, Sumi SM, Streissguth AP, Smith DW. Brain malformations related to prenatal exposure to ethanol. *Journal of Pediatrics* 1978; **92**: 64–7.

4 Squier W, Hope PL, Lindenbaum RH. Neocerebellar hypoplasia in a neonate following intra-uterine exposure to anticonvulsants. *Developmental Medicine and Child Neurology* 1990; **32**: 737–42.

5 Pharoah PO, Connolly KJ. Iodine and brain development. *Developmental Medicine and Child Neurology* 1995; **38**: 464–9.

6 Lima FR, Goncalves N, Gomes FC, de-Freitas MS, Moura NV. Thyroid hormone action on astroglial cells from distinct brain regions during development. *International Journal of Developmental Neuroscience* 1998; **16**: 19–27.

7 Johnston MV, Goldstein GW. Selective vulnerability of the developing brain to lead. *Current Opinion in Neurology* 1998; **11**: 689–93.

8 Janzer RC, Friede RL. Hypotensive brain stem necrosis or cardiac arrest encephalopathy? *Acta Neuropathologica Berlin* 1980; **50**: 53–6.

9 Ferrer I. Cell death in the normal developing brain, and following ionizing radiation, methyl-azoxymethanol acetate, and hypoxia-ischaemia in the rat. *Neuropathology and Applied Neurobiology* 1996; **22**: 489–94.

10 Zellweger H. The cerebro-hepato-renal (Zellweger) syndrome and other peroxisomal disorders. *Developmental Medicine and Child Neurology* 1987; **29**: 821–9.

11 Dobyns WB. Agenesis of the corpus callosum and gyral malformations are frequent manifestations of nonketotic hyperglycinemia. *Neurology* 1989; **39**: 817–20.

12 Yager JY, McClarty BM, Seshia SS. CT-scan findings in an infant with glutaric aciduria type I. *Developmental Medicine and Child Neurology* 1988; **30**: 808–11.

13 Bussel J, Kaplan C. The fetal and neonatal consequences of maternal alloimmune thrombocytopenia. *Baillières Clinical Haematology* 1998; **11**: 391–408.

14 Thorarensen O, Ryan S, Hunter J, Younkin DP. Factor V Leiden mutation: an unrecognized cause of hemiplegic cerebral palsy, neonatal stroke, and placental thrombosis. *Annals of Neurology* 1997; **42**: 372–5.

15 Anderson JM, Milner RD, Strich SJ. Effects of neonatal hypoglycaemia on the nervous system: a pathological study. *Journal of Neurology, Neurosurgery and Psychiatry* 1967; **30**: 295–310.

16 Banker BQ. The neuropathological effects of anoxia and hypoglycemia in the newborn. *Developmental Medicine and Child Neurology* 1967; **9**: 544–50.

17 Auer RN, Wieloch T, Olsson Y, Siesjo BK. The distribution of hypoglycemic brain damage. *Acta Neuropathologica Berlin* 1984; **64**: 177–91.

18 Spar JA, Lewine JD, Orrison-WW J. Neonatal hypoglycemia: CT and MR findings. *American Journal of Neuroradiology* 1994; **15**: 1477–8.

19 Chiu NT, Huang CC, Chang YC, Lin CH, Yao WJ, Yu CY. Technetium-99m-HMPAO brain SPECT in neonates with hypoglycemic encephalopathy. *Journal of Nuclear Medicine* 1998; **39**: 1711–13.

20 Traill Z, Squier M, Anslow P. Brain imaging in neonatal hypoglycaemia. *Archives of Disease in Childhood Fetal and Neonatal Edition* 1998; 79: F145–7.

21 Vannucci RC, Mujsce DJ. Effect of glucose on perinatal hypoxic-ischemic brain damage. *Biology of the Neonate* 1992; **62**: 215–24.

22 Brown GK, Squier MV. Neuropathology and pathogenesis of mitochondrial diseases. *Journal of Inheritable Metabolic Disorders* 1996; **19**: 553–72.

23 Samson JF, Barth PG, de-Vries JI *et al.* Familial mitochondrial encephalopathy with fetal ultrasonographic ventriculomegaly and intracerebral calcifications. *European Journal of Pediatrics* 1994; **153**: 510–16.

24 Toti P, De-Felice C, Palmeri ML, Villanova M, Martin JJ, Buonocore G. Inflammatory pathogenesis of cortical polymicrogyria: an autopsy study. *Pediatric Research* 1998; **44**: 291–6.

25 Leviton A, Paneth N. White matter damage in preterm newborns – an epidemiologic perspective. *Early Human Development* 1990; **24**: 1–22.

26 Yoon BH, Jun JK, Romero R *et al.* Amniotic fluid inflammatory cytokines (interleukin-6, interleukin-1beta, and tumor necrosis factor-alpha), neonatal brain white matter lesions, and cerebral palsy. *American Journal of Obstetrics and Gynecology* 1997; **177**: 19–26.

27 Dammann O, Leviton A. Brain damage in preterm newborns: might enhancement of developmentally regulated endogenous protection open a door for prevention? *Pediatrics* 1999; **104**: 541–50.

28 Kadhim H, Tabarki B, Verellen G, De-Prez C, Rona AM, Sebire G. Inflammatory cytokines in the pathogenesis of periventricular leukomalacia. *Neurology* 2001; **56**: 1278–84.

29 Rutherford MA, Pennock JM, Cowan FM, Dubowitz LM, Hajnal JV, Bydder GM. Does the brain regenerate after perinatal infarction? *European Journal of Paediatric Neurology* 1997; **1**: 13–17.

30 Marin PM. Developmental neuropathology and impact of perinatal brain damage. II: White matter lesions of the neocortex. *Journal of Neuropathology and Experimental Neurology* 1997; **56**: 219–35.

31 Rutherford MA, Pennock JM, Counsell SJ *et al.* Abnormal magnetic resonance signal in the internal capsule predicts poor neurodevelopmental outcome in infants with hypoxic-ischemic encephalopathy. *Pediatrics* 1998; **102**: 323–8.

32 Pettmann B, Henderson CE. Neuronal cell death. *Neuron* 1998; **20**: 633–47.

33 Yue X, Mehmet H, Penrice J *et al.* Apoptosis and necrosis in the newborn piglet brain following transient cerebral hypoxia-ischaemia. *Neuropathology and Applied Neurobiology* 1997; **23**: 16–25.

34 Del-Bigio MR, Becker LE. Microglial aggregation in the dentate gyrus: a marker of mild hypoxic-ischaemic brain insult in human infants. *Neuropathology and Applied Neurobiology* 1994; **20**: 144–51.

35 Roessmann U, Gambetti P. Pathological reaction of astrocytes in perinatal brain injury. Immunohistochemical study. *Acta Neuropathologica Berlin* 1986; **70**: 302–7.

36 Squier M, Chamberlain P, Zaiwalla Z *et al.* Five cases of brain injury following amniocentesis in mid-term pregnancy. *Developmental Medicine and Child Neurology* 2000; **42**: 554–60.

37 Marks KA, Mallard CE, Roberts I, Williams CE, Gluckman PD, Edwards AD. Nitric oxide synthase inhibition attenuates delayed vasodilation and increases injury after cerebral ischemia in fetal sheep. *Pediatric Research* 1996; **40**: 185–91.

38 Mallard EC, Rees S, Stringer M, Cock ML, Harding R. Effects of chronic placental insufficiency on brain development in fetal sheep. *Pediatric Research* 1998; **43**: 262–70.

39 Evrard P, Marret S, Gressens P. Environmental and genetic determinants of neural migration and postmigratory survival. *Acta Paediatrica Supplement* 1997; **422**: 20–6.

40 Marin-Padilla M. Review of perinatal brain damage, repair and neurological sequelae in the premature born infant. *International Pediatrics* 1995; Suppl 1: 26–33.

41 Norman MG, McGillivray MG, Kalousek DK, Hill A, Poskitt KJ. Crossing the midline. In: *Congenital malformations of the brain.* Oxford: Oxford University Press, 1995: 309–31.

42 Walsh CA. Genetic malformations of the human cerebral cortex. *Neuron* 1999; **23**: 19–29.

43 Marques DM, Harmant-van RG, Landrieu P, Lyon G. Prenatal cytomegalovirus disease and cerebral microgyria: evidence for perfusion failure, not disturbance of histogenesis, as the major cause of fetal

cytomegalovirus encephalopathy. *Neuropediatrics* 1984; **15**: 18–24.

44 Mischel PS, Nguyen LP, Vinters HV. Cerebral cortical dysplasia associated with pediatric epilepsy. Review of neuropathologic features and proposal for a grading system. *Journal of Neuropathology and Experimental Neurology* 1995; **54**: 137–53.

45 Barth PG. Disorders of neuronal migration. *Canadian Journal of Neurological Sciences* 1987; **14**: 1–16.

46 Ferrer I, Catala I. Unlayered polymicrogyria: structural and developmental aspects. *Anatomy and Embryology Berlin* 1991; **184**: 517–28.

47 Williams RS, Ferrante RJ, Caviness VSJ. The cellular pathology of microgyria. A Golgi analysis. *Acta Neuropathologica Berlin* 1976; **36**: 269–83.

48 Inder TE, Huppi PS, Zientara GP *et al*. The postmigrational development of polymicrogyria documented by magnetic resonance imaging from 31 weeks' postconceptional age. *Annals of Neurology* 1999; **45**: 798–801.

49 DeReuck J, Chattha AS, Richardson EPJ. Pathogenesis and evolution of periventricular leukomalacia in infancy. *Archives of Neurology* 1972; **27**: 229–36.

50 Kuban KC, Gilles FH. Human telencephalic angiogenesis. *Annals of Neurology* 1985; **17**: 539–48.

51 Borch K, Greisen G. Blood flow distribution in the normal human preterm brain. *Pediatric Research* 1998; **43**: 28–33.

52 Miyawaki T, Matsui K, Takashima S. Developmental characteristics of vessel density in the human fetal and infant brains. *Early Human Development* 1998; **53**: 65–72.

53 McDonald JW, Althomsons SP, Hyrc KL, Choi DW, Goldberg MP. Oligodendrocytes from forebrain are highly vulnerable to AMPA/kainate receptor-mediated excitotoxicity. *Nature Medicine* 1998; **4**: 291–7.

54 Kinney HC, Back SA. Human oligodendroglial development: relationship to periventricular leukomalacia. *Seminars in Pediatric Neurology* 1998; **5**: 180–9.

55 Rutherford M, Pennock J, Schwieso J, Cowan F, Dubowitz L. Hypoxic-ischaemic encephalopathy: early and late magnetic resonance imaging findings in relation to outcome. *Archives of Disease in Childhood Fetal and Neonatal Edition* 1996; **75**: F145–51.

56 Barkovich AJ. MR and CT evaluation of profound neonatal and infantile asphyxia. *American Journal of Neuroradiology* 1992; **13**: 959–72.

57 Azzarelli B, Meade P, Muller J. Hypoxic lesions in areas of primary myelination. A distinct pattern in cerebral palsy. *Child's Brain* 1980; **7**: 132–45.

58 Squier M, Keeling JW. The incidence of prenatal brain injury. *Neuropathology and Applied Neurobiology* 1991; **17**: 29–38.

59 Gaffney G, Squier MV, Johnson A, Flavell V, Sellers S. Clinical associations of prenatal ischaemic white matter injury. *Archives of Disease in Childhood Fetal and Neonatal Edition* 1994; **70**: F101–6.

60 Spinillo A, Capuzzo E, Stronati M, Ometto A, De-Santolo A, Acciano S. Obstetric risk factors for periventricular leukomalacia among preterm infants. *British Journal of Obstetrics and Gynaecology* 1998; **105**: 865–71.

61 Gilles FH, Leviton A, Dooling ED. *The developing human brain, growth and epidemiologic neuropathology.* Boston: John Wright, 1983:

62 de-Vries LS, Dubowitz LM, Pennock JM, Bydder GM. Extensive cystic leucomalacia: correlation of cranial ultrasound, magnetic resonance imaging and clinical findings in sequential studies. *Clinical Radiology* 1989; **40**: 158–66.

63 Erasmus C, Blackwood W, Wilson J. Infantile multicystic encephalomalacia after maternal bee sting anaphylaxis during pregnancy. *Archives of Disease in Childhood* 1982; **57**: 785–7.

64 Larroche JC. Fetal encephalopathies of circulatory origin. *Biology of the Neonate* 1986; **50**: 61–74.

65 Golden JA, Gilles FH, Rudelli R, Leviton A. Frequency of neuropathological abnormalities in very low birth weight infants. *Journal of Neuropathology and Experimental Neurology* 1997; **56**: 472–8.

66 Pryds O, Edwards AD. Cerebral blood flow in the newborn infant. *Archives of Disease in Childhood Fetal and Neonatal Edition* 1996; **74**: F63–9.

67 Meek JH, Tyszczuk L, Elwell CE, Wyatt JS. Low cerebral blood flow is a risk factor for severe intraventricular haemorrhage. *Archives of Disease in Childhood Fetal and Neonatal Edition* 1999; **81**: F15–18.

68 Hansen A, Leviton A, Paneth N *et al*. The correlation between placental pathology and intraventricular hemorrhage in the preterm infant. *Pediatric Research* 1998; **43**: 15–19.

69 de-Vries LS, Rademaker KJ, Groenendaal F *et al*. Correlation between neonatal cranial ultrasound, MRI in infancy and neurodevelopmental outcome in infants with a large intraventricular haemorrhage with or without unilateral parenchymal involvement. *Neuropediatrics* 1998; **29**: 180–8.

70 Volpe JJ. Intraventricular hemorrhage in the premature infant – current concepts. Part I. *Annals of Neurology* 1989; **25**: 3–11.

71 Azzarelli B, Caldemeyer KS, Phillips JP, DeMyer WE. Hypoxic-ischemic encephalopathy in areas of primary myelination: a neuroimaging and PET study. *Pediatric Neurology* 1996; **14**: 108–16.

72 Rutherford MA, Pennock JM, Schwieso JE, Cowan FM, Dubowitz LM. Hypoxic ischaemic encephalopathy: early magnetic resonance imaging findings and their evolution. *Neuropediatrics* 1995; **26**: 183–91.

73 Norman MG. On the morphogenesis of ulegyria. *Acta Neuropathologica Berlin* 1981; **53**: 331–2.

74 Vannucci RC, Vannucci SJ. A model of perinatal hypoxic-ischemic brain damage. *Annals of the New York Academy of Sciences* 1997; **835**: 234–49.

75 Roland EH, Poskitt K, Rodriguez E, Lupton BA, Hill A. Perinatal hypoxic-ischemic thalamic injury:

clinical features and neuroimaging. *Annals of Neurology* 1998; **44**: 161–6.

76 Cohen M, Roessmann U. In utero brain damage: relationship of gestational age to pathological consequences. *Developmental Medicine and Child Neurology* 1994; **36**: 263–8.

77 Barkovich AJ, Sargent SK. Profound asphyxia in the premature infant: imaging findings. *American Journal of Neuroradiology* 1995; **16**: 1837–46.

78 Pasternak JF. Hypoxic-ischemic brain damage in the term infant. Lessons from the laboratory. *Pediatric Clinics of North America* 1993; **40**: 1061–72.

79 Ment LR, Schwartz M, Makuch RW, Stewart WB. Association of chronic sublethal hypoxia with ventriculomegaly in the developing rat brain. *Brain Research and Developmental Brain Research* 1998; **111**: 197–203.

80 Freud S. *Infantile cerebral paralysis* (Translation by Russin LA of *Die Infantile cerebrallahmung*. Wein: A. Holder, 1887). Coral Gables, Florida: University of Miami Press, 1968.

81 Pasternak JF, Gorey MT. The syndrome of acute near-total intrauterine asphyxia in the term infant. *Pediatric Neurology* 1998; **18**: 391–8.

82 Janzer RC, Friede RL. Hypotensive brain stem necrosis or cardiac arrest encephalopathy? *Acta Neuropathologica Berlin* 1980; **50**: 53–6.

83 Dambska M, Laure KM, Liebhart M. Brainstem lesions in the course of chronic fetal asphyxia. *Clinical Neuropathology* 1987; **6**: 110–15.

84 Lipson AH, Gillerot Y, Tannenberg AE, Giurgea S. Two cases of maternal antenatal splenic rupture and hypotension associated with Moebius syndrome and cerebral palsy in offspring. Further evidence for a utero placental vascular aetiology for the Moebius syndrome and some cases of cerebral palsy. *European Journal of Pediatrics* 1996; **155**: 800–4.

85 Baumann RJ, Carr WA, Shuman RM. Patterns of cerebral arterial injury in children with neurological disabilities. *Journal of Child Neurology* 1987; **2**: 298–306.

86 Uvebrant P. Hemiplegic cerebral palsy. Aetiology and outcome. *Acta Paediatrica Scandinavica Supplement* 1988; **345**: 1–100.

87 Larroche JC. *Developmental pathology of the neonate*. Amsterdam: Excerpta Medica, 1977.

88 Yakovlev PI, Wadsworth RC. Schizencephalies: a study of the congenital clefts in the cerebral mantle. I. Clefts with fused lips. *Journal of Neuropathology and Experimental Neurology* 1946; **5**: 116–30.

89 Barkovich AJ, Kjos BO. Nonlissencephalic cortical dysplasias: correlation of imaging findings with clinical deficits. *American Journal of Neuroradiology* 1992; **13**: 95–103.

90 Rorke LB. *Pathology of perinatal brain injury*. New York: Raven Press, 1982.

91 Vergani P, Locatelli A, Strobelt N *et al*. Clinical outcome of mild fetal ventriculomegaly. *American Journal of Obstetrics and Gynecology* 1998; **178**: 218–22.

92 Schwanitz G, Schuler H, Gembruch U, Zerres K. Chromosomal findings in fetuses with ultrasonographically diagnosed ventriculomegaly. *Annals of Genetics* 1993; **36**: 150–3.

93 Roume J, Larroche JC, Razavi EF, Gonzales M, Migne G, Mulliez N. Fetal hydrocephalus. Clinical significance of associated anomalies and genetic counseling: a pathological approach. *Genetic Counseling* 1990; **1**: 185–96.

94 Volpe JJ. Neural tube formation and prosencephalic development. In: *Neurology of the newborn*, 3rd edn. Philadelphia: WB Saunders, 1995: 3–42.

95 Williams B. Aqueduct stenosis. In: Smith W, Cavanagh JB eds. *Recent advances in neuropathology*, 2nd edn. Edinburgh: Churchill Livingstone, 1982.

96 Landrieu P, Ninane J, Ferriere G, Lyon G. Aqueductal stenosis in X-linked hydrocephalus: a secondary phenomenon? *Developmental Medicine and Child Neurology* 1979; **21**: 637–42.

9 Antenatal assessment of fetal health

Paul Chamberlain

The methods used for the antenatal assessment of fetal health have changed dramatically in the last 10–15 years. Collection of maternal urine for estimation of urinary estrogen excretion and measurement of maternal serum human placental lactogen levels have been replaced by dynamic ultrasound-based methods of fetal assessment.[1] Principal among these is real-time ultrasound scanning. Real-time ultrasound scanning allows for assessment of fetal structure, growth, behavioral activity (biophysical profile scoring), and the intrauterine environment (amniotic fluid volume assessment). Additionally, real-time ultrasound can also be used to assess fetal number, gestational age, and presentation, to locate the position of the placenta, and to guide invasive prenatal diagnostic techniques.

In addition, other ultrasound-based methods of fetal assessment are also frequently used for antenatal assessment of fetal well-being. Antenatal recording of fetal heart rate behavior (the cardiotocograph or CTG) is probably the most commonly used method for assessment of fetal health in late pregnancy. Doppler blood flow assessment of a variety of fetal blood vessels has also been reported to have a role to play in the assessment of fetal health, again mainly in late pregnancy.

The purpose of this chapter is to review the methods of fetal health assessment currently in use and to identify newer tests and techniques that may have a role to play in this area in the future.

9.1 REAL-TIME ULTRASOUND ASSESSMENT OF THE FETUS

The development of high-quality real-time ultrasound scanners over the last 15–20 years has revolutionized the practice of obstetrics and has brought about the development of the subspecialty of fetal medicine. With current equipment it is now possible to image the fetus in real-time (e.g. to see movement). Current picture quality allows for the visualization and assessment of fine detail of the fetus (both structural and behavioral).

As noted above, with real-time ultrasound it is now possible to assess a variety of parameters of the fetus. These include the following:

- *Fetal structure* Antenatal identification of structural congenital anomalies is now one of the principal goals of obstetric scanning in the first half of pregnancy.
- *Fetal growth* Antenatal identification of disorders of fetal growth is an important use of real-time ultrasound, particularly in the latter half of pregnancy.

- *Gestational age* Gestational age is uncertain in as many as 20 percent of all obstetric patients.[2] Ultrasound scanning has an important role in clarifying this uncertainty, especially in early pregnancy.
- *Fetal behavior* Documentation of the fetal biophysical profile score (BPS) is one of the commonest investigations used in assessment of fetal risk in high-risk pregnancies. This test, which comprises simultaneous assessment of fetal movement (FM), fetal tone (FT), fetal breathing movements (FBM), amniotic fluid volume (AFV), and the CTG, is used primarily in the latter half of pregnancy.
- *Assessment of placental position and fetal presentation* Antepartum hemorrhage is a not infrequent complication of late pregnancy.[3] It carries significant risks to both mother and fetus. Ultrasound scanning to determine the position of the placenta is the first investigation used in this circumstance. Clinical examination to confirm fetal presentation in late pregnancy is important in order to decide upon the most appropriate method for subsequent delivery. Again ultrasound scanning has a pivotal role in this regard.
- Ultrasound scanning is now a prerequisite when performing *invasive fetal diagnostic procedures* such as amniocentesis, chorion villus sampling (CVS), and fetal blood sampling (FBS). In addition, shunt placement for the treatment of specific fetal abnormalities is also dependent on accurate ultrasound guidance.

Each of the above six uses of ultrasound scanning will be reviewed in more detail.

9.1.1 Antenatal assessment of fetal structure

Congenital abnormality, either structural and/or chromosomal, is one of the principal causes of perinatal death. In screened populations such deaths are the most frequent cause of perinatal mortality.[4] Until the advent of high-resolution real-time ultrasound accurate antenatal identification of the congenitally abnormal fetus was difficult and usually fortuitous. However, nowadays with modern scanning techniques antenatal identification of major (and some minor) congenital abnormalities is the norm.[5] This is particularly so when structural fetal abnormality is considered.

In general, the more obvious the structural defect is postnatally the more likely it is to be diagnosed prenatally. For example, anencephaly, where

Table 9.1 Structures assessed at routine abnormality scanning

Cranial vault
Cerebellum
Cerebral ventricles
Face/lip
Neck and spine
Heart and lungs
Anterior abdominal wall
Stomach and bowel
Kidneys and bladder
Upper and lower limbs
Hands and feet

the fetal cranial vault is absent in whole or in part, is much more likely to be identified prenatally than Down's syndrome, where gross fetal anatomy may be normal. In current obstetric practice, routine screening for structural fetal abnormality by ultrasound scanning is offered to all pregnant women.[6] This examination, termed a routine fetal abnormality scan, is usually performed between 19 and 21 weeks gestation. The examination is performed by trained sonographers (medical, radiography, or nursing) and consists of a detailed and sequenced assessment of fetal anatomy from 'head-to-toes'. The structures/organs listed in Table 9.1 are usually assessed.

Detailed fetal abnormality scanning is a sequenced search to confirm fetal structural normality and to identify fetal structural abnormality, if present. In experienced hands an examination usually takes 15–20 minutes to complete. In addition to the skill and experience of the sonographer, the quality of the scanning equipment, the size of the patient and the position of the fetus all have a bearing on the accuracy of the examination. The larger the patient, the poorer the equipment and the more unfavorable the fetal position in the uterus, the less accurate the examination is likely to be. In addition, as noted above, the greater the deviation from normal fetal anatomy the more likely the defect is to be detected.

Congenital abnormalities open to antenatal diagnosis using ultrasound can be most simply classified by the organ system(s) they affect. Some of the most frequently identified abnormalities are shown in Table 9.2.

In general, the antenatal sonographic appearances of specific structural congenital abnormality are well recognized but wide overlap in scan findings can occur.[6] For example, the absence of the cranial vault on scanning is virtually diagnostic of anencephaly (Fig. 9.1). The presence of an

Table 9.2 Classification of congenital abnormalities most frequently identified at antenatal scanning[a]

Defect category	Example Major	Minor
Neural tube	Anencephaly Spina bifida	Choroid plexus cyst –
Cardiovascular	Hypoplastic left heart syndrome Fallot's tetralogy	Intracardiac echogenic focus Ventricular septal defect
Gastrointestinal	Diaphragmatic hernia Omphalocele	Gastroschisis
Genito-urinary	Multicystic kidney disease Posterior urethral valve syndrome	Hydronephrosis/renal pelvic dilatation
Musculoskeletal	Thanatophoric dysplasia Osteogenesis imperfecta	Talipes Clinodactyly

[a]Many other abnormalities (both major and minor) are open to prenatal diagnosis using ultrasound.

associated spina bifida makes the diagnosis absolute. These findings are associated with a specific recurrence risk (1 in 20 in the absence of vitamin supplementation and specific prophylaxis with folic acid) in future pregnancies.[7] However, sometimes the fetal head may be absent in other conditions (e.g. acardia acephaly) with a significantly different recurrence risk (low). Similarly, the ultrasound appearance of a ventral wall defect such as an omphalocele is well recognized but the prognosis can vary widely depending on associated abnormalities.[8] An uncomplicated omphalocele is usually associated with good long-term outcome following neonatal surgery. Conversely, omphaloceles are known to have an association with chromosome abnormalities (usually trisomy 13 or 18) in approximately 20 percent of cases. If present, an associated chromosomal abnormality significantly alters prognosis. Both trisomies 13 and 18 are lethal conditions.

As noted in Table 9.2 not all structural abnormalities discovered at antenatal scanning are associated with a poor outcome. Gastroschisis, for example, is a minor structural abnormality affecting the umbilicus where small bowel loops float freely in the amniotic fluid. This abnormality usually occurs in young mothers (less than 25 years) and is usually an isolated defect. Prognosis following surgery, which is normally performed within 24 hours of delivery, is, in general, good.[8]

In recent years a number of subtle abnormalities known to be associated with, but not diagnostic of, chromosomal abnormalities have been described. These subtle abnormalities are termed 'soft markers' and include choroid plexus cysts, renal pelvic dilatation, echogenic foci in the heart, nuchal thickening, talipes, and clinodactyly.[9] The finding of these 'soft markers' on anomaly scanning raises the possibility of associated chromosomal abnormality, but in most instances the outcome for the pregnancy will be normal. When present, especially in the older mother, amniocentesis or another form of invasive prenatal diagnosis is usually offered to rule out associated abnormality. 'Soft marker' scanning is a major cause of anxiety in prenatal diagnosis practice and frequently the anxiety generated during early pregnancy is not relieved until after birth or, sometimes, until later in infancy/childhood.[10]

A review of the full range of structural and chromosomal fetal abnormalities open to prenatal diagnosis using ultrasound scanning is beyond the remit of this chapter. Suffice it to say that as experience with the technique increases, the spectrum of abnormality open to prenatal diagnosis also increases. Current research into new genetic techniques, particularly molecular biology, may further increase this spectrum of diagnosable fetal abnormality in the future.

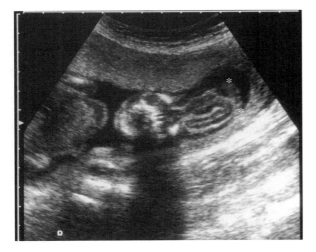

Figure 9.1 Coronal view of the fetal head at 18 weeks gestation. Note brain tissue extruding to the right from the fetal head (marked with *).

9.1.2 Antenatal assessment of fetal growth

Disorders of fetal growth occur primarily in the latter half of pregnancy, usually in the last trimester of pregnancy. Traditionally the antenatal detection of abnormal fetal growth has been based upon clinical examination.[2] The finding of a uterus either smaller or larger than would be expected for the stage of pregnancy is usually the first suggestion that fetal growth may not be normal. Clinical examination is unreliable in making this differentiation in the majority of cases.

With ultrasound scanning it is now possible to measure a number of parameters of fetal growth and to plot them on standard curves throughout gestation.[11–14] Commonly obtained fetal measurements include the biparietal diameter (BPD), head circumference (HC), abdominal circumference (AC), and femur length (FL).[11–14] If gestational age is known, the growth of the fetus as indicated by these growth parameters can be assessed. The importance of accurate knowledge of gestational age in assessment of disorders of fetal growth cannot be overemphasized.

Traditionally, three different types of fetal growth disorder have been recognized, although considerable overlap can occur. These were originally described in newborn infants by Villar and Belizan:[15]

- *Type 1 – Chronic or proportionate intrauterine growth retardation (IUGR) or the normal small fetus* In this type of growth abnormality both the fetal head and abdomen are equally affected so that the fetus is proportionately small. When HC and AC measurements obtained by ultrasound are plotted on standard growth curves both fall below the normal centile ranges. This type of growth abnormality may be seen in fetuses that are small because that is their genetic or constitutional predisposition – both mother and father may also be small. However, this type of growth disturbance may also be seen in fetuses that suffer an early insult that affects ultimate size. Chromosomal abnormalities such as trisomies 13 and 18 and, classically, triploidy may present in this way.
- *Type 2 – Subacute or disproportionate IUGR* In this type of abnormality fetal growth proceeds normally up until approximately 26–30 weeks gestation. At this stage in gestation growth in fetal AC tails off while growth in HC continues. As fetuses achieve two-thirds of their ultimate length and only one-third of their ultimate weight in the first two trimesters of pregnancy these fetuses are long and thin with a relatively large head. This type of growth abnormality may occur in fetuses of mothers who develop severe maternal pregnancy complications (such as pre-eclampsia) in the late mid-trimester of pregnancy.
- *Type 3 – Acute IUGR* Growth in the third trimester is predominantly characterized by increase in fetal weight. Acute IUGR, also termed 'late flattening' growth disorder usually occurs in complicated pregnancies in the late third trimester or even in the post-mature fetus. While growth in length is minimally affected, growth in fetal weight is markedly reduced, resulting in an extremely long, thin fetus. This type of growth disturbance is frequently complicated by oligohydramnios and abnormal cord Doppler indices and can result in unexpected intrauterine fetal death. These associated findings will be discussed later in this chapter.

'Late flattening' type growth abnormalities identified in the late third trimester are usually an indication for serious consideration of early delivery.

9.1.2.1 'Customized' growth curves

More recently, individualized patterns of fetal growth have been described.[16] This method of fetal growth assessment using 'customized fetal growth charts' takes into consideration a variety of maternal physiologic parameters (height, weight at booking, parity, ethnic group, weight, and gestational age at delivery of previous children) specific to individual mothers. The attraction of this method lies in its ability to individualize fetal growth as opposed to the more traditional methods described above which are based upon pooled data from many different patients and different pregnancies. Widespread experience of 'customized fetal growth charts' has not yet been reported and as such it currently remains an attractive research tool.

The accuracy of ultrasound in identification of the abnormally grown fetus varies depending upon the outcome criteria used.[17] Traditionally, a birthweight less than the 10th percentile has been considered as indicative of IUGR. Using this definition sensitivity, specificity, positive and negative predictive values of 84.3 percent, 98.1 percent, 86 percent, and 97.9 percent respectively have been reported.[17] This definition of growth retardation has, however, been seriously criticized as it does not take many important determinants of fetal growth (ethnic group, size, etc.) into consideration. In addition, the interval between the last ultrasound examination and subsequent delivery is important – examinations distant from delivery (greater than 2 weeks) are less likely to identify IUGR accurately than examinations performed more adjacent to delivery.[17]

It is also possible using ultrasound scanning to provide an estimated fetal weight (EFW) with a degree of accuracy that is clinically useful.[18] EFW is determined from formulae incorporating ultrasound measurements, especially AC and, to a lesser degree, HC and FL. Again determinations made close to delivery are likely to be more accurate than more distant observations. EFW is particularly useful in the small fetus (500–2500 g weight range) where estimates are likely to be within 10 percent of actual birthweight in greater than 90 percent of cases if made by an experienced sonographer. EFW in large/macrosomic fetuses is less useful clinically and the degree of error is likely to be greater. This is, in part, due to the technical difficulties encountered when measuring larger fetuses and, in part, due to the limitations in ultrasound transducer size.

Assessment of fetal growth in multiple pregnancy is more complicated than growth assessment in singleton pregnancies. Similar ultrasound measurements are taken in multiple pregnancies as in singleton pregnancies but examinations are usually more difficult. Not uncommonly one fetus might partially obscure its co-twin. Additionally, malpresentation is more frequent than in singleton pregnancies. Similarly, AFV and fetal Doppler examinations are more difficult to perform in multiple pregnancy. In twin pregnancies an inter-twin difference in EFW of >25 percent is usually considered indicative of abnormal growth.[19]

Finally, it is important to recognize that most of the commonly used fetal growth charts were derived from populations of singleton pregnancies. The application of singleton growth charts to multiple pregnancies is not the optimum method for assessment of normal or abnormal fetal growth in multiple pregnancy.

9.1.3 Assessment of gestational age

As noted earlier, gestational age (GA) may be uncertain in as many as 20 percent of all pregnancies.[2] All obstetric decisions are based upon accurate knowledge of how advanced a pregnancy is at any given time. Ultrasound scanning is the principal tool for determination of GA in pregnancies where uncertainty exists. In general, the earlier the assessment of GA is made the more accurate and clinically useful the ultrasound determination will be.[20]

GA is determined by ultrasound scanning from empirically determined relationships between a variety of ultrasound measurements and the duration of pregnancy. Crown–rump length (CRL) is the most accurate measurement for assessment of GA, especially when obtained in the first trimester.[20] In general, CRL is accurate to within 3 days if obtained at this time. Later in pregnancy BPD is the most frequently used measurement to derive GA, although other measurements (HC, FL) can also be used. BPD is accurate to within 10 days if obtained before 20 weeks gestation.[21] Measurements obtained later in pregnancy are less accurate – BPD is only accurate to within 3–4 weeks when obtained in the third trimester.

Accurate assessment of GA is particularly important for many reasons. In early pregnancy, screening tests for Down's syndrome (and other chromosome abnormalities) must be performed at the correct stage of pregnancy.[22] In late pregnancy, inadvertent early delivery is associated with significant complications of prematurity, some of which may be fatal. This is particularly true when elective delivery by cesarean section is planned.

9.1.4 Assessment of fetal behavior – the biophysical profile score

The BPS is one of the most frequently used tests of fetal health in the latter half of pregnancy. This method of fetal assessment is classically used for evaluation of fetal health in high-risk pregnancies, especially those complicated by maternal hypertension/pre-eclampsia, suspected fetal growth retardation, post-maturity, and other maternal medical conditions.

BPS consists of real-time ultrasound documentation of four fetal biophysical variables: fetal movements (FM), fetal tone (FT), fetal breathing movements (FBM), and assessment of amniotic fluid volume (AFV) combined with fetal heart rate activity assessed by cardiotocogram (CTG). This testing method was first described by Manning *et al.* in 1979.[23] Each variable is arbitrarily assigned a score of 2 if normal and 0 if abnormal. A totally normal score is therefore 10 and a totally abnormal score is 0. Intermediate scores of 8, 6, 4 and 2 result,

Table 9.3 Biophysical profile scoring – criteria for normal and abnormal scores[a]

Variable	Normal criteria	Abnormal criteria
Score	2	0
Fetal breathing movements	At least 30 seconds of FBM in a 30-minute interval	Less than 30 seconds FBM
Fetal movement	3 discrete body/limb movements in a 30-minute interval	Less than 3 discrete body/limb movements
Fetal tone	At least 1 episode of active limb/spine extension/flexion	No episodes of limb/spine extension/flexion
Amniotic fluid volume	At least 1 cord-free pocket of amniotic fluid >2 cm	No cord-free pocket of amniotic fluid >2 cm
Cardiotocogram	⩾ 3 accelerations in fetal heart rate of >15 seconds duration and >15 beats per minute (bpm)	<3 accelerations in fetal heart rate of >15 seconds and >15 bpm
Total score	10	0

[a]Revised criteria.[24]

depending on the number of abnormal variables present. The criteria for each variable are shown in Table 9.3.

In contrast to scanning for assessment of fetal structure and growth, both of which are longer-term indices of fetal health and development, BPS testing is best regarded as an immediate method of assessment of fetal well-being. A normal BPS indicates normal fetal health and well-being at the time of testing. Normal fetal structure and growth, in contrast, suggest normal fetal development over a longer term.

BPS testing is primarily used for the day-to-day assessment of fetal health in complicated pregnancies as they approach viability. A normal BPS of 10 or 8 (including normal AFV) is an indication of normal fetal health, and by inference, normal fetal oxygenation.[23,24] Delivery on the basis of a normal BPS is not indicated. In contrast, a BPS of 4 or less is usually interpreted as indicative of fetal compromise and is an indication for serious consideration of delivery, except in cases of extreme prematurity. A BPS of 6 (including normal AFV) is interpreted as an equivocal score and is an indication for re-testing within 24 hours if delivery does not take place.

As noted above, the presence of normal AFV is an integral part of BPS testing. Abnormal AFV regardless of the BPS is an indication for consideration of delivery.[25] This is because of the close association between reduced AFV and abnormal perinatal outcome, especially perinatal death and IUGR.[25] AFV assessment within the context of the BPS involves measurement of the largest cord-free

pocket of amniotic fluid seen at real-time scanning. While other methods of AFV assessment are available, in particular the amniotic fluid index (AFI), wide experience with AFI testing in high-risk obstetric populations has not yet been reported.[26]

There is currently a wide experience of BPS testing in high-risk pregnancy populations. This experience has shown that as the BPS falls from 10 or 8 (including normal AFV) to 0 the incidence of pregnancy complications rises.[27,28] This is true not only for perinatal mortality but also for perinatal morbidity. The incidences of congenital abnormality, fetal asphyxia as indicated by low Apgar scores, meconium aspiration and cord pH at birth, IUGR, and admission to the Special Care Baby Unit all rise as the BPS falls.

Interpretation of the CTG, either alone or within the context of the BPS, will be discussed below.

9.1.5 Assessment of placental position and fetal presentation

9.1.5.1 Placental position

Antepartum hemorrhage (APH) is a frequent complication of pregnancy.[3] Causes of APH include placental abruption, where bleeding occurs from a normally positioned placenta; placenta previa, where bleeding occurs from a placenta implanted in the lower uterine segment or across the internal cervical os; or a local cervical or vaginal cause. Before a vaginal examination is performed following an APH it is important to rule out placenta previa by ultrasound scanning.

The appearances of placenta previa are characteristic, with the placenta occupying the lower uterine segment.[29] With a full maternal bladder the exact relationships between the internal cervical os and the leading (lower) edge of the placenta can be determined. Usually the placenta implants on either the anterior or posterior uterine walls or high in the uterine fundus. If ultrasound scanning shows the lower uterine segment to be free of placental tissue, a placenta previa can be confidently excluded.

Once a placenta previa has been excluded, local vaginal examination can be safely performed to exclude a cervical or vaginal cause. The absence of a local lower genital tract lesion on clinical examination and an ultrasound scan excluding a placenta previa allow a diagnosis of a placental abruption to be made in cases of APH.

APH, whether due to a placenta previa or placental abruption, is a significant complication of pregnancy. Management depends on the cause of the APH, the gestation at which it occurs, and degree of bleeding. APH after fetal lung maturity has been achieved (approximately 36 weeks gestation) is easily managed by delivering the fetus. However, when APH occurs remote from term, conservative management may be appropriate if maternal and fetal conditions are stable. If either maternal or fetal condition is not satisfactory emergency delivery may be required.

The widespread use of ultrasound scanning in recent years has greatly increased our understanding of conditions such as placenta previa and placental abruption. Placental 'migration' during the late second and third trimesters is now widely recognized as a normal event in pregnancy.[30] APH from a placenta previa may occur at 28–30 weeks gestation and ultrasound scanning may reveal a placenta covering the internal cervical os at this gestation. However, with advancing GA, 'migration' of the placenta out of the lower uterine segment in association with development of the lower uterine segment may occur, allowing for normal vaginal delivery at term.

9.1.5.2 Fetal presentation

Similarly, ultrasound scanning in late pregnancy is very useful in confirming fetal presentation at or near term. This is especially so in the obese patient where clinical examination may be difficult or impossible. EFW determination in the clinically large fetus or in cases of breech presentation may also be useful in deciding on the most appropriate mode of delivery. Intrapartum scanning may also be performed to determine fetal presentation after the delivery of the first twin in twin pregnancies.

9.1.6 Invasive prenatal diagnosis

The development of high-quality real-time ultrasound scanners which are portable, relatively cheap, and suitable for near patient care has been directly responsible for the development of the subspecialty of fetal medicine. This is particularly true when the invasive prenatal diagnostic procedures of amniocentesis, fetal blood sampling (FBS), and chorion villus sampling (CVS) are considered. All of these three techniques require accurate needle placement close to the fetus in the amniotic space (amniocentesis), in the fetal umbilical cord (FBS), or in the developing placenta (CVS).[31] These procedures are primarily performed to obtain fetal tissue for karyotyping. The most common reason for karyotyping is for advanced maternal age as the incidence of Down's syndrome increases as maternal age advances. Abnormal ultrasound scan findings, such as those noted previously, are the second most common reason for fetal karyotyping.[10]

The choice of invasive procedure depends in part on the condition suspected and the GA at which the procedure is being performed. For example, maternal age karyotyping is usually performed at 15–18 weeks gestation and at this stage amniocentesis is the safest and most reliable test. Amniocentesis carries a procedure-related loss rate of approximately 1 in 200.[31] Prenatal diagnosis performed earlier in pregnancy is usually done by CVS. This procedure is frequently performed when structural fetal abnormalities are identified in the first trimester (abnormal nuchal translucency) or in patients with a history of being at risk from specific conditions (e.g. cystic fibrosis, spinal muscular atrophy). CVS has a procedure-related loss rate of approximately 1 in 50 and also may occasionally be associated with limb and other abnormalities in the exposed fetus.[32,33] FBS is performed from 18 to 19 weeks gestation onwards and usually again in specific circumstances. The principal indication for FBS is in cases of suspected fetal anemia, especially in Rhesus or other antibody sensitization or in cases of suspected or proven fetal infection (e.g. parvovirus). FBS carries a 1 percent procedure-related loss rate.

Other invasive fetal needling procedures may occasionally be required. Thoraco-amniotic shunt placement may occasionally be of value in treating congenital pleural effusions and vesico-amniotic shunt placement may have a similar small role in treatment of posterior urethral valve syndrome.[34] Such procedures are relatively infrequent in prenatal diagnosis practice and are best confined to a few specialist centers with experience in them.

9.2   THE CARDIOTOCOGRAPH

CTG monitoring is probably the single most frequent test of fetal well-being performed in the third trimester. The test is based upon the demonstration of accelerations in fetal heart rate (FHR) in response to FM. Traditionally, CTG tracings have been interpreted visually and the standard definition of a reactive (normal) trace has been the demonstration of two or more accelerations in FHR of greater than 15 beats per minute and lasting for greater than 15 seconds in a 40-minute interval.[35] Accelerations in FHR in response to FM are interpreted as being indicative of an intact central nervous system and, by definition, of fetal normoxia. Prior to the widespread use and availability of real-time ultrasound scanning, antepartum CTG monitoring was the most widely employed method for assessment of fetal health in high-risk pregnancies. While a normal test result was associated with a very low incidence of abnormal pregnancy outcome the converse of abnormal outcome with an abnormal test was less precise. False-positive test rates of 50–80 percent or higher have been reported, thus significantly limiting the use of CTGs.[36] False-positive tests have in part been due to difficulties or variability in test interpretation by different observers.

In recent years computerized techniques for interpretation of the antenatal FHR have been described.[37] This method of FHR analysis avoids the pitfalls of visual analysis and is based primarily upon assessment of baseline FHR variability. Baseline FHR variability is considered to reflect the moment-to-moment modulation of FHR behavior by higher nervous centers. As with FHR accelerations in visual analysis of CTG traces, normal baseline variability is thought to reflect normal fetal oxygenation and an intact central nervous system. To date, large clinical trials of computerized versus visually analyzed CTGs have not been performed.

9.3   FETAL DOPPLER BLOOD FLOW STUDIES

Most modern ultrasound scanners now also allow for the performance of Doppler blood flow studies on a variety of fetal and maternal blood vessels. The technique, based upon measurement of blood flow velocity waveforms, can be used to assess the relative resistance to blood flow in a variety of fetal vessels. The most commonly measured index is the resistance index (RI) although other indices (e.g. pulsatility index (PI)) have also been studied.

Umbilical blood flow has been the most frequently studied part of the fetal circulation. In normal pregnancy peripheral vascular resistance falls, resulting in a fall in the RI.[38] In complicated pregnancies, especially in IUGR pregnancies, peripheral vascular resistance rises resulting in an increase in the RI. In extreme circumstances blood flow may cease and occasionally be reversed during diastole. A rising RI is an indication for close fetal monitoring; absent or reversed flow should prompt consideration of delivery.[39]

With color-flow Doppler it is also now possible to study blood flow in a variety of other fetal vessels. Cerebral blood flow has been closely assessed, with the middle cerebral artery (MCA) being the most frequently studied intracranial blood vessel.[40] In the normal fetus MCA flow gradually increases with advancing GA and it increases significantly in IUGR. This is thought to explain in part the brain-sparing effect that is frequently seen in that condition. In the hypoxic fetus MCA flow further increases but with advancing hypoxia flow eventually falls. This is thought to indicate developing cerebral edema.[41]

9.4   LITIGATION IN OBSTETRIC SCANNING

Obstetric scanning is now, as noted above, one of the most frequently employed diagnostic tests in clinical practice. In line with the increased usage of scanning there has been a parallel increase in litigation. The principal area where litigation occurs is in cases where congenital abnormality has not been diagnosed prenatally.

In reviewing these cases the following questions should be asked:

1   Was the defect open to identification prenatally?
2   Was the examination performed at the correct time and in the correct manner?

3 Was the person performing the scan appropriately trained and was the equipment optimum?

9.4.1 Defect open to identification prenatally?

In general, the larger the physical defect the more likely it is to be open to accurate diagnosis prenatally. Anencephaly is a prime example of a defect that should be diagnosed antenatally. Conversely, small, low, skin-covered spina bifida lesions are very difficult to diagnose prenatally.

9.4.2 Examination performed at the correct time and in the correct manner?

The optimum time for identifying structural congenital abnormality is at the anomaly scan (19–21 weeks). Examinations performed before this time are more likely to be associated with a missed diagnosis or a misdiagnosis. It is important to remember that sometimes defects may present after the anomaly scan stage. This is particularly true of some intracranial abnormalities (tumors, isolated hydrocephalus) and some congenital diaphragmatic hernias as well as other abnormalities. Additionally, congenital cardiac disease is, in general, poorly detected at routine anomaly scanning.

Recently, the Royal College of Obstetricians and Gynaecologists has produced protocols for the performance of routine obstetric scans in the UK.[42] Recommendations are made both for the manner in which fetal measurements are to be obtained and for the structures to be assessed at individual examinations. These protocols represent a significant attempt by the profession to ensure uniformity of practice and a minimum standard among those professionals who scan. These protocols or similar guidelines should be adopted by all hospitals where obstetric scanning is performed in the near future.

9.4.3 Training and equipment optimum?

It is now widely accepted that people performing obstetric scanning should be appropriately trained and that they should be using appropriate and current equipment. There are recognized courses that both medical and paramedical personnel (nurses, radiographers) should have completed before they scan independently. Appropriate supervision should also be in place. This is usually either by an obstetrician who has specialized in fetal medicine or obtained a postgraduate diploma in obstetric scanning or by a radiologist with a similar postgraduate diploma.

Ultrasound equipment has also undergone many improvements since first introduced into clinical practice 15–20 years ago. The lifespan of current commercially available scanners is approximately 5–7 years and they should be upgraded as necessary.

Other important issues in obstetric scanning include record-keeping and the storage of ultrasound images obtained at examination. In general, images are not routinely taken unless an abnormality is noted. Images are usually obtained on heat-sensitive paper. Occasionally, Polaroid film may be used. As these images only represent a 'snapshot' of what is a dynamic examination, they are, in general, a poor record. There is currently a trend in many scanning units to routinely take images of a variety of fetal structures. This is in part motivated by the possibility of future litigation but also it forms a part of an ongoing internal quality control audit. Should abnormalities be found at delivery the images can be reviewed and the quality of the examination assessed. It is likely in future that all images will be digitally stored and that paper images of the type that are currently taken will cease.

Obstetric scan reports are most frequently either typed or recorded on a pro-forma sheet. This is particularly true of the anomaly scan. The anomaly scan report usually consists of a checklist of structures which are recorded as normal, abnormal, or not seen. The reports are generated directly by the examining sonographer, either medical or radiographer, or other. This is a major difference from radiology practice where all examinations are routinely checked by the supervising consultant before being 'signed out'. Non-medical sonographers are therefore independent practitioners responsible for their own reports. This independence of practice increases the importance that such sonographers are appropriately trained and supervised.

Litigation can occur in other areas of obstetric scanning practice also. Failure to identify multiple pregnancies in the second trimester of pregnancy and failure to accurately diagnose placenta previa have both resulted in litigation. The adoption of clear scanning protocols and the use of up-to-date scanning equipment by appropriately trained staff should help to keep such events to a minimum.

9.5 CONCLUSIONS

It is evident from the above that real-time ultrasound has many roles to play in the antenatal assessment of fetal health. From early in pregnancy GA can be confirmed with a high degree of accuracy and in mid-gestation normal fetal anatomy can be documented. In late pregnancy fetal growth can be assessed, the fetal presentation and the location of the placenta identified. In high-risk pregnancies fetal well-being can be assessed using both the CTG and the BPS, and, if growth is abnormal, by Doppler blood flow studies. Combining tests in this way allows for a more comprehensive assessment of fetal health to be made than is possible using single tests (e.g. CTG only). Combining tests is not only more accurate in identifying fetal ill-health but is also more accurate in identifying the healthy fetus, thus reducing both false-positive and false-negative tests and reducing the incidence of unnecessary intervention.

9.6 REFERENCES

1 Fay T, Grudzinskas G. The biochemical evaluation of placental function. In: Spencer J ed. *Fetal monitoring: physiology and techniques of antenatal and intrapartum assessment*. Kent: Castle House Publications, 1989: 85–90.

2 Dewhurst J. The fetus. In: *Integrated obstetrics and gynaecology*. Oxford: Blackwell Scientific, 1972: 153–4.

3 Dewhurst J. Antepartum haemorrhage. In: *Integrated obstetrics and gynaecology*. Oxford: Blackwell Scientific, 1972: 248–58.

4 Chamberlain P, O'Dwyer E, Slattery M, O'Malley M. Sonographic assessment of fetal health: antenatal identification of the structurally anomalous fetus. *Irish Medical Journal* 1987; **80**: 113–16.

5 Nyberg D, Mahony B, Pretorius D. *Diagnostic ultrasound of fetal anomalies – text and atlas*. St Louis: Mosby-Year Book, 1990.

6 RCOG Working Party. *Routine ultrasound screening in pregnancy – protocol, standards and training, Supplement to ultrasound screening for fetal abnormalities*. London: Royal College of Obstetricians and Gynaecologists, 2000.

7 Daly S, Mills J, Molley A *et al*. Minimum effective dose of folic acid for food. Fortification to prevent neural tube defects. *Lancet* 1997; **350**: 1666–9.

8 Boyd P, Bhattacharjee A, Chamberlain P. Prenatal diagnosis and long term follow-up of anterior abdominal wall defects over 11 years. *Archives of Disease in Childhood Fetal and Neonatal Edition* 1998; **78**: F209–13.

9 Snijders R, Nicolaides K. *Ultrasound markers for fetal chromosomal defects*. London: Parthenon Publishing Group, 1996.

10 Boyd P, Chamberlain P, Hicks N. 6 year experience of prenatal diagnosis in an unselected population in Oxford, UK. *Lancet* 1998; **352**: 1577–81.

11 Altman D, Chitty L. Charts of fetal size: 1. Methodology. *British Journal of Obstetrics and Gynaecology* 1994; **101**: 29–34.

12 Chitty L, Altman D, Henderson A, Campbell S. Charts of fetal size: 2. Head measurements. *British Journal of Obstetrics and Gynaecology* 1994; **101**: 35–43.

13 Chitty L, Altman D, Henderson A, Campbell S. Charts of fetal size: abdominal measurements. *British Journal of Obstetrics and Gynaecology* 1994; **101**: 125–31.

14 Chitty L, Altman D, Henderson A, Campbell S. Charts of fetal size: femur length. *British Journal of Obstetrics and Gynaecology* 1994; **101**: 132–5.

15 Villar J, Belizan J. The timing factor in the pathophysiology of intrauterine growth retardation syndrome. *Obstetrical and Gynecological Survey* 1982; **37**: 499–505.

16 Gardosi J. Customised fetal growth charts. *British Medical Ultrasound Society Bulletin* 1994; **2**: 20–4.

17 Chamberlain P. Composite sonographic assessment of fetal health. *Current Opinion in Obstetrics and Gynecology* 1992; **4**: 256–63.

18 Smith T. A comparison of formulae for the estimation of fetal weight. *British Medical Ultrasound Society Bulletin* 1992; **64**: 36–8.

19 Chamberlain P, Murphy M, Comerford H. How accurate is antenatal sonographic determination of birth weight discordancy in twins? *European Journal of Obstetrics, Gynaecology and Reproductive Biology* 1991; **40**: 91–6.

20 Hadlock F, Shah Y, Kanon D, Lindsey J. Fetal crown-rump length: re-evaluation of relation to menstrual age (5–18 weeks) with high-resolution real-time ultrasound. *Radiology* 1992; **182**: 501–5.

21 Hadlock F, Deter R, Harrist R, Park S. BPD: A critical re-evaluation of the relationship to menstrual age by means of real-time ultrasound. *Journal of Ultrasound Medicine* 1982; **1**: 97–104.

22 Wald N, Cuckle H, Densem J, Kennard A, Smith D. Maternal serum screening for Down's syndrome: the effect of routine ultrasound scan determination of gestationel age and adjustment for maternal weight. *British Journal of Obstetrics and Gynaecology* 1992; **99**: 144–9.

23 Manning F, Platt L, Sipos L. Antepartum fetal evaluation: development of a fetal biophysical profile score. *American Journal of Obstetrics and Gynecology* 1979; **136**: 787–95.

24 Manning F, Harman C, Morrison I *et al*. Fetal assessment based upon fetal biophysical profile scoring. IV.

Analysis of perinatal morbidity and mortality. *American Journal of Obstetrics and Gynecology* 1990; **162**: 703–9.

25 Chamberlain P, Manning F, Morrison I, Harman C, Lange I. Ultrasound evaluation of amniotic fluid volume. 1. The relationship of marginal and decreased amniotic fluid volumes to perinatal outcome. *American Journal of Obstetrics and Gynecology* 1983; **150**: 245–9.

26 Phelan J, Platt L, Yeh S. The role of ultrasound assessment of amniotic fluid volume in postdate pregnancy. *American Journal of Obstetrics and Gynecology* 1985; **139**: 254–8.

27 Manning F, Snidjers R, Harman C, Nicolaides K, Menticoglou S, Morrison I. Fetal Biophysical Profile Score. IV. Correlation with antepartum umbilical venous fetal pH. *American Journal of Obstetrics and Gynecology* 1993; **169**: 755–63.

28 Manning F, Harman C, Morrison I, Menticoglou S. Fetal assessment based on fetal biophysical profile scoring. III. Positive predictive accuracy of the very abnormal test (biophysical profile score = 0). *American Journal of Obstetrics and Gynecology* 1990; **162**: 398–402.

29 Bowie J, Rochester D, Cadkin A, Coohe W, Kunzmann A. Accuracy of placental localisation by ultrasound. *Radiology* 1978; **128**: 177.

30 Laing F. Ultrasound evaluation of obstetric problems relating to the.lower uterine segment and cervix. In: Fleischer A, Romero R, Manning F, Jeanty P, James E eds. *The principles and practice of ultrasonography in obstetrics and gynecology.* Connecticut: Appleton and Lange, 1991: 487–500.

31 Royal College of Obstetricians and Gynaecologists. *Amniocentesis.* Guideline No. 8. London: RCOG, 2000.

32 Crane J. Sonographically guided chorionic villus sampling. In: Fleischer A, Romero R, Manning F, Jeanty P, James E eds. *Ultrasonography in obstetrics and gynecology.* Connecticut: Appleton and Lange, 1991: 429–37.

33 Firth H, Boyd P, Chamberlain P *et al.* Analysis of limb reduction defects in babies exposed to chorionic villus sampling. *Lancet* 1994; **343**: 1069–71.

34 Nicolaides K, Azar G. Thoraco-amniotic shunting. *Fetal Diagnostic Therapy* 1990; **5**: 153–64.

35 *Guidelines for perinatal care*, 4th edn. East Norwalk, Connecticut: V American College of Obstetricians and Gynecologists and American Academy of Pediatrics, 1997: 86–7.

36 Schifrin B, Clement D. Routine antepartum fetal heart rate monitoring. In: Spencer J ed. *Fetal monitoring: physiology and techniques of antenatal and intrapartum assessment.* Kent: Castle House Publications, 1989: 98–103.

37 Steyn D, Odendaal H. Computerised cardiotocography in a high-risk unit in a developing country – its influence on inter-observer variation and duration of recording. *South African Medical Journal* 1996; **86**: 172–5.

38 Gembruch U. Assessment of fetal circulatory state in uteroplacental insufficiency by Doppler ultrasound: which vessels are most practicable? *Ultrasound in Obstetrics and Gynecology* 1996; **8**: 77–81.

39 Ozcan T, Sbracia M, d'Ancona R, Copel J, Mari G. Arterial and venous Doppler velocimetry in the severely growth restricted fetus and associations with adverse perinatal outcome. *Ultrasound in Obstetrics and Gynecology* 1998; **12**: 39–44.

40 Twining P. Color flow Doppler in obstetrics. *British Medical Ultrasound Society Bulletin* 1992; **64**: 22–5.

41 Vyas S, Nicolaides K, Bower S, Campbell S. Middle cerebral artery flow velocity waveforms in fetal hypoxia. *British Journal of Obstetrics and Gynaecology* 1990; **97**: 797–803.

42 Royal College of Obstetricians and Gynaecologists. *Routine ultrasound screening in pregnancy – protocol, standards and training.* London: RCOG, 2000.

10 Clinical assessment of the neonate

David Evans and Malcolm Levene

Assessment of the neonate is based upon careful clinical examination as well as the use of sophisticated investigations and imaging techniques.

Clinical manifestations of cerebral injury differ in term and preterm infants due to the differing vulnerability of the brain to damage at different stages of development.

The extent of investigation may be limited in the very sick neonate, especially the sick preterm, by the condition of the infant and particularly if transfer to another unit is required.

Careful observation is a prerequisite to predicting outcome. Similarly, careful and detailed recording of all neonatal observations is essential for retrospective determination of the role of perinatal factors in children who subsequently suffer neurological impairment. The validity of predictive values and likelihood ratios in assessing outcome is discussed below.

10.1 HYPOXIC-ISCHEMIC INJURY

Hypoxia-ischemia describes a process characterized by hypoxemia with tissue ischemia and resultant hypercarbia and acidosis. Labor is a stressful time for the fetus, and an hypoxic-ischemic insult can occur when the physiological stress of labor is compounded by additional stresses, overwhelming the ability of the normal fetus to adapt. This situation can arise as a consequence of a number of etiologies: interruption of the umbilical circulation, altered placental gas exchange, reduced maternal perfusion or oxygenation, or failure to establish neonatal cardiopulmonary circulation after birth. When mature infants suffer intrapartum hypoxic-ischemic injury in this manner, it gives rise to a clinical syndrome recognized as 'birth asphyxia'. A similar presentation may occur in a previously compromised fetus unable to adapt to the physiological stresses of a normal labor. This is discussed in more detail later.

In the term infant, hypoxic-ischemic insults can result in a number of recognized patterns of infarction of the cortex, basal ganglion, and white matter.

Hypoxic-ischemic insults are poorly defined in the preterm infant. They are less likely to reflect solely intrapartum insults and are more likely to cause additional neurological compromise during antenatal and postnatal periods. An hypoxic-ischemic insult acting upon the immature brain is less likely to produce cortical injury and therefore the clinical features of encephalopathy. Moreover, the preterm neonate is at risk from additional insults arising in the perinatal period, such as infection, placental insufficiency, and neonatal cerebrovascular disturbances. These insults may confound or potentiate the influence of hypoxia-ischemia. Different pathological patterns of injury are found in the premature infant; in particular, the periventricular white matter appears more vulnerable to hypoxic-ischemic injury.

For these reasons, the section on hypoxic-ischemic injury will concentrate upon the clinical features manifest by a mature infant. Injuries occurring predominantly in the preterm infant will be described in the later sections on periventricular leukomalacia and germinal matrix hemorrhage-intraventricular hemorrhage.

10.1.1 Clinical features

10.1.1.1 Condition at birth

Virginia Apgar proposed a scoring system as a method of assessing an infant's condition at 1 minute of life.[1] This was later extended and involved reassessment at 5 minutes,[2] followed by repeated assessments every 5 minutes, if necessary. An hypoxic-ischemic insult in the period immediately preceding delivery can cause a depression of neonatal vital signs, resulting in a low or depressed Apgar score. Equating a low Apgar score with a significant hypoxic-ischemic injury in the majority of infants is unjustified and may be misleading for a number of reasons.

1 A transient episode of hypoxic-ischemic insult preceding delivery is common and the normal fetus is well adapted to cope with such 'physiological stress'. Many of these infants may only require minimal neonatal resuscitation and such transient insults are unlikely to result in significant injuries. This is borne out by the long-term follow-up studies of infants with transiently depressed Apgar scores demonstrating no increased risk of later neurodevelopmental impairment.[3]

2 Factors other than hypoxic-ischemic insults can cause depression of Apgar scores, for example prematurity, maternal anesthetic or analgesia.

3 Importantly, a normal Apgar score does not exclude significant hypoxic-ischemic injury, particularly if the insult occurs before the period immediately preceding delivery. The majority of children with cerebral palsy have normal Apgar scores of 7–10 at 5 minutes of life.

Nevertheless, as the period of depression of the Apgar score after birth becomes more prolonged, its specificity and predictive value in predicting subsequent death or neurodevelopmental impairment increase (Table 10.1).

10.1.1.2 Neonatal encephalopathy

Mature infants exposed to an hypoxic-ischemic insult demonstrate a stereotyped sequence of neurological features. The severity and the duration of this hypoxic-ischemic encephalopathy (HIE) appear to be related to the severity of the hypoxic-ischemic insult. Sarnat and Sarnat were the first to devise a clinical staging system, combined with EEG activity,[4] detailed in Table 10.2. Subsequently, a number of methods based upon the Sarnat scheme have been described, all of which use a similar three-stage scale.[5–8]

It is unclear to what extent preterm infants can manifest similar clinical features following hypoxic-ischemic insults, compared to term infants, although clinical features of HIE have been described in an infant of 31 weeks gestation.[9]

10.1.1.2.1 Mild (grade I) encephalopathy

There is no alteration in the conscious level although these infants may appear 'hyperalert', with staring (decreased frequency of blinking),

Table 10.1 Outcome associated with latest[a] very low Apgar score (0–3) in infants of birthweight >2500 g

Time (min)	Number liveborn	Death by 1 year (%)	Number known to 7 years	Cerebral palsy (%)	Predictive value for poor outcome (%)	Likelihood ratio
1	1729	3.1	1330	0.7	3.6	2.5
5	286	7.7	217	0.9	8.4	6.0
10	66	18.2	43	4.7	21.2	17.7
15	23	47.8	11	9.1	52.2	71.7
20	39	59.0	14	57.1	79.5	254

Overall prevalence of death and cerebral palsy = 1.5 percent.
Adapted from Nelson and Ellenberg.[3]
[a]Counts at each time include only those children with very low Apgar scores at that time and no later very low Apgar score.

Table 10.2 Sarnat staging system for hypoxic-ischemic encephalopathy[4]

	Mild (I)	Moderate (II)	Severe (III)
Level of consciousness	Hyperalert	Lethargic	Stuporose
Neuromuscular control			
Muscle tone	Normal	Mild hypotonia	Flaccid
Posture	Mild distal flexion	Strong distal flexion	Intermittent decerebration
Stretch reflexes	Overactive	Overactive	Decreased or absent
Segmental myoclonus	Present	Present	Absent
Complex reflexes			
Suck	Weak	Weak or absent	Absent
Moro	Strong: low threshold	Weak: incomplete; high threshold	Absent
Oculovestibular	Normal	Overactive	Weak or absent
Tonic neck	Slight	Strong	Absent
Autonomic dysfunction	Generalized sympathetic	Generalized parasympathetic	Both systems depressed
Pupils	Mydriasis	Miosis	Variable; often unequal; poor light reflex
Heart rate	Tachycardia	Bradycardia	Variable
Bronchial and salivary secretions	Sparse	Profuse	Variable
Gastrointestinal motility	Normal or decreased	Increased: diarrhea	Variable
Seizures	None	Common; focal or multifocal	Uncommon (excluding decerebration)

normal or decreased spontaneous motor activity and a lower threshold for all stimuli including the easily elicited Moro reflex. Passive limb tone is normal but the neck extensor muscle tone is increased relative to the flexors. The sucking reflex may be weak and encouragement to complete feeds may be necessary. Clinically apparent seizures do not occur. Recovery usually occurs within 48 hours, although Amiel-Tison and Ellison allow up to 7 days.[5]

10.1.1.2.2   Moderate (grade II) encephalopathy

Seizures occur commonly, beginning within the first 24 hours. They may be subtle or fragmentary but are relatively easily controlled. There is lethargy, hypotonia with reduced spontaneous movements and a higher threshold for primitive reflexes. A consistent feature is differential tone between the upper and lower limbs with the arms being relatively hypotonic and showing less spontaneous movement compared with the legs.[10] Autonomic dysfunction occurs with mainly parasympathetic responses including a relative bradycardia and constricted pupils. The sucking reflex is poor and tube feeding is often necessary. If recovery occurs, it may take several weeks, although some improvement is usual by the end of the first week.

10.1.1.2.3   Severe (grade III) encephalopathy

These neonates are comatose with hypotonia and no spontaneous movements. Respiratory support is often required because of poor respiratory effort. Tendon reflexes, primitive reflexes, and the suck reflex are often absent. The pupils are fixed and dilated. Seizures may be frequent, prolonged, and difficult to control pharmacologically, although in the most severe cases there may be no seizure activity and an isoelectric EEG. In the infants that do recover, a progression from hypotonia to extensor hypertonicity is observed.

10.1.1.2.4   Progression of encephalopathy

Infants with moderate and severe HIE follow a progression of clinical signs. Initially, the infant may breathe spontaneously at first and show increased tone and motor activity, before hypotonia becomes evident. Seizures appear, subtle at first, becoming more overt and the length of time they continue depends upon the severity of encephalopathy. Subsequently, signs of clinical recovery occur in some infants.

It may be necessary to exclude other conditions that can produce encephalopathic features, a number of which may coexist with hypoxia-ischemia (Table 10.3).

10.1.1.3   Multi-organ involvement

During hypoxia-ischemia, blood flow is redistributed in order to preserve circulation to the most vital organs, namely the brain, heart, and adrenals, at the expense of the kidneys, liver, and gastrointestinal tract. Therefore important systemic

Table 10.3 Differential diagnosis of early neonatal encephalopathy

Etiology	Investigation
Hypoxia-ischemia	
Infection	
Neonatal meningitis	Lumbar puncture, infection screen
Drug-related	
Maternal anesthesia/analgesia	
Maternal drug abuse	Maternal and neonatal urine for toxicology
CNS malformations	Ultrasound, MRI
Intracranial hemorrhage	CT, MRI
Metabolic	
Hypoglycemia	Glucose
Hyponatremia/hypocalcemia	Electrolytes
Amino acid and organic acidemias	Urine/plasma chromatography
Lactate acidemias	Serum/CSF lactate
Urea cycle disorders	Serum ammonia
Pyridoxine dependency	Therapeutic trial of pyridoxine (with EEG)

abnormalities often accompany hypoxic-ischemic encephalopathy and serve as a further marker of such an insult (Table 10.4). In a prospective study of 35 term infants with Apgar scores of 5 or less at 5 minutes and umbilical cord pH <7.20, 85 percent had evidence of non-CNS organ involvement; renal and cardiac dysfunctions were most commonly observed.[11]

10.1.2 Investigations

This section concentrates upon investigations that are of particular relevance to hypoxic-ischemic injury in term infants. Cerebral artery infarction and intracranial hemorrhage will be described in later sections.

10.1.2.1 Cranial ultrasound

Ultrasound is a readily portable cotside technique that can be used repeatedly on neonates without disrupting ongoing intensive care. Although it is most useful in the detection of germinal matrix hemorrhage-intraventricular hemorrhage and periventricular ischemic lesions, ultrasound can provide valuable information following an hypoxic-ischemic insult. Initially cerebral edema is recognized by a generalized increase in subcortical and periventricular echogenicity, indistinct sulci, and compression of the lateral ventricles. It is recognized that compression of the lateral ventricles alone is not abnormal at term; it has been reported in 60 percent of infants[12] but is considered abnor-

Table 10.4 Manifestations of non-CNS organ injury following an hypoxic-ischemic insult

System	Manifestation	Approximate incidence (%)[11]
Renal	Acute renal failure	55
	Hematuria/myoglobinuria	
	Transient oliguria/raised serum creatinine	
Cardiovascular	Reduced ventricular function	35
	Myocardial ischemia (ECG)	
	Papillary muscle necrosis	
Pulmonary	Persistent pulmonary hypertension	25
	Meconium aspiration	
Gastrointestinal	Abnormal motility and feed intolerance	
	Necrotizing enterocolitis	
Hematological	Disseminated intravascular coagulation	
Metabolic	Hyponatremia/inappropriate ADH	
	Hypoglycemia/hypocalcemia	
	Elevated liver enzymes/ammonia	
	Metabolic acidosis	

mal if persisting for more than 36 hours. The presence of cerebral edema may indicate a cerebral insult but the ultrasound appearances are of little prognostic significance. Ultrasound findings of more predictive value are seen following resolution of the cerebral edema. These include uniformly echogenic basal ganglia, representing severe basal ganglia injury,[13] and diffuse parenchymal echodensities which represent selective neuronal necrosis. With severe white matter injury, subcortical or periventricular cystic changes may become apparent by the second week (Fig. 10.1). Resolution of these cysts and ventricular dilatation secondary to subcortical and cortical atrophy occur over a period of months in surviving infants.[12] In a study using ultrasound examinations during the neonatal period in hypoxic-ischemic encephalopathy, the presence of patchy parenchymal echodensities, echogenic basal ganglia, cystic or early atrophic changes were associated with severe neurodevelopmental impairment.[14]

One of the major limitations of this technique is its inability to assess peripheral cortical injury,[12] particularly the occipital cortex. These limitations can be addressed to some extent by the ability of the occipital cortex to be imaged through the posterior fontanel[15] and the increased resolution of 10-MHz probes in detecting cortical echodensities associated with hypoxic-ischemic injury.[16]

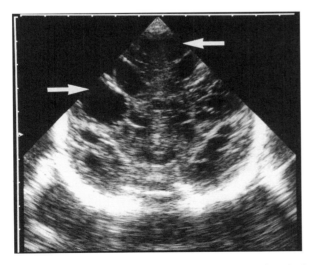

Figure 10.1 Hypoxic-ischemic injury. Ultrasound (coronal section) performed 3 weeks following a severe intrapartum hypoxic-ischemic insult showing extensive subcortical and periventricular cystic change.

10.1.2.2   Cerebral blood flow velocity (CBFV)

Using pulsed-wave duplex Doppler, blood flow velocity in an artery can be determined by analysis of the back scattered signal. It is practically difficult to estimate the angle of insonation and therefore difficult to calculate the absolute value of blood flow velocity. It is possible, however, to calculate ratios of systolic and diastolic values without measuring this angle. The Pourcelot's Resistivity Index (PRI) is most commonly calculated, which is the ratio between the difference in systolic (S) and diastolic (D) velocities to the systolic velocity (PRI = $[S - D]/S$). Using this technique to measure CBFVs in the cerebral arteries of asphyxiated neonates (usually the anterior cerebral artery), the PRI is taken as a measure of cerebrovascular resistance. A decrease in the cerebrovascular resistance, with a relative increase in the end diastolic flow velocity, is associated with a poor outcome, presumably reflecting an hypoxic-ischemic insult which has disrupted cerebrovascular autoregulation.[17,18] The predictive value of a PRI ratio less than 0.55 is high and appears by 24 hours of age,[17] although the prognostic value is much less if performed earlier.[19]

10.1.2.3   Magnetic resonance imaging (MRI)

MRI has only relatively recently emerged as a valuable neuro-imaging modality in neonates, compared with the enormous impact it has already had upon adult neurology. The neonatal brain has a relatively high water content, the T1 and T2 relaxation times are longer, which reduces the contrast between gray and white matter. Over the last 10 years, however, there have been considerable improvements in MRI systems performance, particularly the use of turbo-spin echo sequences with longer effective echo times. These have led to improved signal-to-noise ratios and enhanced gray/white matter differentiation.

In the first week following an hypoxic-ischemic insult, there is evidence of cerebral edema which, on T1-weighted sequences, is manifest by loss of gray/white matter contrast, loss of sulcal markings and extracerebral space and compression of the lateral ventricles. High signal intensity in the cortex on T1 ('cortical highlighting'), abnormal signal intensity in the subcortical white matter (low T1, high T2), and the basal ganglia abnormalities (high T1) can also be seen during the first

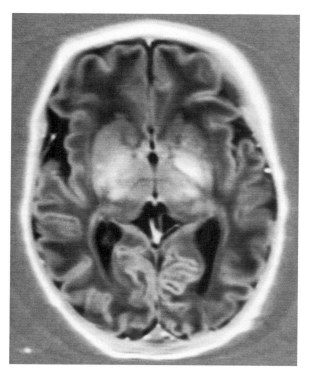

Figure 10.2 Hypoxic-ischemic injury. MR inversion recovery sequence (axial section) at 7 days of age. Abnormal high signal intensity is present in the basal ganglia; the subcortical white matter is of abnormally low signal intensity.

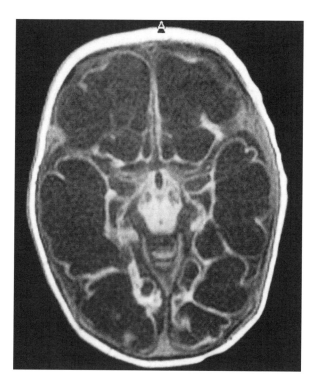

Figure 10.3 Hypoxic-ischemic injury. MR T1-weighted sequence (axial section) at 3 weeks of age. There is extensive cystic change throughout the white matter and shrinkage of the basal ganglia.

week (Fig. 10.2); these changes become more obvious at the end of the first week as the cerebral edema resolves.[20,21] Cortical highlighting, thought to represent neuronal necrosis, and abnormalities of the basal ganglia, particularly around the posterior limb of the internal capsule, are associated with progression to atrophic changes at 3 months and later adverse neurodevelopmental outcome.[22–24] Basal ganglia enhancement following the administration of MR contrast agent indicates a severe injury and is associated with a particularly poor outcome.[25] The appearance of early MRI abnormalities can be enhanced further by using diffusion-weighted techniques.[26]

In the second week, further loss of white matter occurs with subcortical breakdown and cyst formation.[21] The basal ganglia may also show breakdown, shrinkage, and cyst formation (Fig. 10.3). MRI is also excellent at demonstrating other pathologies associated with hypoxia-ischemia and birth trauma, such as focal cerebral infarction and intracranial hemorrhage, described in later sections.

Late MRI findings associated with a poor prognosis are: delayed myelination, reduction in white matter volume and ventricular dilatation, thinning of the corpus callosum, cortical atrophy, persisting basal ganglia signal change and extensive white matter signal change.[27] Patchy white matter abnormalities have recently been demonstrated in infants who are normal at 2 years, but who had mild (grade I) HIE, and may represent an injury which could have implications for school performance.[23]

10.1.2.4   Computerized tomography (CT)

CT provides important diagnostic information in identification of diffuse cortical injury (neuronal necrosis) and injury to the basal ganglia, although the superior anatomical definition provided by MRI is likely to lead to CT becoming less frequently used for this indication. The most important CT appearance in the second week following hypoxia-ischemia is a diffuse or global pattern of decreased density, thought to represent neuronal necrosis. In a study of 43 term asphyxiated infants, cerebral CT scans were performed in the first 2 weeks and the appearances classified as normal or decreased density (subdivided into patchy, diffuse or global).[28,29] Diffuse or global decreased density indicates a poor prognosis. Other studies have shown little correlation unless the scans are performed after the first week when cerebral edema, which has similar appearances but different prognostic implications, has subsided.[30,31]

The CT appearances of basal ganglia injury are areas of increased attenuation, particularly in the thalami. These may be due to infarction, edema, hemorrhage, or later calcification, some of which have been described pathologically.[32,33] In some cases, the thalamic areas show enhancement after contrast administration, suggestive of post-hypoxic-ischemic hypervascularity.[34] CT is an effective means of demonstrating any intracerebral hemorrhage that may coexist with hypoxic-ischemic injury.

10.1.2.5 *Electroencephalography (EEG) and evoked potentials (EPs)*

The EEG is useful for detecting seizures but it is the background, inter-ictal EEG activity which appears to have most bearing upon post-hypoxic-ischemic prognosis. Activities associated with a poor prognosis are: discontinuous, or burst-suppression, persistently low voltage states and status epilepticus.[35] Continuous computer EEG analyses, allowing quantification of the background activity, have demonstrated that the more discontinuous the activity, the worse the outcome.[36] Care must be taken when interpreting the EEGs of premature infants, however, as these normally show discontinuous activity with long interburst intervals, the duration of which is dependent upon gestational age.[37]

Unfortunately, access to EEG monitoring for extended periods is very limited in most clinical settings and the interpretation is very observer dependent, requiring considerable experience. A more convenient form of continuously monitoring seizure and background activity is to use the modified amplitude-integrated EEG or cerebral function monitor (CFM).[38,39] Cerebral activity is recorded from three electrodes and printed out on a compressed time-scale at the cot side. Seizures can be recognized by a period of higher voltage activity with a narrow range of voltages, compared to background activity (Fig. 10.4). CFM output needs to be interpreted with caution as artefacts, such as movement, will be erroneously recorded as cerebral activity, transient disturbances may be overlooked because of the compressed time-scale, and low-frequency seizures may be filtered. Several studies have used CFM within the first 6 hours following hypoxia-ischemia and have found the background activity to have a high predictive value for a poor prognosis.[40,41] Thus CFM is one of the earliest useful indicators of future outcome.

Evoked potentials (EPs) are a measure of the integrity of the sensory pathways being stimulated. In an asphyxiated infant, persistently absent auditory brainstem-evoked responses (ABRs) and visual evoked potentials (VEPs) are predictive of sensorineural hearing loss and visual impairment, respectively.[42,43] Although technically difficult, somatosensory evoked potentials (SEPs) are useful in predicting motor impairment because of the close proximity of the motor and sensory axons in the

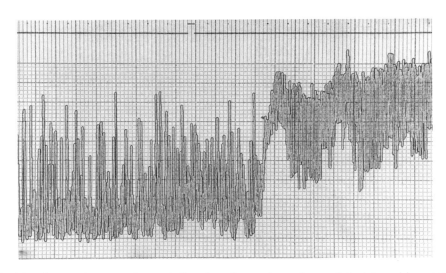

Figure 10.4 Cerebral function monitor trace demonstrating discontinuous low-voltage activity followed by a period of high-voltage seizure activity.

Table 10.5   Evidence for intrapartum hypoxic-ischemic injury

Evidence for hypoxic-ischemic insult	Electronic fetal monitoring (multiple late decelerations, decreased variability)
	Fetal acidosis
	Meconium-stained liquor
	History of intrapartum insult (e.g. cord prolapse, abruption, etc.)
	Depressed Apgar scores
	Delayed onset of respiration, requiring resuscitation
	Hypoxic-ischemic encephalopathy (excluding other causes of neonatal encephalopathy)
	Multi-organ dysfunction
Supporting evidence	MRI features compatible with recognized pattern of injury
	Head growth (normal fetal brain growth until birth, followed by failure of normal brain growth after birth)
Pattern of disability	Spastic quadriplegia
	Dyskinetic cerebral palsy

periventricular white matter. An absent median nerve SEP during the first 24 hours following a hypoxic-ischemic insult is predictive of death or major handicap, whereas a normal SEP is reassuring.[44]

10.1.2.6   *Magnetic resonance spectroscopy (MRS)*

Phosphorus (^{31}P) MRS can be used to study the intracellular energy status of neonatal brain following hypoxia-ischemia, using the spectral peaks attributable to phosphocreatine (PCr) and inorganic phosphate (Pi). The PCr/Pi ratio is a measure of the phosphorylated energy status and a PCr/Pi ratio below the normal range is associated with a poor prognosis following hypoxia-ischemia.[45–47] Using ^{31}P-MRS, the outcome of neonates with moderate (grade II) HIE could be predicted more accurately by adding the information from ^{31}P-MRS to the neurological score, but not vice versa.[48]

Proton (^{1}H) MRS demonstrates peaks that can be assigned to *N*-acetylaspartate (NAA: taken as a marker of neuronal integrity), choline-containing compounds (Cho), and lactate.[49] A low NAA/Cho ratio[50] and a high lactate/NAA ratio[51,52] are associated with a poor outcome. These changes in the ^{1}H-MR spectra occur at a time when the ^{31}P spectra have yet to change[53] and therefore ^{1}H-MRS gives valuable prognostic information at an earlier stage of neuronal injury.

10.1.3   Nature and time of hypoxic-ischemic injury

10.1.3.1   *Defining 'birth asphyxia'*

There are no uniformly accepted diagnostic criteria, but rather the definition rests upon the weight of evidence that can be accumulated pointing to an intrapartum hypoxic-ischemic insult causing a recognized pattern of neurological injury. The suggestive markers are given in Table 10.5. Early neonatal encephalopathy is mandatory for the diagnosis and therefore it is extremely important to exclude other causes of disturbed conscious level (Table 10.3). Careful consideration must also be given to the nature and timing of the injury. Injuries more usually seen in preterm infants and those in an already advanced state of evolution imply a causative insult during the antenatal period.

A damaging antenatal neurological insult may impair the ability of the fetus to adapt to the physiological stress of a normal labor, resulting in a clinical presentation similar to birth asphyxia, although correct obstetric intrapartum intervention may not prevent an abnormal outcome.

10.1.4   Prognosis

Using the Sarnat staging system or similar three-stage scales referring to mild, moderate, or severe abnormality, studies have demonstrated that the maximal stage of HIE is a predictor of death or severe neurodevelopmental impairment. In a review of five studies examining the outcome of neonates with different HIE grades,[11] it appears that grade I (mild) HIE does not confer any increased risk of death or disability. Of those infants with grade II (moderate) HIE, 6 percent will die and 20 percent will have severe disability. Sixty-one percent of infants with grade III (severe) HIE will die and 72 percent of survivors will develop severe disability.

Table 10.6 demonstrates the usefulness of the encephalopathy grades in predicting outcome

Table 10.6 Hypoxic-ischemic insult grades and adverse outcome

HIE grade	Number of infants	Outcome: death (prevalence 13%)		Outcome: death + handicap (prevalence 25%)	
		Predictive value (%)	Likelihood ratio (95% CIs)	Predictive value (%)	Likelihood ratio (95% CIs)
Mild	196	1.3	0.09 (0.03–0.30)	1.6	0.05 (0.02–0.15)
Moderate	153	5.6	0.39 (0.21–0.71)	24	0.94 (0.71–1.23)
Severe	74	61	11.0 (7.56–15.9)	78	10.7 (6.71–17.1)

Data from Peliowski and Finer.[54]

from these studies.[54] From the table one can see that the clinician can be reassuring to parents that if their infant has shown only signs of mild encephalopathy, he or she stands no additional risk for death or disability. Infants with severe HIE, however, are at considerable risk of either death or surviving with severe neurodevelopmental impairments.

In contrast to grade I (mild) or grade III (severe) HIE, the prognosis of infants with grade II (moderate) HIE in terms of disability is not clear from the clinical signs alone. There is also a suggestion that, even if the infant with grade II HIE survives without a major disability, there is a risk of the child having a reduced IQ when assessed at 8 years of age.[55] This makes counseling parents of these infants problematic without additional investigations.

Amiel-Tison and Ellison have attempted to overcome this problem by subdividing the mild, moderate, and severe grades each into two levels of severity.[5] The subdivision is based upon the length of time that signs are present in grade I, on the presence or absence of seizures in grade II, and on the presence or absence of brainstem signs in grade III. It remains to be seen from follow-up studies whether these subdivisions confer any greater predictive value upon grade II (moderate) HIE.

In practice, most clinicians continue to use the Sarnat staging scheme and integrate the clinical findings with the results of further investigations in those infants with moderate (grade II) or severe (grade III) HIE. Investigations aid determination of the prognosis in those infants with moderate (grade II) HIE. They are also useful in confirming the poor prognosis of infants with severe (grade III) HIE at an early enough stage to consider discontinuation of ventilatory support. The predictive values, likelihood ratios, and the times at which they can be defined for the various investigations are given in Table 10.7. Severe basal ganglia injury is associated with severe spastic quadriplegia with pronounced

feeding difficulties and convulsions; infants with mainly white matter and cortical abnormalities have less severe problems.[23]

The best early predictors of poor outcome are sustained low-voltage states and discontinuous activity on continuous EEG or cerebral function monitoring, appearing by 6 hours, and abnormal Doppler cerebral blood flow velocities, appearing by 24 hours. If the results of these investigations are unequivocal on two separate occasions after the first 24 hours, the poor prognosis should be explained to the parents and consideration given to withdrawing ventilatory support.

10.2 CEREBRAL ISCHEMIC LESIONS

This section will deal with the more specific condition of cerebral ischemia associated with vascular compromise in arterial watershed areas, which can occur either following cerebral artery infarction or in leukomalacia. Parenchymal venous infarction will also be considered as it is largely ischemic in nature.

10.2.1 Cerebral artery infarction

Unilateral cerebral infarction, most commonly arising in the territory of the middle cerebral artery, has been reported as a causative factor in 12 percent of neonatal seizures.[56] Its etiology remains obscure, although hypoxia-ischemia is the most common association[57,58] and studies suggest a perinatal insult in most cases.[59]

10.2.1.1 Clinical features

The incidence of unilateral cerebral infarction is 0.02 percent livebirths;[60] 80 percent of such infants present with seizures, often focal and usually on the first postnatal day. The neonatal signs may be

Table 10.7 Prediction of death and severe disability following intrapartum hypoxic-ischemic insult at term

Test	Time assessed	Positive predictive value (%)	Negative predictive value (%)	Likelihood ratio	Reference
Apgar 0–3	5 min	8	–	6.0	3
	10 min	21	–	17.7	
	20 min	80	–	254	
Cerebral function monitor Burst suppression, low voltage or flat	1–6 hours	86	96	9.2	41
HIE					
Mild	6–72 hours	1.6	–	0.05	57
Moderate		24	–	0.94	
Severe		78	–	10.7	
Doppler CBFV PRI <0.55	24 hours	67	100	5.0	17
EEG Burst suppression, low voltage or flat	1–4 days	84	88	7.6	41
MRI Diffuse hyperintensity of cerebral hemispheres, basal ganglia changes (moderate–severe)	5–14 days	70	100	12.3	22
CT Diffuse/global decreased density	7–14 days	90	86	4.8	28

subtle and transient but by 6 months of age the signs of a hemiparesis may become apparent, contralateral to the side of the arterial occlusion.[61] If the lesion is in the territory of the middle cerebral artery, the hemiparesis will involve the face and upper limbs, the legs being relatively unaffected. The subtlety of the neonatal presentation suggests that this condition may be underdiagnosed as a perinatal cause of a spastic hemiplegia.

10.2.1.2 Imaging and timing

In the first week of life, cranial ultrasound is an insensitive method of detecting infarction. The infarcted region can be recognized as an echodensity but this may take a week to become apparent.[59] Color Doppler and power Doppler ultrasonography may show an increase in the size and number of visible vessels in the periphery of the infarct ('luxury perfusion').[62,63] Generally, MRI is superior at demonstrating the presence and extent of the lesion within the first 5 days of postnatal life (Fig. 10.5).[59] The appearance of early MRI abnormalities can be enhanced further by using diffusion-weighted techniques.[26] Diffusion-weighted images can detect ischemic regions within hours after injury, becoming less abnormal towards the end of the first week, by which time ischemic

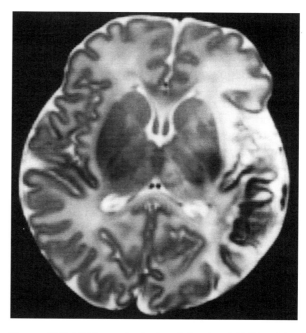

Figure 10.5 Middle cerebral artery infarction. MR T2-weighted sequence (axial section) at 6 days of age. Abnormal high signal intensity in the white matter and low signal intensity in the cortex are present in the territory of the left middle cerebral artery.

lesions can be more easily seen on conventional MR images.[64] This enables the timing of the injury to be estimated and studies using this technique suggest a perinatal insult in most cases.[59] Proton magnetic resonance spectroscopy imaging (^{1}H-MRSI) is able to detect persisting lactate resonances, normally absent in the brain after term, in the area of infarction.[65]

10.2.1.3 Prognosis

The published data regarding outcome following unilateral cerebral infarction are contradictory. The incidence of a spastic hemiplegia varies in published studies from the majority[65,66] to approximately 10 percent.[56,67] Later childhood seizure disorders can occur.[68] Cognitive impairment and effects upon language have been reported, although the involvement of language bears no relationship to the side of the infarction.[66,69] Impairment of visual function has been reported, although the severity could not be predicted from the site and extent of the lesion seen on neonatal MRI.[70] Other studies have not detected visual or hearing problems in early childhood.[56]

The variable prognosis reported following neonatal cerebral infarction may reflect that, between studies, there may be differing etiologies with varying degrees of associated cerebral compromise not detected by neonatal imaging. Earlier studies may bias reporting towards more severe clinical presentations, later studies may use more sensitive imaging and therefore report the outcome of a less clinically severe cohort.

10.2.2 Leukomalacia

Periventricular leukomalacia (PVL) has been considered to be related to hypoperfusion of the boundary zones between the ventriculofugal and ventriculopetal arteries in preterm infants. There is recent evidence for other etiologies, particularly materno-fetal infection. Subcortical leukomalacia (SCL) arises in the watershed areas between the major cerebral arteries in the white matter at the depths of the sulci.[71] SCL is more likely to occur in more mature infants, although both PVL and SCL can coexist in preterm infants. The insult responsible for such injuries may occur in the antenatal, intrapartum, or neonatal periods, although establishing the exact timing is difficult.

10.2.2.1 Clinical features

If leukomalacia is secondary to hypoperfusion, it may be expected that many cases of PVL occur in preterm infants with a history of neonatal hypotension. In a large retrospective case note analysis, however, only 21 percent of cases of cystic PVL had overt hypotension in the immediate neonatal period; most cases were associated with relatively benign clinical courses and were only detected by routine ultrasound screening.[72] Ischemic lesions occur at greater frequency in certain neonatal clinical conditions, such as a surviving monozygotic twin[73] and non-immune hydrops,[74] although these represent the minority. Perinatal infection, particularly associated with prolonged rupture of the membranes and chorioamnionitis, is emerging as a major risk factor.[72,75]

The early clinical features associated with leukomalacia in the preterm infant are ill-defined. This reflects partly the chronic perinatal nature of the insult and partly the fact that, until recovery occurs from any initial respiratory illness, complete neurological examination may not be possible. Hypotonia and decreased visual alertness have been described within the first few weeks of life.[76] An increase in upper limb flexor tone, adducted thumbs, increased lower limb extensor tone, and poor head and trunk control are evident by term. A normal neurological examination at term, in combination with a normal cerebral ultrasound examination, correlates well with a favorable outcome.[77] The characteristic signs of spasticity and cerebral palsy may take between 6 and 36 months to become apparent, depending upon the nature and severity of the initial insult.

10.2.2.2 Imaging and timing

10.2.2.2.1 Cerebral ultrasound

Over the last 15 years, ultrasound has evolved into a useful technique in the detection of ischemic injury in preterm infants. Its major advantage over other imaging modalities is that it can be performed at the cot side with minimal physiological disturbance to the infant and is therefore readily repeatable. The resolution is limited, although technological advances have led to improvement.

Areas of increased echodensity are demonstrated by ultrasound within 24–48 hours of an ischemic insult (Fig. 10.6). At first, these were thought to correspond to hemorrhage into previously ischemic tissue,[78] but subsequent studies have shown that non-hemorrhage infarction can also produce such appearances.[79–81] These echodensities may undergo cystic change within a period of 7–14 days; the cysts appear in clusters within the area of previous echodensity (Fig. 10.7).[82] The cysts become smaller

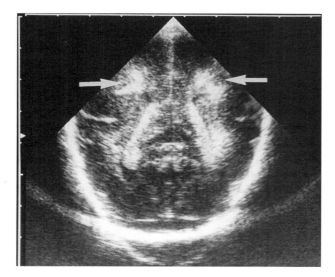

Figure 10.6 Periventricular leukomalacia: pre-cystic phase. Ultrasound (coronal section) at 48 hours of age showing echodense areas within the periventricular white matter.

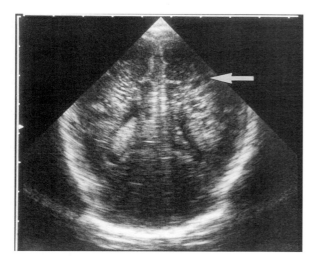

Figure 10.7 Cystic periventricular leukomalacia. Ultrasound (coronal section) at 3 weeks of age, in the same patient as Figure 10.6. Cysts have now formed in the previously echodense regions.

and are not usually visualized on ultrasound once the infant is over 2–3 months of age, although dilatation of the lateral ventricles may be noted,[83] which is thought to represent periventricular white matter atrophy.[81] The periventricular echodensities (PVEDs) may also persist for a variable period before resolution occurs without cystic degeneration. PVEDs persisting for more than 14 days have been associated with gliosis at post-mortem and therefore probably represent a milder degree of PVL.[81,84,85]

Extensive cystic lesions in the subcortical white matter have been described using ultrasound.[86–88]

These arise in the watershed areas between the major cerebral arteries in the white matter at the depths of the sulci.[71] Such lesions are termed subcortical leukomalacia (SCL) and are more likely to occur in the period from 40 weeks to 3 months postmenstrual age. SCL has been described in association with PVL and in preterm infants following a clinical deterioration in the neonatal period.[89] Cystic change occurs within 2–3 weeks of the insult. The cysts tend to be larger in diameter than cysts of PVL and persist much longer.

Knowledge of the evolution of these ultrasound appearances enables some inference as to the timing of the insult. It is known from pathological studies that PVL can occur *in utero*.[90,91] and cysts have been demonstrated using fetal cerebral ultrasound.[92] Cystic change appearing within 7 days of postnatal age suggests a prenatal insult.[93,94] It appears that the majority of cystic PVL occurs in the perinatal period[95] but any later severe deterioration in the condition of the infant up to 40 weeks of postmenstrual age can still lead to PVL and SCL.[89,96]

As most cases of cystic PVL occur in preterm infants with relatively benign clinical courses, all preterm infants and term infants at risk from cerebral ischemic insults should undergo routine ultrasound examinations. The first should be shortly after birth and subsequent examinations should be carried out at regular intervals, continued until 40 weeks postmenstrual age or 2–3 weeks following an episode of clinical deterioration, whichever is later. Restricting the examinations to the immediate postnatal period limits the sensitivity of ultrasound in detecting ischemic lesions.[97]

10.2.2.2.2 Magnetic resonance imaging (MRI)

Several studies have demonstrated that delayed myelination, white matter gliosis, and ventriculomegaly, seen on MRI performed outside the neonatal period but within the first year, are associated with adverse outcome.[98–100] MRI abnormalities of the optic radiation or visual cortex are associated with later visual impairment.[101,102] Although there appears to be a good correlation between the degree of PVL, diagnosed using cerebral ultrasound, and the extent of the MRI changes noted in infancy,[103] it is unclear whether the presence of such MRI changes provides any additional prognostic information compared with cerebral ultrasound.[104,105]

MRI is able to identify leukomalacia in the neonatal period. Cystic PVL and SCL can be readily

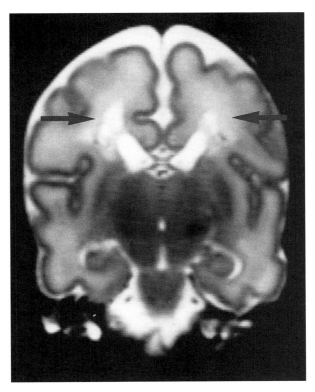

Figure 10.8 Cystic periventricular leukomalacia. MR T2-weighted sequence (coronal section) performed on the same day as the ultrasound in Figure 10.7. Cysts of the same signal intensity as the CSF are seen above the lateral ventricles.

observed and the cysts contain fluid of similar signal intensity to CSF (low T1, high T2; Fig. 10.8). Patchy areas of altered signal intensity may be seen in the periventricular white matter (high T1, low T2) and these may represent non-cystic PVL. MRI affords greater anatomical definition of acute preterm white matter injury but it remains to be seen whether neonatal MRI will improve prediction of later neurodevelopmental impairment.

10.2.2.2.3   Evoked potentials (EPs)

Somatosensory evoked potentials (SEPs) provide functional information regarding the integrity of the sensory pathways contiguous to areas involved in motor development. A prolonged short latency (N_1 peak) component of the SEP, following median nerve stimulation, was found to be predictive of an adverse outcome in a cohort of preterm infants with abnormalities on cerebral ultrasound.[106] Another study using a larger cohort of preterm infants with cystic PVL on cerebral ultrasound failed to demonstrate that median nerve SEPs had any advantage over cerebral ultra-

sound in prediction of outcome.[107] These earlier studies recorded SEPs around term, since normal preterm infants can have values outside the normal range during the first week of life.[108] Posterior tibial nerve SEPs were found to have a higher sensitivity than median nerve stimulation in prediction of outcome in preterm infants (negative predictive value 96 percent),[109] although the technique can be difficult and time-consuming.[110] Performing SEPs during the second and third weeks, combined with serial measurements, may improve predictive power.[111]

10.2.2.3   Prognosis

Several studies on populations of preterm infants have been carried out in order to determine the prognostic value of neonatal cerebral ultrasound examinations. The incidence of PVL and the prevalence of neurodevelopmental impairment vary between studies, reflecting the differing maturity of the populations studied and the different definitions of impairment. The initial reports suggested that extensive cystic PVL was predictive of a poor neurodevelopmental outcome, although few infants were studied.[83,112–114] More recently, several larger prospective cohort studies have examined the relationship between ultrasound findings and subsequent outcome, paying particular attention to the nature of the lesion (Table 10.8).

Certain ultrasound studies have demonstrated that the size of the cysts are significantly associated with outcome. Cysts greater than 5–10 mm diameter are associated with motor deficits.[120,121] Infants with small focal cystic change, when assessed at 5 years, do not have cerebral palsy but have subtle motor abnormalities, attention deficit disorders and cognitive impairment.[122] The position of the cystic change appears of great importance in predicting poor outcome. Isolated frontal cystic PVL is associated with normal development; infants with frontal-parietal cysts may develop cerebral palsy (spastic diplegia) and motor impairment, whereas extensive cystic change involving the occipital white matter is strongly predictive of cerebral palsy and cognitive impairment (Table 10.9).[116,117] Other studies have suggested features predictive of adverse outcome to be cystic PVL involving multiple areas and cysts developing later in neonatal life.[120,123] Many infants with extensive cystic PVL have associated visual problems, in particular squints and reduced acuity.[114,124,125] These visual problems are especially severe in the more mature infants (35–37 weeks)

Table 10.8 Evidence from prospective cohort ultrasound screening studies differentiating between hemorrhagic and ischemic lesions with assessment of neurodevelopment at 1–3 years in the whole cohort

Selection	Szymonowicz[115] <1251 g	Fawer[116] <35 weeks	Graham[117] <1501 g	Nwaesei[97] <33 weeks	Bozynski[118] <1201 g	Fazzi[119] <1501 g	Predictive value (%) (95% CIs)	Likelihood ratio
Number at birth	50	120	200	150	–	203		
Number at follow-up	32	82	156	110	116	122		
Mean gestation (weeks)	27	31	29	30	29	30		
Mean birthweight (g)	880	1465	1200	1322	977	1175		
Age at follow-up (months)	24	18	18	12	12–18	12–36		
Prevalence of disability[a] (%)	19	10	8	17	10	21		
Predictive values (%)								
Major ultrasound abnormality[b]	100	33	64	100	43	54	55 (46–64)	7.5
Cystic PVL	100	28	62	100	–	71	61 (47–74)	9.6
Minor ultrasound abnormality[b]	17	0	1	–	0	12	4 (1–6)	0.26
Normal ultrasound	0	0	5	8	5	7	5 (3–8)	0.34

[a]Major disability: non-ambulant cerebral palsy/mental retardation/severe visual or sensorineural hearing impairments.

[b]Ultrasound abnormality: major; cystic PVL/SCL/parenchymal venous infarction/persistent PVED; minor: GMH/IVH/transient PVED.

GMH, geminal matrix hemorrhage; IVH, intraventricular hemorrhage; PVED, periventricular echodensities; PVL, periventricular leukomalacia; SCL, subcortical leukomalacia.

Table 10.9 Cystic periventricular leukomalacia (PVL): position of cysts and subsequent major disability in infants <35 weeks[116]

	Number	Positive predictive value (%)	Likelihood ratio
Infants prospectively enrolled	120		
Infants followed up	82		
Cystic PVL	18	28	3.5
Frontal cysts	10	0	0
Fronto-parietal cysts	5	40	6.0
Fronto-parieto-occipital cysts	3	100	∞
Prevalence of major disability	10%		

with cystic PVL extending into the deep subcortical white matter (SCL).[126] As a group, infants with SCL also appear to have more severe motor impairments (spastic quadriplegia) and mental retardation.[87,127]

Generally, the presence of cystic PVL on ultrasound is useful in predicting subsequent motor impairment but is less effective in predicting cognitive impairment and mental disability. The presence of subcortical cysts, however, confers a high risk of motor, cognitive and visual problems.

There are several reports of infants with periventricular echodensities (PVEDs) developing cerebral palsy, although the predictive power is low since the majority of infants with PVEDs did not have major motor impairments.[128–130] In a large cohort of 59 preterm infants with PVEDs matched with preterm infants with normal ultrasound examinations, a higher prevalence of spastic diplegia and transient dystonia was found on initial follow-up.[131] The risk of abnormality was greatest if the PVED was in the area of the trigone and persisted for more than 10 days. When this cohort was later assessed at 6 years, the degree of motor impairment was related to the duration of echodensity, although there were no differences in cognitive abilities.[132]

It therefore appears that persistent PVEDs represent a less severe injury than cystic PVL or SCL and rarely result in major handicap but may lead to more subtle motor impairment, detectable on longer term follow-up.

To date, no prospective neonatal MRI screening studies have been reported similar to the large-scale cerebral ultrasound studies of the 1980s, and therefore no conclusions can yet be drawn regarding the predictive values of neonatal MRI abnormalities. It remains to be seen whether MRI will enable more accurate prediction of both cognitive impairment and minor motor dysfunction than ultrasound.

Abnormal VEPs predict visual impairment in preterm infants with extensive cystic PVL. They do not provide any more reliable information than cerebral ultrasound[127,133] and are of no greater value in the prediction of neurodevelopmental impairment.[134]

10.2.3 Parenchymal venous infarction

Parenchymal hemorrhage into the periventricular white matter has been observed in association with germinal matrix-intraventricular hemorrhage (GMH-IVH).[135] Originally, the periventricular bleed was believed to arise from direct extension of an intraventricular hemorrhage. Subsequently, this was thought unlikely as the GMH-IVH probably arises from low-pressure capillary rupture[136] and thus an ischemic process was proposed as an alternative hypothesis.[137] Histopathological studies suggest that hemorrhagic necrosis results from a venous infarction following obstruction of the terminal veins by a GMH-IVH.[138,139]

The neonatal clinical features associated with a parenchymal venous infarction are similar to those arising from GMH-IVH and are therefore described in this later section. The late features of neurological injury secondary to parenchymal venous infarction are of spastic hemiparesis, with leg involvement greater than arm involvement.

10.2.3.1 Imaging

Parenchymal venous infarctions initially appear echogenic on cerebral ultrasound due to the presence of venous congestion and hemorrhage within the periventricular white matter. They are markedly asymmetrical, invariably occur on the same side as a GMH-IVH, and develop and progress after the occurrence of GMH-IVH.[140] The

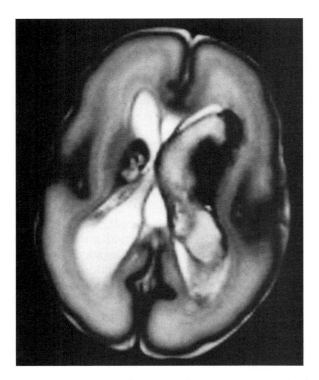

Figure 10.9 Parenchymal venous infarction. MR T2-weighted sequence (axial section). The left parenchymal venous infarction is seen as an area of low signal intensity and is associated with a left intraventricular hemorrhage. There is also a small right germinal matrix hemorrhage, of low signal intensity.

echogenic area is replaced by a single large porencephalic cyst over a period of 7–14 days, reflecting the ischemic nature of the injury. Porencephalic cysts, arising as a result of a parenchymal venous infarction, differ from cysts of PVL in that the former are usually solitary, of large diameter, unilateral or grossly asymmetrical, are commonly more anteriorly located in the frontal or parietal regions and often communicate with the lateral ventricle. The later appearances of ventriculomegaly with an irregular lateral ventricular wall result from white matter atrophy of the ischemic region. Ultrasound suggests that parenchymal venous infarction is less frequent than PVL, occurring in 3 percent of surviving neonates of 32 weeks gestation or less[97,115,117] compared with 6 percent for cystic changes.[97,115–117,119]

CT and MRI are also able to demonstrate the presence of blood in the parenchyma (Fig. 10.9) and the gradual resolution of this hematoma with porencephalic cyst formation, although the practical difficulties in transporting unstable preterm infants for early imaging have, as yet, prevented either CT or MRI superseding cerebral ultrasound as the standard imaging modality.

10.2.3.2 Prognosis

Follow-up studies of infants with parenchymal venous infarction suggest there may be a high incidence of neurodevelopmental impairment. It is difficult to distinguish between venous infarction and early PVL until the evolution into porencephaly or multiple cystic degeneration. Therefore early ultrasound appearances are less predictive than later appearances.[141] The prognosis for porencephaly is controversial. A poor outcome with cerebral palsy and developmental impairment has been reported.[140,141] Other studies suggest that, although there is a high risk of hemiplegic cerebral palsy, cognitive function is relatively spared.[142,143] Following parenchymal venous infarction and porencephaly, 81 percent of children were found to have cerebral palsy at follow-up, whereas only 19 percent had severe cognitive impairment.[143] The differences in reported prognosis from these studies may reflect differences in the ultrasound definition of parenchymal venous infarction because of the difficulty in distinguishing it from echogenic phase of PVL.

10.3 INTRACRANIAL HEMORRHAGE

10.3.1 Germinal matrix hemorrhage-intraventricular hemorrhage (GMH-IVH)

Prior to the introduction of routine neonatal imaging, GMH-IVH was thought to be a devastating condition with obvious neurological signs, either a catastrophic syndrome (coma, generalized tonic convulsions, decerebrate posturing and flaccid quadriparesis), or a more subtle saltatory syndrome (altered consciousness, hypotonia, abnormal eye position and movements).[144] With the availability of scanning techniques, it has been recognized that the majority of infants with GMH-IVH show no obvious clinical signs,[145] although a variety of subtle signs are correlated with the presence of GMH-IVH on ultrasound, including impaired visual tracking, hypertonicity of the lower limbs with a reduced popliteal angle and later development of roving eye movements.[146] If post-hemorrhagic hydrocephalus develops, it may present later with a rapidly enlarging head circumference, bulging anterior fontanel and signs of raised intracranial pressure.

10.3.1.1 Imaging

CT was first used to diagnose GMH-IVH in 1976[147] but its use was superseded by cerebral ultrasound.

With ultrasound, a GMH appears as an echogenic area at the head of the caudate nucleus, separate from the choroid plexus. IVHs are characterized by the presence of echogenic hematoma in the body of the ventricle. Autopsy verification of ultrasound diagnosis shows that the sensitivities for detecting germinal matrix hemorrhages and intraventricular hemorrhages are 61 percent and 91 percent respectively.[148] These values fall for the detection of lesions less than 0.5 cm diameter.[149] MRI may have a higher sensitivity in the detection of smaller hemorrhages.

The first classification of intraventricular hemorrhage was devised from CT appearances and comprised four grades:[150] (I) germinal matrix hemorrhage, (II) intraventricular hemorrhage without ventricular distension, (III) intraventricular hemorrhage with blood distending the lateral ventricle, and (IV) parenchymal hemorrhage. This was adapted for use with cerebral ultrasound although the distinction between grades II and III may be difficult. For this reason, and the fact that parenchymal hemorrhages are thought to represent venous infarction, not extensions of intraventricular hemorrhages, it is preferable to describe the hemorrhage as either germinal matrix (GMH) or intraventricular (IVH) and use the term germinal matrix-intraventicular hemorrhage (GMH-IVH) to describe the pathophysiological concept.

10.3.1.2 Timing

Using cerebral ultrasound, cohort screening studies report incidences of GMH and IVH to be 8 percent and 10 percent respectively in infants less than 29 weeks gestation, the incidence falling with increasing maturity.[151] The majority of GMH-IVH occur within 72 hours of birth,[152] although further progression can occur over the following 48 hours.[153] Hemorrhage visible on ultrasound within 6 hours of birth is suggestive of a prenatal event.[154] MRI may have a role in determining the age of the hematoma. In the first few days, hemorrhage is isointense on T1- and hypointense on T2-weighted images. In the following days, the hemorrhage becomes hyperintense on T1- and markedly hypointense on T2-weighted images. By 2 weeks the hematoma remains of high signal intensity on T1 and is of low signal intensity in the center, surrounded by high signal, on T2-weighted sequences.[155] It is difficult to be any more precise in MRI dating of hemorrhage because of the many factors influencing its MR signal intensity, such as the protein concentration of the hematoma, the presence of paramagnetic forms of hemoglobin (deoxy- and methemoglobin), and the heterogeneity of the internal structure of the hematoma.[156]

10.3.1.3 Prognosis

Information regarding prognosis is derived from prospective studies using ultrasound in cohorts of preterm infants. These studies suggest that the presence of a GMH-IVH alone is not associated with an increased risk of later neurodevelopmental disability (Table 10.8).

Ventriculomegaly, with the lateral ventricular indices more than 4 mm above the 97th centile,[157] can occur following GMH-IVH. Enlargement of the ventricles may be secondary to obstruction to CSF resorption at the arachnoid granulations or cerebral atrophy following parenchymal injury. About half of the infants with ventriculomegaly will develop progressive hydrocephalus and require neurosurgical drainage, usually by placement of a ventriculo-peritoneal shunt.[158] CSF aspiration by spinal or ventricular tap may transiently relieve symptoms and signs of raised intracranial pressure (apnea, vomiting, rapidly enlarging head

Table 10.10 Prognosis following post-hemorrhagic ventricular dilatation: results from the Ventriculomegaly Trial Group[158,159]

Outcome	Total cohort	With parenchymal lesions	Without parenchymal lesions
Infants at trial entry	157	101	56
Deaths prior to follow-up	32 (20%)	24 (24%)	8 (14%)
Loss to follow-up	13 (8%)	9 (9%)	4 (7%)
Number assessed at 30 months	112 (71%)	68 (67%)	44 (79%)
Mean gestational age	28.4 weeks		
Mean birthweight	1267 g		
Marked disability	85 (54%)	61 (60%)	24 (43%)
Normal	10 (6%)	3 (3%)	7 (13%)

circumference, divarification of the sutures) but does not prevent the need for neurosurgery or the ultimate neurodevelopmental outcome (Table 10.10).[158,159] The prognosis following post-hemorrhagic ventricular dilatation is particularly poor in infants with associated parenchymal echodensities[159] and in those who require repeated shunt revision.[160]

10.3.2   Subdural hemorrhage

Fifty years ago, subdural hemorrhage (SDH) was commonly seen at post-mortem, associated with obstetric trauma.[161] This is now less common. Although this is largely due to improvements in obstetric practice, many cases may remain undiagnosed since small hemorrhages are associated with few clinical signs. Extensive SDH may be precipitated by excessive neck extension causing occipital osteodiastasis during breech extraction[162] and dural tears secondary to mechanical stress. Rupture of the superior cerebral bridging veins produces a less extensive convexity hemorrhage.[163] There have been numerous recent cases of symptomatic tentorial tears associated with vacuum extraction.[164–167] SDH is not invariably caused by obstetric trauma; many infants with SDH have a normal vaginal delivery[168] and fetal SDH has been identified on antenatal ultrasound examination.[169]

Tentorial laceration with massive infratentorial SDH presents from birth with coma, lateral deviation of the eyes and unequal pupils; there may be associated signs of shock or coexistent signs of hypoxia-ischemia. Less severe posterior fossa SDH resulting from smaller tears presents hours, or even days, after birth with signs of raised intracranial pressure, brainstem compression and seizures. A convexity SDH may present with generalized or multifocal seizures, occasionally with signs suggestive of third cranial nerve compression,[170] or with no clinical signs.

10.3.2.1   *Imaging*

Ultrasound will detect SDH if large enough to produce midline shift or ventricular compression but is unreliable at demonstrating small hemorrhages.[167] CT and MRI are the imaging modalities of choice. CT is useful in detecting acute hemorrhage. MRI is more effective at demonstrating small hemorrhages, particularly in the posterior fossa (Fig. 10.10).[171] MRI may have a future role in dating the hemorrhage, once the differential susceptibility effects of hemoglobin breakdown on

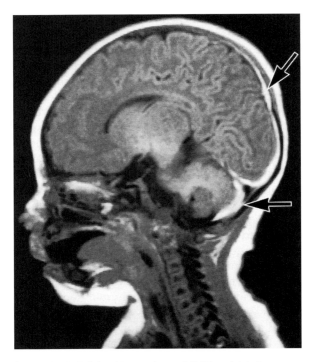

Figure 10.10 Subdural hemorrhage. MR T1-weighted sequence (sagittal section). The hematoma is seen as the area of high signal intensity around the occipital lobe and in the posterior fossa. This was an incidental finding in an asymptomatic infant, 6 days following delivery by ventouse extraction.

T1 and T2 relaxation times have been fully elucidated.

10.3.2.2   *Prognosis*

Most infants with major tentorial lacerations die. Smaller posterior fossa SDH is associated with a variable prognosis, depending upon the extent of the hematoma, the speed of any surgical intervention, and the presence of associated hypoxic-ischemic injury. Surgical decompression is required if there are signs of brainstem compression and raised intracranial pressure.[167] The prognosis with convexity hemorrhages is relatively good; a subdural tap is occasionally required if there is midline shift. Approximately 75 percent of infants with symptomatic convexity SDH are normal on follow-up.[168]

10.3.3   Primary subarachnoid hemorrhage

This is probably the most common type of hemorrhage occurring in neonates and is seen more frequently in premature than term infants. The pathogenesis is incompletely understood but the majority are thought to arise from trauma or hypoxic-ischemic insults. Primary subarachnoid hemorrhage (SAH) can be due to rupture of the veins bridging the subarachnoid space.[172] An extensive convexity SAH causing compression to the underlying temporal lobe has also been described.[173] A secondary SAH can arise from blood tracking following an intraventricular hemorrhage.

The majority of infants with primary SAH are asymptomatic. Primary SAH can result in convulsions. These are usually generalized and multifocal but the infants characteristically behave and feed normally between seizures. There may be other features of hypoxia-ischemia accompanying symptomatic SAH. Massive convexity SAH may cause similar symptoms to massive SDH, with circulatory collapse, coma and signs of raised intracranial pressure; most of these infants will have also sustained a severe hypoxic-ischemic injury and few survive.

10.3.3.1 *Imaging*

Ultrasound has little role in the diagnosis or exclusion of SAH.[174] CT and MRI demonstrate the blood in the subarachnoid space. The distinction between subarachnoid and subdural hematoma is more readily made using MRI.

10.3.3.2 *Prognosis*

The majority of primary SAHs are asymptomatic in infants without serious traumatic or hypoxic-ischemic injury and therefore are associated with a normal outcome. Infants with symptomatic SAH that survive the neonatal period were thought to have a normal outcome in 90 percent of cases[175] but a more recent study suggests a more guarded prognosis, with only 50 percent normal at follow-up.[176]

10.3.4 Intracerebellar hemorrhage

Primary intracerebellar hemorrhages are thought to arise from within the cerebellar cortex or in the subependymal layer of the roof of the fourth ventricle.[163] They may occur spontaneously or secondary to trauma and are more common in preterm infants. Secondary intracerebellar hemorrhages have been described in association with occipital osteodiastasis and breech delivery[162] or secondary to occipital compression during certain neonatal maneuvers, for example bag and mask

resuscitation, intubation, and placement of intravenous canulae in scalp veins.[172]

The prevalence of intracerebellar hemorrhage in post-mortem studies of preterm infants has been reported to be as high as 10 percent, although CT studies of living preterm neonates following hypoxia-ischemia have only demonstrated hemorrhages in 1 percent.[177] Onset of clinical features varies from the first postnatal day to 2–3 weeks of age and the features include signs of brainstem compression: apnea, respiratory irregularities, obstruction to CSF flow, skew deviation of the eyes and facial paresis.[178–180]

10.3.4.1 *Imaging*

CT and MRI demonstrate the lesions, although distinguishing them from posterior fossa SDH may be difficult.[181]

10.3.4.2 *Prognosis*

The prognosis for preterm infants is usually very poor; the outcome for term infants is more favorable, although the indications for surgical evacuation of the hematoma are not clear. A number of reports document survival in term infants following posterior fossa craniotomy and evacuation;[182] others document a similar neurological outcome associated with medical support alone.[180] Insertion of a ventriculoperitoneal shunt may be necessary in infants with acute obstructive hydrocephalus before hematoma resolution.[180]

10.3.5 Thalamic hemorrhage

A primary intrathalamic hemorrhage may occur with secondary rupture into the lateral ventricles.[183,184] It can be associated with perinatal asphyxia.[185] The presentation is characteristically in the second week of life with seizures occurring in an otherwise normal infant.[186] An acute facial nerve palsy may be seen and eye deviation may occur: downwards and outwards to the side of the thalamic hematoma.

10.3.5.1 *Imaging*

The hemorrhage can be demonstrated using ultrasound or MRI.[185]

10.3.5.2 *Prognosis*

The prognosis is reported to be generally good, although recent experience suggests that moderate cognitive impairment is seen in a significant proportion of these infants. This lesion represents a separate entity from the bilateral thalamic densities associated with severe hypoxic-ischemic injury.

10.4 SUMMARY

10.4.1 Prediction of outcome

The ability of any prognostic test to predict subsequent neurodevelopmental impairment is best summarized by the likelihood ratio. The likelihood ratio is the ratio of the post-test odds to the pre-test odds. The higher the likelihood ratio, the more predictive the test. Interpretation of a ratio of odds is not intuitive and many clinicians find the positive predictive value useful (the proportion of subjects testing positive who later develop impairment). The positive predictive value depends upon the prevalence of impairment in the population in which the test was evaluated, whereas the likelihood ratio does not. Therefore, predictive abilities of prognostic tests should be compared by means of their likelihood ratios and not be positive predictive values derived from different studies with varying prevalence of impairment.

10.4.2 Term infants

The likelihood ratios for various prognostic indicators following an intrapartum hypoxic-ischemic insult are given in Table 10.7. For example, in suspected intrapartum asphyxia, an Apgar score of 0–3 at 20 minutes has an extremely strong association with subsequent disability (likelihood ratio 254), whereas moderate hypoxic-ischemic encephalopathy has a relatively weak association (likelihood ratio 0.94). Thus, in a child with cerebral palsy who had suffered moderate HIE, there would be only weak evidence that the neonatal events were associated with the observed disability, compared with the much stronger evidence of an association had the infant had a severely depressed Apgar score at 20 minutes.

Although many of the indicators listed in Table 10.7 have good predictive power, the sensitivity is low for the detection of neurodevelopmental disability in the population as a whole, reflecting the fact that intrapartum hypoxic-ischemic insults only account for 5–12 percent of cerebral palsy.[187–189]

10.4.3 Preterm infants

The prevalence of cerebral palsy in preterm infants of birthweight <1500 g is over 70 per 1000 survivors, compared with 1.4 per 1000 for normal birthweight infants.[190] Therefore preterm infants are at high risk of neurodevelopmental impairment, making the neonatal period an important time during which to screen for brain injuries capable of causing future disability.

Clinical examination in the early neonatal period may not be practicable if the infant is too sick and unstable. When the infant reaches 40 weeks corrected age, however, a normal neurological examination, combined with normal cerebral ultrasonography, correlates well with a favorable outcome.[191]

In the immediate neonatal period, cerebral ultrasound provides the most accurate prognostic information. A normal cerebral ultrasound predicts a good outcome in 95 percent of cases (Table 10.8) and an entirely normal outcome in 88 percent of cases.[192] Minor ultrasound abnormalities (germinal matrix hemorrhage-intraventricular hemorrhage, transient PVED) are not associated with an increased risk of disability. Cystic leukomalacia and parenchymal venous infarction carry the worst prognosis, particularly if the cystic changes involve the occipital periventricular or subcortical white matter (Tables 10.8 and 10.9). The predictive value of early MRI in the preterm infant has yet to be established. Delayed myelination and white matter atrophy, demonstrated on MRI performed beyond the neonatal period, are associated with adverse outcome. Somatosensory evoked potentials (SEPs) can provide additional prognostic information but are rarely used outside research study.

10.5 REFERENCES

1 Apgar V. A proposal for a new method of evaluation of the newborn infant. *Anesthesia and Analgesia* 1953; **32**: 260–7.

2 Drage JS, Kennedy C, Schwarz BK. The Apgar score as an index of neonatal mortality: a report from the collaborative study of cerebral palsy. *Obstetrics and Gynecology* 1964; **24**: 222–30.

3 Nelson KB, Ellenberg JH. Apgar scores as predictors of chronic neurologic disability. *Pediatrics* 1981; **68**: 36–44.

4 Sarnat HB, Sarnat MS. Neonatal encephalopathy following fetal distress. *Archives of Neurology* 1976; **33**: 696–705.

5 Amiel-Tison C, Ellison P. Birth asphyxia in the fullterm newborn: early assessment and outcome.

Developmental Medicine and Child Neurology 1986; **28**: 671–82.

6 Fenichel GM. Hypoxic-ischemic encephalopathy in the newborn. *Archives of Neurology* 1983; **40**: 261–6.

7 Finer NN, Roberston CM, Richards RT, Pinnell LE, Peters KL. Hypoxic-ischemic encephalopathy in term neonates: perinatal factors and outcome. *Journal of Pediatrics* 1981; **98**: 112–17.

8 Levene MI, Kornberg J, Williams THC. The incidence and severity of post-asphyxial encephalopathy in full-term infants. *Early Human Development* 1985; **11**: 21–6.

9 Niijima S, Levene MI. Post-asphyxial encephalopathy in a preterm infant. *Developmental Medicine and Child Neurology* 1989; **31**: 391–7.

10 Volpe JJ, Pasternak JF. Parasagittal cerebral injury in neonatal hypoxic-ischemic encephalopathy, clinical and neuroradiologic features. *Journal of Pediatrics* 1977; **91**: 472–6.

11 Perlman JM, Tack ED, Martin T, Shackelford G, Amon E. Acute systemic organ injury in term infants after asphyxia. *American Journal of Diseases in Children* 1989; **143**: 617–20.

12 Siegel MJ, Shackelford GD, Perlman GM, Fulling KH. Hypoxic-ischaemic encephalopathy in term infants: diagnosis and prognosis evaluated by ultrasound. *Radiology* 1984; **152**: 395–9.

13 Connolly B, Kelehan P, O'Brien N *et al.* The echogenic thalamus in hypoxic-ischaemic encephalopathy. *Pediatric Radiology* 1994; **24**: 268–71.

14 Rutherford MA, Pennock JM, Dubowitz LM. Cranial ultrasound and magnetic resonance imaging in hypoxic-ischaemic encephalopathy: a comparison with outcome. *Developmental Medicine and Child Neurology* 1994; **36**: 813–25.

15 de Vries LS, Eken P, Beek E, Groenendaal F, Meiners LC. The posterior fontanelle: a neglected acoustic window. *Neuropediatrics* 1996; **27**: 101–4.

16 Eken P, Jansen GH, Groenendaal F, Rademaker KJ, de Vries LS. Intracranial lesions in the fullterm infant with hypoxic-ischaemic encephalopathy: ultrasound and autospy correlation. *Neuropediatrics* 1994; **25**: 301–7.

17 Archer LNJ, Levene MI, Evans DH. Cerebral artery Doppler ultrasonography for prediction of outcome after perinatal asphyxia. *Lancet* 1986; **ii**: 1116–18.

18 Stark JE, Seibert JJ. Cerebral artery Doppler ultrasonography for prediction of outcome after perinatal asphyxia. *Journal of Ultrasound Medicine* 1994; **13**: 595–600.

19 Eken P, Toet MC, Groenendaal F, de Vries LS. Predictive value of early neuroimaging, pulsed Doppler and neurophysiology in full term infants with hypoxic-ischaemic encephalopathy. *Archives of Disease in Childhood* 1995; **73**: F75–80.

20 Barkovich AJ, Westmark K, Partridge C, Sola A, Ferriero DM. Perinatal asphyxia: MR findings in the first 10 days. *AJNR: American Journal of Neuroradiology* 1995; **16**: 427–38.

21 Cristophe C, Clercx A, Blum D, Hasaerts D, Segebarth C, Perlmutter N. Early MR detection of cortical and subcortical hypoxic-ischemic encephalopathy in full-term infants. *Pediatric Radiology* 1994; **24**: 581–4.

22 Kuenzle C, Baenziger O, Martin E *et al.* Prognostic value of early MR imaging in term infants with severe perinatal asphyxia. *Neuropediatrics* 1994; **25**: 191–200.

23 Rutherford M, Pennock J, Schwieso J, Cowan F, Dubowitz L. Hypoxic-ischaemic encephalopathy: early and late magnetic resonance imaging findings in relation to outcome. *Archives of Disease in Childhood* 1996; **75**: F145–51.

24 Rutherford MA, Pennock JM, Schwieso JE, Cowan FM, Dubowitz LM. Hypoxic-ischaemic encephalopathy: early magnetic resonance imaging findings and their evolution. *Neuropediatrics* 1995; **26**: 183–91.

25 Westmark KD, Barkovich AJ, Sola A, Ferriero D, Partridge JC. Patterns and implications of MR contrast enhancement in perinatal asphyxia: a preliminary report. *AJNR: American Journal of Neuroradiology* 1995; **16**: 685–92.

26 Cowan FM, Pennock JM, Hanrahan JD, Manji KP, Edwards AD. Early detection of cerebral infarction and hypoxic-ischemic encephalopathy in neonates using diffusion-weighted magnetic resonance imaging. *Neuropediatrics* 1994; **25**: 172–5.

27 Byrne P, Welch R, Johnson MA, Darrah J, Piper M. Serial magnetic resonance imaging in neonatal hypoxic-ischemic encephalopathy. *Journal of Pediatrics* 1990; **117**: 694–700.

28 Adsett DB, Fitz CR, Hill A. Hypoxic-ischaemic cerebral injury in the term newborn: correlation of CT findings with neurological outcome. *Developmental Medicine and Child Neurology* 1985; **27**: 155–60.

29 Fitzhardinge PM, Flodmark O, Fitz CR, Ashby S. The prognostic value of computed tomography as an adjunct to assessment of the term infant with postasphyxial encephalopathy. *Journal of Pediatrics* 1981; **99**: 777–81.

30 Lipp-Zwahlen AE, Deonna T, Chrzanowski R, Micheli JL, Calame A. Temporal evolution of hypoxic-ischaemic brain lesions in the asphyxiated full-term newborns assessed by computerized tomography. *Neuroradiology* 1985; **27**: 138–44.

31 Lipp-Zwahlen AE, Deonna T, Micheli JL, Calame A, Chrzanowski R, Cetre E. Prognostic value of neonatal CT scans in asphyxiated term babies: low density score compared with neonatal neurological signs. *Neuropediatrics* 1985; **16**: 209–17.

32 Ansari MQ, Chincanchan CA, Armstrong DL. Brain calcification in hypoxic-ischemic lesions: an autopsy review. *Pediatric Neurology* 1990; **6**: 94–101.

33 Kotagal S, Toce SS, Kotagal P, Archer CR. Symmetric bithalamic and striatal hemorrhage following perinatal hypoxia in a term infant. *Journal of Computer Assisted Tomography* 1983; **7**: 353–5.

34 Shewmon DA, Fine M, Masdeu JC, Palacios E. Postischemic hypervascularity of infancy: a stage in the evolution of ischemic brain damage with characteristic CT scan. *Annals of Neurology* 1981; **9**: 358–65.

35 Takeuchi T, Watanabe K. The EEG evolution and neurological prognosis of perinatal hypoxia in neonates. *Brain Development* 1988; **11**: 115–20.

36 Wertheim D, Mercuri E, Faundez JC, Rutherford M, Acolet D, Dubowitz L. Prognostic value of continuous electroencephalographic recording in full term infants with hypoxic ischaemic encephalopathy. *Archives of Disease in Childhood* 1994; **71**: F97–102.

37 Connell J, Oozeer RC, Dubovitz V. Continuous 4 channel EEG monitoring: a guide to interpretation, with normal values, in preterm infants. *Neuropediatrics* 1987; **18**: 138–45.

38 Murdoch Eaton DG, Connell J, Dubowitz L, Dubowitz V. Monitoring of the electroencephalogram during intensive care. *Clinics in Developmental Medicine* 1992; **120**: 48–65.

39 Thornberg E, Ekstrom-Jobal B. Cerebral function monitoring: a method of predicting outcome in term neonates after severe perinatal asphyxia. *Acta Paediatrica* 1994; **83**: 596–601.

40 Eken P, Toet MC, Groenendaal F, de Vries LS. Predictive value of early neuroimaging, pulsed Doppler and neurophysiology in full term infants with hypoxic-ischaemic encephalopathy. *Archives of Disease in Childhood* 1995; **73**: F75–80.

41 Hellstrom-Westas L, Rosen I, Svenningsen NW. Predictive value of early continuous amplitude integrated EEG recordings on outcome after severe birth asphyxia in full term infants. *Archives of Disease in Childhood* 1995; **72**: F34–8.

42 Stockard JE, Stockard JJ, Kleinberg F, Westmoreland BF. Prognostic value of brainstem auditory evoked potentials in neonates. *Archives of Neurology* 1983; **40**: 360–5.

43 Muttitt SC, Taylor MJ, Kobyashi JS, MacMillan L, Whyte HE. Serial evoked visual potentials and outcome in full term birth asphyxia. *Pediatric Neurology* 1991; **7**: 86–90.

44 De Vries LS. Somatosensory evoked potential in term neonates with postasphyxial encephalopathy. *Clinics in Perinatology* 1993; **20**: 463–82.

45 Hope PL, Costello AM, Cady EB *et al.* Cerebral energy metabolism studied with phosphorous NMR spectroscopy in normal and birth-asphyxiated infants. *Lancet* 1984; **ii**: 366–70.

46 Azzopardi D, Wyatt JS, Cady EB *et al.* Prognosis of newborn infants with hypoxic-ischemic brain injury assessed by phosphorus magnetic resonance spectroscopy. *Pediatric Research* 1989; **25**: 445–51.

47 Moorcraft J, Bolas NM, Ives NK *et al.* Global and depth resolved phosphorus magnetic resonance spectroscopy to predict outcome after birth asphyxia. *Archives of Disease in Childhood* 1991; **66**: 1119–23.

48 Martin E, Buchli R, Ritter S *et al.* Diagnostic and prognostic value of cerebral 31P magnetic resonance spectroscopy in neonates with perinatal asphyxia. *Pediatric Research* 1996; **40**: 749–58.

49 Peden CJ, Cowan FM, Bryant DJ *et al.* Proton MR spectroscopy of the brain in infants. *Journal of Computer Assissted Tomography* 1990; **14**: 886–94.

50 Peden CJ, Rutherford MA, Sargentoni J, Cox IJ, Bryant DJ, Dubowitz LMS. Proton spectroscopy of the neonatal brain following hypoxic-ischaemic injury. *Developmental Medicine and Child Neurology* 1993; **35**: 502–10.

51 Groenendaal F, Veenhoven RH, van der Grond J, Jansen GH, Witkamp TD, de Vries LS. Cerebral lactate and N-acetyl-aspartate/choline ratios in asphyxiated full-term neonates demonstrated in vivo using proton magnetic resonance spectroscopy. *Pediatric Research* 1994; **35**: 148–51.

52 Penrice J, Cady EB, Lorek A *et al.* Proton magnetic resonance spectroscopy of the brain in normal preterm and term infants, and early changes after perinatal hypoxia-ischemia. *Pediatric Research* 1996; **40**: 6–14.

53 Hanrahan JD, Sargentoni J, Azzopardi D *et al.* Cerebral metabolism within 18 hours of birth asphyxia: a proton magnetic resonance spectroscopy study. *Pediatric Research* 1996; **39**: 584–90.

54 Peliowski A, Finer NN. Birth asphyxia in the term infant. In: Sinclair JC, Bracken MB eds. *Effective care of the newborn infant.* Oxford: Oxford University Press, 1992: 249–79.

55 Roberston CMT, Finer NN, Grace MGA. School performance of survivors of neonatal encephalopathy associated with birth asphyxia at term. *Journal of Pediatrics* 1989; **114**: 753–60.

56 Estan J, Hope P. Unilateral neonatal cerebral infarction in full term infants. *Archives of Disease in Childhood* 1996; **76**: F88–93.

57 Voorhies TM, Ehrlich ME, Frayer W, Lee B, Vannucci RC. Occlusive vascular disease in perinatal cerebral hypoxia-ischemia. *American Journal of Perinatology* 1983; **1**: 1–5.

58 Volpe JJ. Hypoxic-ischemic encephalopathy: neuropathology and pathogenesis. In: Volpe JJ ed. *Neurology of the newborn*, 3rd edn. Philadelphia: Saunders, 1995: 279–313.

59 Mercuri E, Cowan F, Rutherford M, Acolet D, Pennock J, Dubowitz L. Ischaemic and haemorrhagic brain lesions in newborns with seizures and normal Apgar scores. *Archives of Disease in Childhood* 1995; **73**: F67–74.

60 Perlman JM, Rollins NK, Evans D. Neonatal stroke: clinical characteristics and cerebral blood flow velocity measurements. *Pediatric Neurology* 1994; **11**: 281–4.

61 Bouza H, Rutherford M, Acolet D, Pennock JM, Dubowitz LM. Evolution of early hemiplegic signs in full-term infants with unilateral brain lesions in the neonatal period: a prospective study. *Neuropediatrics* 1994; **25**: 201–7.

62 Taylor GA. Alterations in regional cerebral blood flow in neonatal stroke: preliminary findings with color Doppler sonography. *Pediatric Radiology* 1994; **24**: 111–15.

63 Steventon DM, John PR. Power Doppler ultrasound appearances of neonatal ischaemic brain injury. *Pediatric Radiology* 1997; **27**: 147–9.

64 Moseley ME, Kucharczyk J, Mintorovitch J *et al*. Diffusion weighted MR imaging of acute stroke: correlation with T2 weighted and magnetic susceptibility enhanced MR imaging in cats. *AJNR: American Journal of Neuroradiology* 1990; **11**: 423–9.

65 Groenendaal F, van der Grond J, Witkamp TD, de Vries LS. Proton magnetic resonance spectroscopic imaging in neonatal stroke. *Neuropediatrics* 1995; **26**: 243–8.

66 Wulfeck BB, Trauner DA, Tallal PA. Neurologic, cognitive, and linguistic features of infants after early stroke. *Pediatric Neurology* 1991; **7**: 266–9.

67 Clancy R, Malin S, Laraque D, Baumgart S, Younkin D. Focal motor seizures heralding stroke in full-term neonates. *American Journal of Diseases in Children* 1985; **139**: 601–6.

68 Sran SK, Baumann RJ. Outcome of neonatal strokes. *American Journal of Diseases in Children* 1988; **142**: 1086–8.

69 Feldman HM, Holland AL, Kemp SS, Janosky JE. Language development after unilateral brain injury. *Brain and Language* 1992; **42**: 89–102.

70 Mercuri E, Atkinson J, Braddick O *et al*. Visual function and perinatal focal cerebral infarction. *Archives of Disease in Childhood* 1996; **75**: F76–81.

71 Takashima S, Armstrong DL, Becker LE. Subcortical leukomalacia. Relationship to development of the cerebral sulcus and its vascular supply. *Archives of Neurology* 1978; **35**: 470–2.

72 Perlman JM, Risser R, Broyles RS. Bilateral cystic periventricular leukomalacia in the premature infant: associated risk factors. *Pediatrics* 1996; **97**: 822–7.

73 Szymonowicz W, Preston H, Yu VYH. The surviving monozygotic twin. *Archives of Disease in Childhood* 1986; **61**: 454–8.

74 Larroche J-C, Aubry M-C, Narcy F. Intrauterine brain damage in nonimmune hydrops fetalis. *Biology of the Neonate* 1992; **61**: 273–80.

75 Zupan V, Gonzalez P, Lacaze-Masmonteil T. Periventricular leukomalacia: risk factors revisited. *Developmental Medicine and Child Neurology* 1996; **38**: 1061–7.

76 Dubowitz LMS, Bydder GM, Mushin J. Developmental sequence of periventricular leukomalacia. *Archives of Disease in Childhood* 1985; **60**: 349–55.

77 Stewart A, Hope PL, Hamilton P *et al*. Prediction in very preterm infants of satisfactory neurodevelopmental progress at 12 months. *Developmental Medicine and Child Neurology* 1988; **30**: 53–63.

78 Hill A, Melson GL, Clark HB, Volpe JJ. Hemorrhagic periventricular leucomalacia: diagnosis by real time ultrasound and correlation with autopsy findings. *Pediatrics* 1982; **69**: 282–4.

79 Nwaesei CG, Pape KE, Martin DJ, Becker LE, Fitz CR. Periventricular infarction diagnosed by ultrasound: a postmortem correlation. *Journal of Pediatrics* 1984; **105**: 106–10.

80 Martin DJ, Hill A, Fitz CR, Daneman A, Havill DA, Becker LE. Hypoxic/ischaemic cerebral injury in the neonatal brain. A report of sonographic features with computed tomographic correlation. *Pediatric Radiology* 1983; **13**: 307–12.

81 Trounce JQ, Rutter N, Levene MI. Periventricular leucomalacia and intraventricular haemorrhage in the preterm neonate. *Archives of Disease in Childhood* 1986; **61**: 1196–202.

82 Levene MI, Wigglesworth JS, Dubowitz V. Hemorrhagic periventricular leukomalacia in the neonate: a real-time ultrasound study. *Pediatrics* 1983; **71**: 794–7.

83 Bozynski ME, Nelson MN, Matalon TA *et al*. Cavitary periventricular leukomalacia: incidence and short-term outcome in infants weighing less than or equal to 1200 grams at birth. *Developmental Medicine and Child Neurology* 1985; **27**: 572–7.

84 Fawar C-L, Calame A, Perentes E, Anderegg A. Periventricular leukomalacia: a correlation study between real-time ultrasound and autopsy findings. *Neuroradiology* 1985; **27**: 292–300.

85 de Vries LS, Wigglesworth JS, Regev R, Dubowitz LMS. Evolution of periventricular leukomalacia during the neonatal period and infancy: correlation of imaging and postmortem findings. *Early Human Development* 1988; **17**: 205–19.

86 Pfister-Goedeke L, Boltshauser E. Postnatale Entwicklung einer multilokularen zystischen Enzephalopathie beim Neugeborenen. Ultraschall-Verlaufskontrolle multipler Hirninfarkte. Postnatal development of muticystic encephlopathy in a newborn infant. [Ultrasound study of the evolution of multiple cerebral infarctions]. *Helvetica Paediatrica Acta* 1982; **37**: 59–65.

87 Trounce JQ, Levene MI. Diagnosis and outcome of subcortical leucomalacia. *Archives of Disease in Childhood* 1985; **60**: 1041–4.

88 de Vries L, Dubowitz LMS. Cystic leucomalacia in preterm infants: site of lesion in relation to prognosis. *Lancet* 1985; **ii**: 1075–6.

89 de Vries LS, Regev R, Dubowitz LM. Late onset cystic leucomalacia. *Archives of Disease in Childhood* 1986; **61**: 298–9.

90 Larroche J-C. Fetal encephalopathies of circulatory origin. *Biology of the Neonate* 1986; **50**: 61–74.

91 Nakamura Y, Fujiyoshi Y, Fukuda S *et al*. Cystic brain lesion in utero. *Acta Pathologica Japonica* 1986; **36**: 613–20.

92 Achiron R, Pinchas OH, Reichman B *et al*. Fetal intracranial haemorrhage: clinical significance of in utero ultrasonographic diagnosis. *British Journal of Obstetrics and Gynaecology* 1993; **100**: 995–9.

93 Bejar R, Coen RW, Merrit TA *et al*. Focal necrosis of the white matter (periventricular leukomalacia): sonographic, pathologic, and electroencephalographic features. *AJNR: American Journal of Neuroradiology* 1986; **7**: 1073–9.

94 Bejar R, Wozniak P, Allard M *et al*. Antenatal origin of neurologic damage in newborn infants. I. Preterm infants. *American Journal of Obstetrics and Gynecology* 1988; **159**: 357–63.

95 Goetz MC, Gretebeck RJ, Oh KS, Shaffer D, Hermansen MC. Incidence, timing, and follow-up of periventricular leukomalacia. *American Journal of Pathology* 1995; **12**: 325–7.

96 Rushton DI, Preston PR, Durbin GM. Structure and evolution of echodense lesions in the neonatal brain. *Archives of Disease in Childhood* 1985; **60**: 798–808.

97 Nwaesei CG, Allen AC, Vincer MJ *et al*. Effect of timing of cerebral ultrasonography on the prediction of later neurodevelopmental outcome in high-risk preterm infants. *Journal of Pediatrics* 1988; **112**: 970–5.

98 Dubowitz LM, Bydder GM, Mushin J. Developmental sequence of periventricular leukomalacia. Correlation of ultrasound, clinical, and nuclear magnetic resonance functions. *Archives of Disease in Childhood* 1985; **60**: 349–55.

99 Wilson DA, Steiner RE. Periventricular leukomalacia: evaluation with MR imaging. *Radiology* 1986; **160**: 507–11.

100 de Vries LS, Dubowitz LM, Pennock JM, Bydder GM. Extensive cystic leukomalacia: correlation of cranial ultrasound, magnetic resonance imaging and clinical findings in sequential studies. *Clinical Radiology* 1989; **40**: 158–66.

101 Eken P, de Vries LS, van der Graaf Y, Meiners LC, van Nieuwenhuizen O. Haemorrhagic-ischaemic lesions of the neonatal brain: correlation between cerebral visual impairment, neurodevelopmental outcome and MRI in infancy. *Developmental Medicine and Child Neurology* 1995; **37**: 41–55.

102 Eken P, de Vries LS, van Nieuwenhuizen O, Schalij-Delfos NE, Reits D, Spekreijse H. Early predictors of cerebral visual impairment in infants with cystic leukomalacia. *Neuropediatrics* 1996; **27**: 16–25.

103 de Vries LS, Eken P, Groenendaal F, van Haastert IC, Meiners LC. Correlation between the degree of periventricular leukomalacia diagnosed using cranial ultrasound and MRI later in infancy in children with cerebral palsy. *Neuropediatrics* 1993; **24**: 263–8.

104 Guit GL, van der Bor M, den Ouden L, Wondergem JH. Prediction of neurodevelopmental outcome in the preterm infant: MR-staged myelination compared with cranial ultrasound. *Radiology* 1990; **175**: 107–9.

105 van der Bor M, den Ouden L, Guit GL. Value of cranial ultrasound and magnetic resonance imaging in predicting neurodevelopmental outcome in preterm infants. *Pediatrics* 1992; **90**: 196–9.

106 Klimach VJ, Cooke RW. Short-latency cortical somatosensory evoked responses of preterm infants with ultrasound abnormality of the brain. *Developmental Medicine and Child Neurology* 1988; **30**: 215–21.

107 de Vries LS, Eken P, Pierrat V, Daniels H, Casaer P. Prediction of neurodevelopmental outcome in the preterm infant: short latency cortical somatosensory evoked potentials compared with cranial ultrasound. *Archives of Disease in Childhood* 1992; **67**: 1177–81.

108 Pierrat V, de Vries LS, Minami T, Caesar P. Somatosensory evoked potentials and adaptation to extrauterine life: a longitudinal study. *Brain Development* 1990; **12**: 376–80.

109 White CP, Cooke RW. Somatosensory evoked potentials following posterior tibial nerve stimulation predict later motor outcome. *Developmental Medicine and Child Neurology* 1994; **36**: 34–40.

110 Gilmore R, Brock J, Hermansen MC, Baumann R. Development of lumbar spinal cord and cortical evoked potentials after tibial nerve stimulation in the preterm infant: effects of gestational age and other factors. *Electroencephalography and Clinical Neurophysiology* 1987; **68**: 28–39.

111 Taylor MJ, Saliba E, Laugier J. Use of evoked potentials in preterm neonates. *Archives of Disease in Childhood* 1996; **74**: F70–6.

112 Bowerman RA, Donn SM, DiPetro MA, D'Amato CJ, Hicks SP. Periventricular leukomalacia in the preterm newborn infant: sonographic and clinical features. *Radiology* 1984; **151**: 383–8.

113 Weindling AM, Rochefort MJ, Calvert SA, Fok T-F, Wilkinson A. Development of cerebral palsy after sonographic detection of periventricular cysts in the newborn. *Developmental Medicine and Child Neurology* 1985; **27**: 800–6.

114 Calvert SA, Hoskins EM, Fong KW, Forsyth SC. Periventricular leukomalacia: ultrasonic diagnosis and neurological outcome. *Acta Paediatrica Scandinavica* 1986; **76**: 254–59.

115 Szymonowicz W, Yu VYH, Bajuk B, Astbury J. Neurodevelopmental outcome of periventricular haemorrhage and leukomalacia in infants 1250g or less at birth. *Early Human Development* 1986; **14**: 1–7.

116 Fawer CL, Diebold P, Calame A. Periventricular leukomalacia and neurodevelopmental outcome in preterm infants. *Archives of Disease in Childhood* 1987; **62**: 30–6.

117 Graham M, Levene MI, Trounce JQ, Rutter N. Prediction of cerebral palsy in very low birthweight infants: prospective ultrasound study. *Lancet* 1987; **ii**: 593–6.

118 Bozynski MEA, Nelson MN, Genaze D *et al*. Cranial ultrasound and the prediction of cerebral palsy in infants weighing 1200 grams or less at birth. *Developmental Medicine and Child Neurology* 1988; **30**: 342–8.

119 Fazzi E, Lanzi G, Gerardo A, Ometto A, Orcesi S, Rondini G. Neurodevelopmental outcome in very-low-birthweight infants with or without periventricular haemorrhage and/or leucomalacia. *Acta Paediatrica* 1992; **81**: 808–11.

120 Shortland D, Levene MI, Trounce J, Ng Y, Graham M. The evolution and outcome of cavitating periventricular leukomalacia in infancy: a study of 46 cases. *Journal of Perinatal Medicine* 1988; **16**: 241–7.

121 Fazzi E, Orcesi S, Caffi L, *et al*. Neurodevelopmental outcome at 5–7 years in preterm infants with periventricular leukomalacia. *Neuropediatrics* 1994; **25**: 134–9.

122 Fawar CL, Calame A. Significance of ultrasound appearances in the neurological development and

cognitive abilities of preterm infants at 5 years. *European Journal of Pediatrics* 1991; **150**: 515–20.

123 Monset-Couchard M, de Bethmann O, Radvanyi-Bouvet MF, Papin C, Bordarier C, Relier JP. Neurodevelopmental outcome in cystic periventricular leukomalacia (CPVL) (30 cases). *Neuropediatrics* 1988; **19**: 124–31.

124 de Vries LS, Dubowitz LM, Dubowitz V *et al.* Predictive value of cranial ultrasound in the newborn baby: a reappraisal. *Lancet* 1985; **ii**: 137–40.

125 Scher MS, Dobson V, Carpenter NA, Guthrie RD. Visual and neurological outcome of infants with periventricular leukomalacia. *Developmental Medicine and Child Neurology* 1989; **31**: 353–65.

126 Eken P, Nieuwenhuizen O, van der Graaf Y, Schalij-Delfos NE, de Vries LS. Relation between neonatal cranial ultrasound abnormalities and cerebral visual impairment in infancy. *Developmental Medicine and Child Neurology* 1994; **36**: 3–15.

127 De Vries LS, Connell JA, Dubowitz LM, Oozeer RC, Dubowitz V, Pennock JM. Neurological electrophysiological and MRI abnormalities in infants with extensive cystic leukomalacia. *Neuropediatrics* 1987; **18**: 61–6.

128 Appleton RE, Lee RE, Hey EN. Neurodevelopmental outcome of transient neonatal intracerebral echodensities. *Archives of Disease in Childhood* 1990; **65**: 27–9.

129 McMenamin JB, Shackelford GD, Volpe JJ. Outcome of neonatal intraventricular hemorrhage with periventricular echodense lesions. *Annals of Neurology* 1984; **15**: 285–90.

130 Levene M, Dowling S, Graham M, Fogelman K, Galton M, Phillips M. Impaired motor function (clumsiness) in 5 year old children: correlation with neonatal ultrasound scans. *Archives of Disease in Childhood* 1992; **67**: 687–90.

131 De Vries LS, Regev R, Pennock JM, Wigglesworth JS, Dubowitz LM. Ultrasound evolution and later outcome of infants with periventricular densities. *Early Human Development* 1988; **16**: 225–33.

132 Jongmans M, Henderson S, de Vries L, Dubowitz L. Duration of periventricular echodensities in preterm infants and neurological outcome at 6 years of age. *Archives of Disease in Childhood* 1993; **69**: 9–13.

133 Eken P, de Vries LS, van Nieuwenhuizen O, Schalij-Delfos NE, Reits D, Spekreijse H. Early predictors of cerebral visual impairment in infants with cystic leukomalacia. *Neuropediatrics* 1996; **27**: 16–25.

134 Ekert PG, Keenan NK, Whyte HE, Boulton J, Taylor MJ. Visual evoked potentials for prediction of neuro developmental outcome in preterm infants. *Biology of the Neonate* 1997; **71**: 148–55.

135 Papile L-A, Burstein J, Burstein R, Koffler H. Incidence and evolution of subependymal and intraventricular hemorrhage: a study of infants with birth weight less than 1500 g. *Journal of Pediatrics* 1978; **92**: 529–34.

136 Hambleton G, Wigglesworth JS. Origin of intraventricular haemorrhage in the preterm infant. *Archives of Disease in Childhood* 1976; **51**: 651–9.

137 Rushton DI, Preston PR, Durbin GM. Structure and evolution of echodense lesions in the neonatal brain: a combined ultrasound and necropsy study. *Archives of Disease in Childhood* 1985; **60**: 798–808.

138 Takashima S, Mito T, Ando Y. Pathogenesis of periventricular white matter hemorrhages in preterm infants. *Brain Development* 1986; **8**: 25–30.

139 Gould SJ, Howard S, Hope PL, Reynolds EO. Periventricular intraparenchymal cerebral haemorrhage in preterm infants: the role of venous infarction. *Journal of Pathology* 1987; **151**: 197–202.

140 Guzzetta F, Shackelford GD, Volpe S, Perlman JM, Volpe JJ. Periventricular intraparenchymal echodensities in the premature newborn: critical determinant of neurologic outcome. *Pediatrics* 1986; **78**: 995–1006.

141 Cooke RWI. Early and late cranial ultrasonographic appearances and outcome in very low birthweight infants. *Archives of Disease in Childhood* 1987; **62**: 931–7.

142 Fawer C-L, Levene MI, Dubowitz LMS. Intraventricular haemorrhage in a preterm neonate: discordance between clinical course and ultrasound scan. *Neuropediatrics* 1983; **14**: 242–4.

143 Blackman JA, McGuinness GA, Bale JF Jr, Smith WL Jr. Large postnatally acquired porencephalic cysts: unexpected developmental outcomes. *Journal of Child Neurology* 1991; **6**: 58–64.

144 Volpe JJ. Neonatal intracranial hemorrhage: pathophysiology, neuropathology, and clinical features. *Clinical Perinatology* 1977; **4**: 77–102.

145 Burstein J, Papile LA, Burstein R. Intraventricular hemorrhage in premature newborns: a prospective study with CT. *American Journal of Roentgenology* 1979; **132**: 631–5.

146 Dubowitz LMS, Levene MI, Morante A, Palmer P, Dubowitz V. Neurologic signs in neonatal intraventricular hemorrhage: a correlation with real time ultrasound. *Journal of Paediatrics* 1981; **99**: 127–33.

147 Pevsner PH, Garcia-Bunuel R, Leeds N, Finkelstein M. Subependymal and intraventricular hemorrhage in neonates: early diagnosis by computed tomography. *Radiology* 1976; **119**: 111–14.

148 Hope PL, Gould SJ, Howard S, Hamilton PA, Costello AM de L, Reynolds EOR. Precision of ultrasound diagnosis of pathologically verified lesions in the brains of very preterm infants. *Developmental Medicine and Child Neurology* 1988; **30**: 457–71.

149 Carson SC, Hertzberg BS, Bowie JD, Burger PC. Value of sonography in the diagnosis of intracranial hemorrhage and periventricular leukomalacia: a postmortem study of 35 cases. *AJR American Journal of Radiology* 1990; **155**: 595–601.

150 Papile L-A, Burstein J, Burstein R, Koffler H. Incidence and evolution of subependymal and intraventricular hemorrhage: a study of infants with birthweight <1500 g. *Journal of Pediatrics* 1978; **92**: 529–34.

151 Claris O, Besnier S, Lapillonne A, Picaud JC, Salle BL. Incidence of ischemic-hemorrhagic

cerebral lesions in premature infants of gestational age < or = 28 weeks: a prospective ultrasound study. *Biology of the Neonate* 1996; **70**: 29–34.

152 Szymonowicz W, Yu VYH. Timing and evolution of periventricular haemorrhage in infants weighing less than 1250g at birth. *Archives of Disease in Childhood* 1984; **59**: 7–12.

153 Levene MI, de Vries LS. Extension of neonatal intraventricular haemorrhage. *Archives of Disease in Childhood* 1984; **57**: 631–6.

154 de Vries LS, Eken P, Dubowitz LM. The spectrum of leukomalacia using cranial ultrasound. *Behavioural Brain Research* 1992; **49**: 1–6.

155 Zuerrer M, Martin E, Bolthauser E. MR imaging of intracranial hemorrhage in neonates and infants at 2.35 Tesla. *Neuroradiology* 1992; **33**: 233–9.

156 Taber KH, Hayman LA, Herrick RC, Kirkpatrick JB. Importance of clot structure in gradient-echo magnetic resonance imaging of hematoma. *Journal of Magnetic Resonance Imaging* 1996; **6**: 878–83.

157 Levene MI. Measurement of the growth of the lateral ventricles in pre-term infants with real time ultrasound. *Archives of Disease in Childhood* 1981; **56**: 900–4.

158 Anonymous. Randomised trial of early tapping in neonatal posthaemorrhagic ventricular dilatation. Ventriculomegaly Trial Group. *Archives of Disease in Childhood* 1990; **65**: 3–10.

159 Anonymous. Randomised trial of early tapping in neonatal posthaemorrhagic ventricular dilatation: results at 30 months. Ventriculomegaly Trial Group. *Archives of Disease in Childhood* 1994; **70**: F129–36.

160 Shankaran S, Keopke T, Woldt E *et al*. Outcome after posthemorrhagic ventriculomegaly in comparison with mild hemorrhage without ventriculomegaly. *Journal of Pediatrics* 1989; **114**: 109–14.

161 Craig WS. Intracranial haemorrhage in the newborn. *Archives of Disease in Childhood* 1938; **13**: 89–124.

162 Wigglesworth JS, Husemeyer RP. Intracranial birth trauma in vaginal breech delivery: the continued importance of injury to the occipital bone. *British Journal of Obstetrics and Gynaecology* 1977; **84**: 684–91.

163 Pape KE, Wigglesworth JS. Haemorrhage, ischaemia and the perinatal brain. *Clinics in Developmental Medicine* **69/70**. London: Spastics International Medical Publications, 1979.

164 Avrahami E, Frishman E, Minz M. CT demonstration of intracranial haemorrhage in term newborn following vacuum extractor delivery. *Neuroradiology* 1993; **35**: 107–8.

165 Castillo M, Fordham LA. MR of neurologically symptomatic newborns after vacuum extraction delivery. *AJNR: American Journal of Neuroradiology* 1995; **16**: 816–18.

166 Hanigan WC, Morgan AM, Stahlberg LK, Hiller JL. Tentorial hemorrhage associated with vacuum extraction. *Pediatrics* 1990; **85**: 534–9.

167 Huang CC, Shen EY. Tentorial subdural hemorrhage in term neonates: ultrasonographic diagnosis and clinical correlates. *Pediatric Neurology* 1991; **7**: 171–7.

168 Hayashi T, Hashimoto T, Fukuda S, Ohshima Y, Moritaka K. Neonatal subdural hematoma secondary to birth injury. Clinical analysis of 48 survivors. *Child's Nervous System* 1987; **3**: 23–9.

169 Rotmensch S, Grannum PA, Nores JA *et al*. In utero diagnosis and management of fetal subdural hematoma. *American Journal of Obstetrics and Gynecology* 1991; **164**: 1246–8.

170 Volpe JJ. Neonatal intracranial haemorrhage. Pathophysiology, neuropathology, and clinical features. *Clinics in Perinatology* 1977; **4**: 77–102.

171 Keeney SE, Adcock EW, McArdle CB. Prospective observations of 100 high-risk neonates by high-field (1.5 tesla) magnetic resonance imaging of the central nervous system. I. Intraventricular and extracerebral lesions. *Pediatrics* 1991; **87**: 421–9.

172 Pape KE, Wigglesworth JS. *Haemorrhage, ischaemia and the perinatal brain*. Philadelphia: JB Lippincott, 1979.

173 Larroche J-C. *Developmental pathology of the neonate*. Amsterdam: Excerpta Medica, 1977.

174 Levene MI, Williams JL, Fawer C-L. Ultrasound of the infant brain. *Clinics in Developmental Medicine* **92**. Oxford: Blackwell Scientific, 1985.

175 Rose AL, Lombroso CT. A study of clinical, pathological, and electroencephalographic features in 137 full-term babies with a long-term follow up. *Pediatrics* 1970; **45**: 404–25.

176 Palmer TW, Donn SM. Symptomatic subarachnoid haemorrhage in the term newborn. *Journal of Perinatology* 1991; **11**: 112–16.

177 Flodmark O, Becker LE, Harwood-Nash DC, Fitzhardinge PM, Fitz CR, Chuang SH. Correlation between computed tomography and autopsy in premature and full-term neonates that have suffered perinatal asphyxia. *Radiology* 1980; **137**: 93–103.

178 Grunnet ML, Shields WD. Cerebellar hemorrhage in the premature infant. *Journal of Pediatrics* 1976; **88**: 605–8.

179 Perlman JM, Nelson JS, McAlister WH, Volpe JJ. Intracerebellar hemorrhage in a premature newborn: diagnosis by real-time ultrasound and correlation with autopsy findings. *Pediatrics* 1983; **71**: 159–62.

180 Williamson WD, Percy AK, Fishman MA *et al*. Cerebellar hemorrhage in the term neonate: developmental and neurologic outcome. *Pediatric Neurology* 1985; **1**: 356–60.

181 Scotti G, Flodmark O, Harwood-Nash DC, Humphries RP. Posterior fossa hemorrhages in the newborn. *Journal of Computer Assisted Tomography* 1981; **5**: 68–72.

182 Rom S, Serfontein GL, Humphreys RP. Intracerebellar hematoma in the neonate. *Journal of Pediatrics* 1978; **93**: 486–8.

183 Trounce JQ, Dodd KL, Fawer CL, Fielder AR, Punt J, Levene MI. Primary thalamic haemorrhage in the newborn: a new clinical entity. *Lancet* 1985; **i**: 190–2.

184 Roland EH, Flodmark O, Hill A. Thalamic hemorrhage with intraventricular hemorrhage in the full-term newborn. *Pediatrics* 1993; **91**: 1219–20.

185 De Vries LS, Smet M, Goemans N, Wilms G, Devlieger H, Casaer P. Unilateral thalamic haemorrhage in the pre-term and full-term newborn. *Neuropediatrics* 1992; **23**: 153–6.

186 Adams C, Hochhauser L, Logan WJ. Primary thalamic and caudate hemorrhage in term neonates presenting with seizures. *Pediatric Neurology* 1988; **4**: 175–7.

187 Blair E, Stanley FJ. Intrapartum asphyxia: a rare cause of cerebral palsy. *Journal of Pediatrics* 1988; **112**: 515–19.

188 Nelson KB. What proportion of cerebral palsy is related to birth asphyxia? *Journal of Pediatrics* 1988; **112**: 572–3.

189 Truwit CL, Barkovich AJ, Koch TK, Ferriero DM. Cerebral palsy: MR findings in 40 patients. *AJNR: American Journal of Neuroradiology* 1992; **13**: 67–78.

190 Pharoah POD, Platt MJ, Cooke T. The changing epidemiology of cerebral palsy. *Archives of Disease in Childhood* 1996; **75**: F169–73.

191 Stewart A, Hope PL, Hamilton P *et al.* Prediction in very preterm infants of satisfactory neurodevelopmental progress at 12 months. *Developmental Medicine and Child Neurology* 1988; **30**: 53–63.

192 Ng PC, Dear PRF. The predictive value of a normal ultrasound scan in the preterm baby – a meta-analysis. *Acta Paediatrica* 1990; **79**: 286–91.

11 Magnetic resonance imaging of injury to the immature brain

Mary A Rutherford

11.1 DEFINITIONS

Hypoxic-ischemic encephalopathy (HIE) – For the purposes of the cases and images presented in this chapter the criteria were:

1 fetal distress on cardiotocogram, late decelerations or bradycardia, with or without meconium-stained liquor,

2 low Apgar scores with a need for resuscitation,
3 an encephalopathy from birth, although this may become more obvious over 24 hours,
4 absence of congenital malformations, metabolic disorder, or congenital infection.

The term HIE is being slowly replaced by neonatal encephalopathy, which covers a wider spectrum of disorders and does not presume a specific etiology.

This change in terminology reflects the inherent problems in proving that a fetus has suffered a severe hypoxic-ischemic event. It also allows for the fact that dual pathologies may occur within an infant, e.g. sepsis and ischemia. HIE may be graded and the following signs used as a guide to severity:

Grade I – Transient abnormalities in tone
Grade II – Abnormalities in tone, convulsions, difficulties feeding
Grade III – Altered consiousness, abnormalities in tone, ventilatory disturbance, with or without convulsions.

Term infant – Infant born at a gestation of greater than 37 completed weeks.
Preterm infant – Infant born at a gestation of less than 37 completed weeks.
Perinatal – This term has been used somewhat arbitrarily here to imply the period just prior to delivery and immediately after. It has been used to imply that the timing of the lesion is related to delivery and has not occurred more than a day prior to onset of labor or a day after delivery.

11.2   PURPOSE

This chapter will describe the magnetic resonance (MR) imaging appearances of brain injury in the immature brain. These appearances may be very specific to a particular insult at a given time and can often be used to predict the later neurodevelopmental outcome for the child.

11.3   MAGNETIC RESONANCE IMAGING – BASIC PRINCIPLES

MR imaging relies on the presence of protons (hydrogen nuclei) within the water of the body. A proton can be regarded as a small, freely suspended bar magnet, which spins rapidly around its own axis. When placed in a static magnetic field (B_0), the magnetization of the protons within the body lines up with the applied field. As a result, in a strong magnetic field there is a net nuclear magnetization, with the protons rotating or 'processing' about the direction of the main magnetic field. If a pulse of radiofrequency magnetic field rotating at the same frequency as the protons (B_1) generated by a coil is then applied to these protons there is a strong resonance or interaction. This can be used to rotate the net magnetization, which is par-

allel to the main magnetic field through any angle, depending on the strength and duration of the applied pulse. The usual choice is 90° or 180° so that the net nuclear magnetization becomes perpendicular or opposite in direction to the original static magnetic field.

Once the applied pulse is switched off, the protons tend to realign with the main magnetic field; this changing magnetization, perpendicular to B_0, induces a small voltage in a receiver coil which is placed around the patient. This electrical signal (voltage or current) is known as free induction decay (FID). The initial magnitude of FID is determined by the nuclear relaxation times. It decays with the constant T2, the transverse relaxation time, which reflects the interaction of nuclei with one another. After the net magnetization has been rotated into the transverse plane, the longitudinal magnetization parallel to B_0 recovers with the time constant T1, the longitudinal relaxation time. There is a wide range of values of T1 and T2 for different tissues, but in general terms, there is a relationship with viscosity: liquids have long T1 and long T2 values, soft tissues have shorter T1 and T2 values, and solids have very short T2 and very long T1 values.

MR pulse sequences consist of radiofrequency pulses and gradient magnetic fields that are applied to nuclei within the main static magnetic field in a systematic way with the FID signal or a variant of it collected at specific times. The pulse sequence incorporates methods of localizing the signal to specific voxels. Changes to tissues can often be detected as a result of changes in T1 and T2 and other parameters. More detail is available elsewhere.[1,2]

11.4   TECHNICAL ISSUES

Most MR scanners have been made for imaging adults and are also suitable for older children, but it is usually necessary to modify the approach when imaging the newborn. Adjustments need to be made to coils, sequences and monitoring equipment to insure good-quality images with maximum safety. Many different magnet systems may be used. Most commercially available scanners have a strength of 1 or 1.5 T (tesla), although open 0.7 T systems are now being produced and 3 T systems are being developed for clinical use.

Signal-to-noise ratios are approximately proportional to field strength but with increasing strength there are increased artefacts from chemical shift, patient motion, susceptibility, and flow.

The signal-to-noise ratio of an MR image is greatly improved by using the smallest receiver coil appropriate for the body part being examined. A dedicated infant coil will improve signal-to-noise ratio, shorten scanning times, and allow easier positioning of the infant.

With the advent of fast imaging sequences that allow non-motion artefacted images of the fetus, the identification and description of antenatally acquired brain damage are feasible prior to delivery. Fetal imaging may be performed on any system that has a sufficiently wide bore to accommodate the pregnant mother, suitable surface coils to place over the abdomen, and the ability to perform fast imaging. Single shots of the fetal brain can be taken in less than a second. Image quality is not yet as good as *ex-utero* scans but improvements will undoubtedly occur over the next few years.

11.5   PULSE SEQUENCES

Sequences need to be adjusted to allow for the different composition of the immature brain. The neonatal brain is approximately 92–95 percent water. This decreases over the first 2 years of life to adult values of 80–85 percent. The increased water content of the neonatal brain is associated with a marked increase in T1 and T2 and the standard sequences used for adults are not always suitable. The choice of sequences used for an examination is also limited by their availability within an MR system and their duration. Infants may be clinically unstable or sedation may wear off, and for those reasons faster sequences are preferred but image quality and anatomical detail must still be acceptable. We routinely use a T1-weighted conventional spin-echo sequence (SE 860/20 [TR/TE]), a conventional T2-weighted sequence (SE 2700/120 [TR/TE]) or a fast spin-echo T2-weighted sequence (FSE 3000/208$_{ef}$ [TR/TE]) and an inversion recovery sequence (IR 3800/30/950 [TR/TE/TI]).

Diffusion-weighted (DW) imaging is now being used more frequently. DW imaging is the method of choice for identifying areas of acute white matter infarction but spatial resolution using fast DW may be limited. DW abnormalities decrease with time from the insult, and are usually no longer evident 2 weeks after the insult. DW imaging has been disappointing for identifying early changes within the basal ganglia and thalami. Imaging with three different sensitization directions may show abnormalities within the posterior limb of the internal capsule (PLIC); however, these changes may

appear no earlier than they do with conventional images. Measurements of apparent diffusion coefficients within different regions of the brain may provide earlier detection of injury and help characterize its nature. Protocols that provide fast diffusion and perfusion sequences are available and have been used with good result in adult stroke patients but the role of perfusion-weighted imaging in the neonate has yet to be established.

There is little information available about the value of contrast enhancement in infants with hypoxic-ischemic injury. The appearances of the normal neonatal brain following contrast have been described.[3] Contrast administration may enhance changes within the cortex, so-called 'cortical highlighting' in HIE. As in the adult patient, contrast should always be used in cases of suspected infection. This would enhance parenchymal lesions and also infected meninges. The fluid attenuated inversion recovery (FLAIR) sequence has been used to identify both subarachnoid and intraventricular hemorrhage in adult patients[4,5] and is frequently used in infants with suspected non-accidental brain injury. There are few reports on the use of the FLAIR sequence in neonates with HIE[6] but it is often used after the first year of life for identifying abnormally increased T2, consistent with glial tissue (see Fig. 11.25).

Proton density images may be useful in the first few days after delivery as abnormalities within the basal ganglia and thalami may be detected earlier than with other sequences.[7] The proton density sequence may also provide early information on 'cortical edema'[7] or loss of gray/white matter differentiation.

11.6   PREPARATION FOR IMAGING

Neonates may often be scanned without sedation during natural sleep. However, any movement of the head, even with rather labored or noisy breathing, can render the images difficult to interpret. Infants over the age of 3 months will almost always require sedation and we usually use chloral hydrate orally or via suppository. It is rarely necessary to use general anesthesia to image a child under 2 years old. In our unit, all neonates and infants undergoing MR scanning are monitored with ECG and pulse oximetry and a pediatrician is in attendance throughout. Infants who require assisted ventilation can be imaged in an MR scanner providing MR-compatible ventilation and monitoring equipment are available.

11.7   TIMING THE MR IMAGE EXAMINATION

The ideal time to image depends on the information required but is often constrained by the resources available for imaging sick neonates. Conventional scans performed within the first 24 hours may appear normal even when there has been severe perinatal injury to the brain (see Fig. 11.4b). Further studies to evaluate the role of very early diffusion-weighted imaging, the use of contrast and the FLAIR sequence are needed but are hampered by the difficulties of transferring acutely ill infants into the scanner very soon after delivery. Early imaging will, however, help to differentiate antenatal from perinatal lesions although repeat imaging may then be required to see the extent of the latter.

Perinatally acquired abnormalities 'mature' and become easier to identify by the end of the first week. For information on the exact pattern of injury a scan between 1 and 2 weeks of age is ideal. After 2 weeks there may be signs of cystic breakdown and atrophy, which may make the initial pattern of injury more difficult to define. Later imaging usually provides valuable information if the images are interpreted with a knowledge of both the spectrum of lesions seen following perinatal events and their evolution.

11.8   IMAGE INTERPRETATION

A knowledge of the normal MR appearances (Figs 11.1, 11.2a, and 11.3a) at different gestations is essential as clinically significant pathology can be relatively subtle. A normal finding for 36 weeks may be abnormal at 40 weeks. Imaging appearances are also influenced by the strength of magnet, the sequences used, the angle of acquisition and the windowing used. There are many sources of artefact when producing an image and these may sometimes be difficult to differentiate from pathological lesions. As a general rule, if images are obtained in at least two planes and with at least two sequences it is possible to distinguish most artefacts from pathological lesions.

Images should always be interpreted with knowledge of the gestation, age from birth and clinical course of the infant. A normal scan following perinatal asphyxia carries a good prognosis but in an infant with an atypical clinical course, suggestive of a metabolic disorder, a normal scan may have no prognostic power at all.

- Infants with a clinical picture of HIE should be imaged between the first and second week for maximum information about the sites of injury and therefore for prognosis.
- Very early imaging (less than 48 hours) may be helpful in deciding on management and whether intensive life support should be withdrawn. It will also help to exclude antenatally acquired lesions.
- Late imaging (over 1 month) needs cautious interpretation with a full knowledge of the spectrum of antenatally or perinatally acquired lesions and with their evolution.

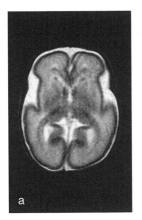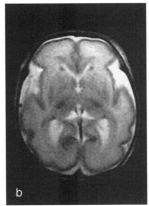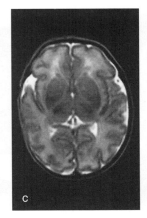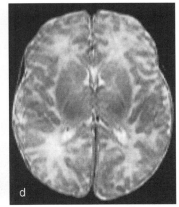

Figure 11.1 Normal appearances with increasing gestation. T2-weighted spin-echo sequences: (a) 25 weeks gestation, (b) 28 weeks gestation, (c) 34 weeks, (d) 40 weeks gestation. The cortex is seen as low signal intensity. The cerebrospinal fluid is high signal intensity. The most striking change is the rapid increase in cortical folding that occurs during this period.

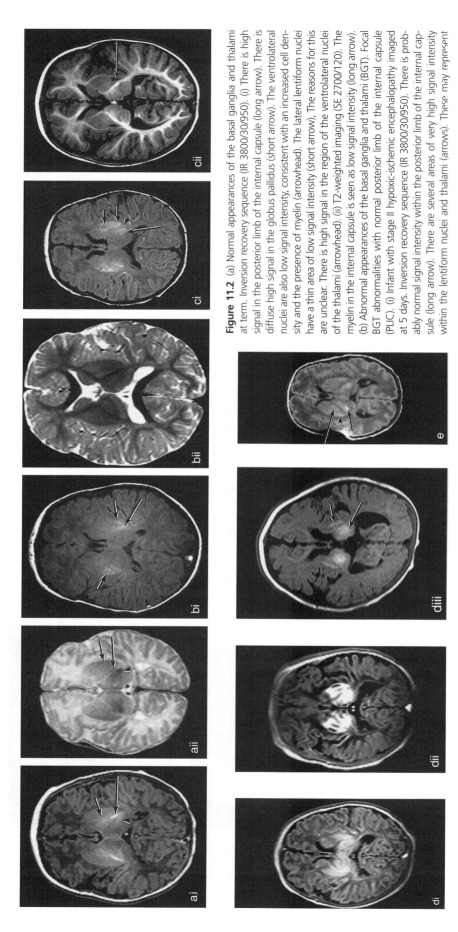

Figure 11.2 (a) Normal appearances of the basal ganglia and thalami at term. Inversion recovery sequence (IR 3800/30/950). (i) There is high signal in the posterior limb of the internal capsule (long arrow). There is diffuse high signal in the globus pallidus (short arrow). The ventrolateral nuclei are also low signal intensity, consistent with an increased cell density and the presence of myelin (arrowhead). The lateral lentiform nuclei have a thin area of low signal intensity (short arrow). The reasons for this are unclear. There is high signal in the region of the ventrolateral nuclei of the thalami (arrowhead). (ii) T2-weighted imaging (SE 2700/120). The myelin in the internal capsule is seen as low signal intensity (long arrow). Focal BGT abnormalities with normal posterior limb of the internal capsule (PLIC). (i) Infant with stage II hypoxic-ischemic encephalopathy imaged at 5 days. Inversion recovery sequence (IR 3800/30/950). There is probably normal signal intensity within the posterior limb of the internal capsule (long arrow). There are several areas of very high signal intensity within the lentiform nuclei and thalami (arrows). These may represent

small hemorrhages. (ii) T2-weighted spin-echo sequence (SE 2700/70). There are no abnormal signal intensities on follow-up imaging at 15 months when the infant had normal motor development. (c) (i) Focal BGT abnormalities with abnormal signal intensity (SI) in the PLIC. Inversion recovery sequence (IR 3800/30/950). There are focal abnormal high signal intensity areas in the lentiform nucleus (short arrows) and an exaggeration of the normal high signal in the lateral thalami (long arrow). There is no high signal from myelin within the PLIC (arrowhead). (ii) At 1 year of age there are characteristic focal low signal intensity cysts in the posterior part of the putamen (arrow). This infant developed an athetoid quadriplegia. (d) (i) Severe BGT abnormalities. Infant with stage II hypoxic-ischemic encephalopathy imaged at 5 days. There are widespread abnormal high SI throughout the basal ganglia and thalami. (ii) The same infant at 18 days. There is a further increase in high signal intensity. There are now additional low signal intensity lesions consistent with cyst formation. The high signal intensity is probably due to capillary proliferation. There is no obvious myelin within the PLIC. (iii) The same infant aged 7 months. Inversion recovery sequence (IR 3600/30/950). There has been marked atrophy of the basal ganglia and thalami. There is abnormal high signal intensity, which is most obvious in the thalami (long arrow). There is a linear abnormal high signal intensity within the lentiform nucleus (short arrow). This may represent abnormal myelination, so-called 'status marmoratus'. There is additional white matter atrophy. The child had developed microcephaly and a severe extensor spastic quadriplegia. She had persistent convulsions and made no real developmental progress. She died at 3 years of age from respiratory complications. (e) BGT abnormalities in the preterm brain. Preterm infant, gestation 28 weeks, who had a cardiorespiratory arrest at 2 weeks of age in association with clinical deterioration presumed to be septic in origin. Inversion recovery sequence (IR FSE 3500/30/950) at 32 weeks. This image has a left-sided superficial artefact. There is abnormal high signal intensity in the lateral thalamus (short arrow), the lateral lentiform (arrowhead) and the globus pallidus (long arrow). This was found to be infarction on post-mortem. The very bright signal intensity within the thalami (short arrow) corresponded to areas of neuronal mineralization.

In addition to a thorough knowledge of the normal appearances, an understanding of the evolution of pathological changes is necessary, although this may not be straightforward. The evolution of infarcted tissue is discussed later. MR imaging is exquisitely sensitive to hemorrhage. The appearances of hemorrhage change dramatically but not always predictably with time. Most studies on the evolution of hemorrhage are from adult patients. Hemorrhage in the immature brain sometimes behaves differently (Table 11.1). Despite popular belief, it is not always easy to date hemorrhage on MRI and it is not correct to assume that hemorrhagic areas of different signal intensity are always of different ages. The rate of evolution of hemorrhage may be due to factors other than the time of onset, such as the size and site of the lesion and whether there is associated infarction.

11.9   GESTATIONAL AGE AND BRAIN INJURY

All aspects of brain injury can be influenced by the gestation of the infant at the time of the insult. Gestational age may influence the type of insult sustained, the vulnerability of a specific structure to damage and the response of the brain to that damage. An infant is termed preterm if born at less than 37 weeks gestation and term if born after 37 weeks gestation. However, the majority of pathology in the preterm infant is seen at gestations of less than 32 weeks. Preterm patterns of damage may be found in infants who are subsequently born at term and can be confirmed as antenatal in origin by early imaging. In addition, occasionally preterm infants sustain an acute severe injury postnatally at a more mature age (Fig. 11.2e).

For the purposes of this chapter, the imaging patterns are divided according to the predominant site of the brain involved for both term and preterm infants.

11.10   LESIONS WITHIN THE BASAL GANGLIA AND THALAMI

11.10.1   Bilateral basal ganglia and thalamic lesions

Bilateral lesions within the basal ganglia and thalami (BGT) are often associated with later impairment but may result from a variety of insults.

11.10.1.1   Severe acute asphyxia

BGT lesions are responsible for the majority of cases of cerebral palsy in term-born infants with perinatal brain injury. BGT lesions are seen as a consequence of a severe acute hypoxic-ischemic insult.[8-16] In term infants they are typically found after events such as uterine rupture or placental abruption associated with severe fetal distress and a necessity for resuscitation at birth. Occasionally, severe BGT lesions are seen with less obvious precipitating events. This may reflect our failure to recognize the severity of asphyxia or an individual susceptibility to damage, perhaps because of previous hypoxic-ischemic events or because of an underlying metabolic or thrombotic disorder. In some neonates a lack of fetal distress and need for resuscitation is associated with bilateral BGT lesions that are well established and have occurred a few days prior to delivery, giving the fetus time to 'recover'. BGT lesions that occur many weeks before term delivery have been described following attempted maternal suicide (Fig. 11.3c).[17] These antenatal BGT lesions may result in a clinical picture of arthrogryposis in the fetus and may be confused with a primary neuromuscular disorder.

Table 11.1 Evolution of signal intensity from hemorrhage (adult data, idealized)

Age of parenchymal hemorrhage	T1-weighted image	T2-weighted image	Hemoglobin state
Hyperacute (<3 hours)	nil	nil	Oxyhemoglobin
Acute (3 hours–3 days)	isointense	low SI	Intracellular deoxyhemoglobin
Early subacute (3 days–10 days)	high SI	low SI	Intracellular methemoglobin
Late subacute (10 days–3 weeks)	high SI	high SI	Extracellular methemoglobin
Chronic (3 weeks plus)	nil/low SI	low SI	Hemosiderin

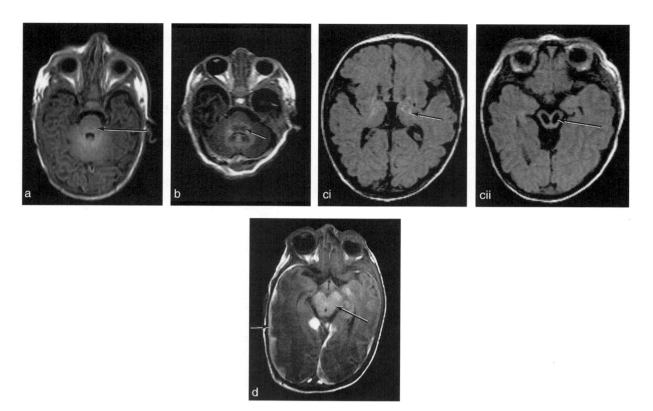

Figure 11.3 Brainstem. (a) Normal control infant at term. T1-weighted spin-echo (SE 860/20) sequence. There is a small area of focal high signal intensity (arrow) bilaterally consistent with myelin in the medial lemnisci of the pons There is a thin low SI region dorsal to the tracts. (b) Term infant with stage III hypoxic-ischemic encephalopathy. T1-weighted spin-echo sequence (SE 860/20). There are large bilateral abnormal low signal intensity lesions within the dorsal pons (arrow). Histology confirmed the presence of bilateral infarcts. (c) Female infant born at 27 weeks with arthrogryposis. There was a failed attempt at maternal suicide during the pregnancy at 22 weeks. Inversion recovery sequence (IR FSE 3500/30/950) at 5 days. (i) There is atrophy of the basal ganglia and thalami and abnormal high signal intensity within the thalamus (arrow). (ii) There is bilateral low signal intensity consistent with infarction in the mesencephalon. (d) Infant with stage III hypoxic-ischemic encephalopathy aged 8 days. There is a diffuse high signal within the mesencephalon bilaterally (long arrow). This image also shows extensive subdural hemorrhage (short arrow).

Term infants with perinatally acquired BGT lesions usually present with hypoxic-ischemic encephalopathy (HIE).[18]

The BGT are susceptible to injury because they are metabolically very active in the immature brain.[19] This is in part due to ongoing myelination. They also possess a high concentration of excitatory receptors. The changes seen on MR imaging are thought to be secondary to ischemia although the signal intensity abnormalities are such that they were originally described as hemorrhagic. Bilateral basal ganglia hemorrhage is very rare and the bilateral damage seen in HIE is presumed to be ischemic in etiology. The short T1 and T2 signal intensities seen as the lesions evolve (Fig. 11.2) are probably due to capillary proliferation and later to mineralization. Occasionally, small focal lesions are seen early on which may represent hemorrhage (Fig. 11.2bi). A distinction may be important as these

hemorrhages seem to evolve without atrophy or cyst formation and the infants do not develop major motor impairment (Fig. 11.2bii). These lesions are not, however, like the more classic large thalamic hemorrhages, which are usually unilateral (see Plate 27).

In term infants with HIE the main sites of abnormality are the posterior and lateral lentiform nucleus and the ventrolateral nuclei of thalami (Fig. 11.2c). More extensive lesions may involve all of the basal ganglia and medial areas of thalami (Fig. 11.2d) and there may be spread downwards to involve the midbrain and the dorsal aspects of the pons and medulla (Fig. 11.3b,c,d). Infants with such extensive lesions usually have stage III HIE and die within days or weeks of birth. In the preterm brain there may be predominantly thalamic involvement following severe asphyxia with less involvement of the lateral lentiform nuclei (Fig. 11.2e).[9]

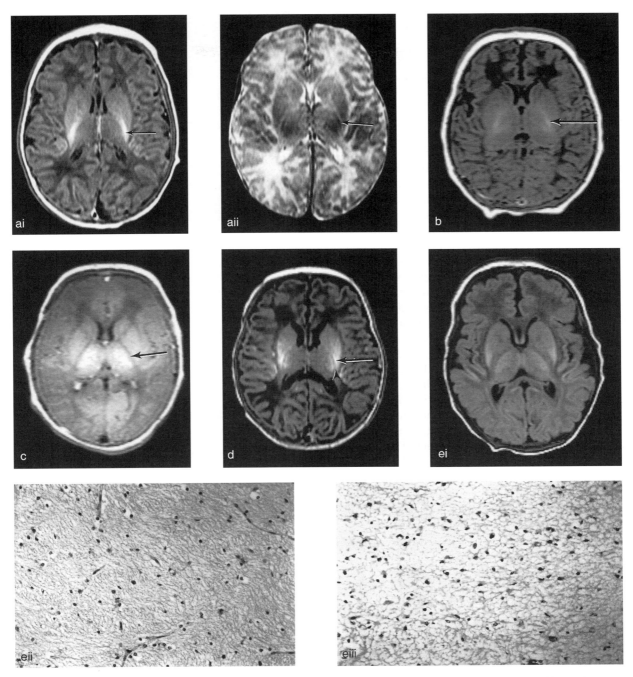

Figure 11.4 Posterior limb of the internal capsule. (a) Normal term infant born at 40 weeks gestation aged 2 days. (i) Inversion recovery sequence (IR 3800/30/950). Myelin is demonstrated in the posterior third of the posterior limb of the internal capsule (arrow). (ii) T2-weighted spin-echo sequence (SE 2700/120). The low signal intensity from myelin is less obvious (arrow). (b,c) Delayed loss of signal intensity in an infant with stage III hypoxic-ischemic encephalopathy who subsequently died. At 2 days of age there is a normal appearance to the myelin (b) (arrow). At 4 days there is a complete loss of signal intensity (c) (arrow). (d) Infant with stage II hypoxic-ischemic encephalopathy aged 5 days. Inversion recovery sequence (IR 3800/30/950). There is loss of the normal signal from myelin in the posterior limb but there are areas of abnormal high signal intensity running parallel to the internal capsule (arrow). (e) Infant with stage III hypoxic-ischemic encephalopathy who died at 14 days of age. Inversion recovery sequence (IR 3800/30/950) aged 12 days. (i) There is loss of the normal high signal intensity from myelin. There are additional abnormal high signal intensity areas within the basal ganglia and thalami. (ii) Normal histological appearances of the posterior limb of the internal capsule. (iii) The same infant as in (ei) who died at 14 days of age. There is edema and nuclear pyknosis throughout the internal capsule. (H&E from Dr W Squier, Oxford, with permission.)

11.10.1.2 Posterior limb of the internal capsule

In the term infant the most clinically useful association with BGT lesions is the signal intensity (SI) within the posterior limb of the internal capsule. In the normal brain at term there should be evidence of myelin in the posterior third to half of the internal capsule (Fig. 11.3a). Myelination is usually first evident at around 37 weeks gestation and slightly earlier in infants born preterm. Absence of the normal SI in infants >37 weeks gestation is often seen with severe BGT lesions (Fig. 11.2c,d) and it is able to predict the neurodevelopmental outcome in term infants with HIE with a sensitivity of 0.9 and a specificity of 1.0.[13] Its advantage for predicting outcome is that it may appear before abnormal SI within other areas of the brain. However, it may still take up to 48 hours to become abnormal in some infants (Fig. 11.4b,c). The appearances of the abnormal internal capsule can vary and may sometimes be difficult to interpret (Fig. 11.4d). The long T1 and long T2 seen on imaging are consistent with edema or early infarction (Fig. 11.4e). Histological comparisons have confirmed the presence of edema throughout the posterior limb (Fig. 11.4e). Infants with abnormal SI within the PLIC on conventional imaging may have abnormal increased SI on diffusion-weighted imaging in all planes of sensitization, consistent with restricted diffusion of the protons within water. This implies that the

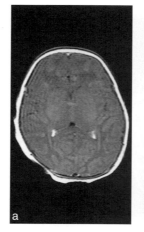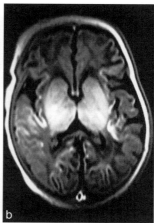

Figure 11.5 Brain swelling. T1-weighted spin-echo sequence (SE 860/20). (a) Post-contrast image showing severe brain swelling at 2 days of age in an infant with stage II hypoxic-ischemic encephalopathy. There are slit-like ventricles, a narrowed extra-cerebral space, interhemispheric fissure, and sulcal spaces. There is some loss of gray/white matter differentiation. (b) At 3 weeks of age the infant has developed widespread cortical and white matter abnormalities.

edema is cytotoxic and that there is irreversible infarction within the PLIC.

11.10.1.3 Additional abnormalities associated with BGT lesions

Term-born infants with BGT lesions in association with HIE may also have early brain swelling,

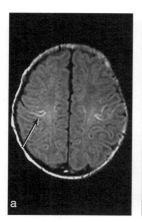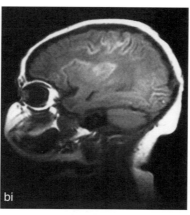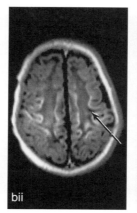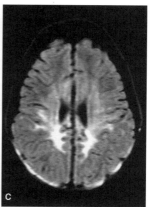

Figure 11.6 Abnormal 'highlighting' of the cortex. Inversion recovery sequence (IR 3800/30/950). (a) There is cortical highlighting around the central fissure (arrow). (b,c) Infant with stage II hypoxic-ischemic encephalopathy whose mother had repeated episodes of PV bleeding in pregnancy. Delivery was precipitated by an acute severe antepartum hemorrhage. Imaging was performed at 17 days. (b) T1-weighted spin-echo sequence (SE 860/20). (i) Sagittal plane. There is widespread cortical highlighting involving the cortex around the central sulcus, the insula, and in the occipital lobes. The highlighting is maximum at the depths of sulci. (ii) Level of the centrum semiovale. There is low signal intensity (arrow) developing in the subcortical white matter adjacent to areas of cortical highlighting. (c) Fluid attenuated inversion recovery (FLAIR) sequence aged 2.5 years. There is marked white matter atrophy and marked abnormal increased signal intensity at the site of the previous subcortical white matter infarction. This child had a global developmental delay and a spastic diplegia.

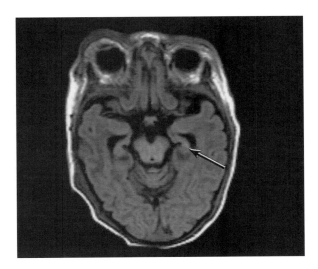

Figure 11.7 Hippocampal abnormalities. Infant with stage III hypoxic-ischemic encephalopathy aged 12 days. Inversion recovery sequence (IR 3800/300/950). There is abnormal high signal intensity in the hippocampal region (arrow). There is already some dilatation of the temporal horn of the lateral ventricle consistent with atrophy. This infant had additional diffuse changes throughout the basal ganglia and thalami on imaging and at postmortem.

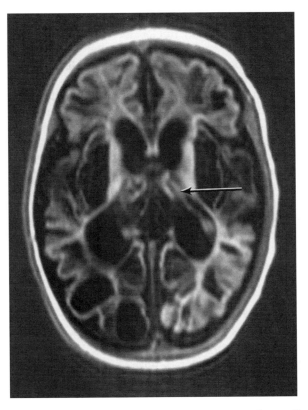

Figure 11.8 Severe basal ganglia and white matter abnormalities. Inversion recovery sequence (IR 3800/30/950). Infant with stage II hypoxic-ischemic encephalopathy at 4 weeks of age. There is atrophy and cystic breakdown throughout the basal ganglia and thalami (arrow). There is cystic breakdown of the entire white matter.

although this may not be severe and rarely lasts longer than a week (Fig. 11.5). Abnormal mainly short T1 appearances in the cortex, so-called 'cortical highlighting', almost always accompany significant BGT lesions at term. The predominant sites are the central fissure, the interhemispheric fissure and the insula (Fig. 11.6). The depths of the cortical sulci are preferentially affected (Fig. 11.6). The abnormal SI may take several days to evolve, being seen most clearly during the second week, by which time the adjacent subcortical white matter has developed abnormal SI consistent with infarction (Fig. 11.6). Cortical highlighting may not be present in the preterm infant with BGT lesions.[9] The highlighting is consistent with capillary proliferation occurring as a result of infarction in the deepest layers of cortex.

Severe BGT lesions are also associated with abnormalities in the medial temporal lobe. These are not immediately obvious but by the end of the second week there are definite short T1 areas within the hippocampal region and dilatation of the temporal horn as a result of adjacent tissue atrophy (Fig. 11.7).

In some infants with severe BGT there are additional widespread abnormalities in the white matter consistent with infarction giving rise to so-called multicystic leukomalacia (Fig. 11.8). In

infants with HIE who develop both BGT and early white matter infarction there may be compounding factors that prime the white matter. These factors include a more chronic or repetitive ischemic insult, infection, or an inherent susceptibility to ischemia.

11.10.1.4 Long-term evolution

In severe lesions the BGT may atrophy within 3 weeks. Late images usually have areas of long T2 within the atrophied basal ganglia. Abnormal high SI on T1-weighted images may no longer be evident but if present may represent status marmoratus (Fig. 11.2diii).[20] In infants with severe BGT the white matter also atrophies. Some of this atrophy can be explained by the subcortical white matter infarction seen in association with the initial cortical abnormalities. White matter atrophy may occur as a secondary phenomenon because of axonal interruption as a result of damage to the BGT.

In less severe focal BGT damage, cysts in the posterior lentiform nuclei are usually visible on 6–9 months scans (Fig. 11.2cii). Between 3 and 9 months the BGT may look remarkably normal even in the presence of injury severe enough to result in motor impairment. Mild atrophy of the BGT in these infants is difficult to detect on visual analysis of the images alone although sometimes the lentiform nuclei may have a flattened lateral border. Minor focal BGT lesions may leave no obvious MR abnormality outside of the neonatal period (Fig. 11.2bi,ii).

The normal SI from myelin in the PLIC returns in all but the most severe lesions, although it may have a thin and irregular appearance. The speed of return appears to reflect the degree of damage within the BGT.

11.10.1.5 Neurodevelopmental outcome

The clinical outcome of the child is dependent on the severity of the BGT lesions. Severe BGT lesions are associated with a severe spastic or mixed dystonic/spastic quadriplegia, secondary microcephaly, and severe intellectual impairment. There are usually persistent feeding difficulties and these children often require a gastrostomy to avoid long-term nasogastric tube feeding. These children make little developmental progress and may have seizures, which are difficult to control. Early death is common, usually as a result of respiratory complications (Fig. 11.2d). In infants with a combination of BGT and multicystic leukoencephalopathy (Fig. 11.8), the neurodevelopmental outcome is determined mainly by the severity of the BGT, particularly in terms of motor impairment. Less severe BGT lesions (Fig. 11.2c) are associated with the development of an athetoid quadriplegia, usually with good preservation of intellect and normal head growth. Mild BGT lesions may be associated with late-onset tremor and mild but often transient abnormalities of tone.

11.10.1.6 Posterior cerebral artery infarction

Bilateral lesions may be seen in the medial thalami in association with brainstem and cerebellar lesions (Fig. 11.9). This medial thalamic syndrome is well described in adults and is probably due to interruption of the posterior cerebral artery by either spasm or embolus.

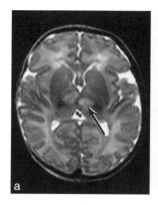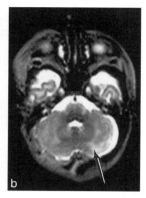

Figure 11.9 Medial thalamic lesions. Term-born infant presenting with convulsions on day 2 following a vacuum extraction. Apgar scores were normal. Imaging was performed on day 2. T2-eighted spin-echo sequence (SE 2700/120). (a) Low ventricular level. There are bilateral areas of abnormal high signal intensity within the medial thalami (arrow). There is a normal low signal intensity from myelin within the posterior limb of the internal capsule. (b) There is an area of abnormal high signal intensity within the left cerebellar hemisphere (arrow).

11.10.1.7 Sinus thrombosis

Bilateral lesions within the thalami may also be seen in the presence of straight sinus thrombosis (See Fig. 11.41).

11.10.1.8 Kernicterus

Infants with a history of bilirubinemia may show bilateral abnormal signal intensity within the basal ganglia although the distribution is different from that seen in HIE. Safe levels for serum bilirubin are well established in term infants but these are less easy to predict in the sick preterm infant.[21] MR abnormalities are seen in the globus pallidus and may also be detected in the subthalamic nuclei (Fig. 11.10). However, visualization of the latter is dependent on the angle of acquisition of the images. The abnormalities may be quite subtle initially as the globus pallidus has a similar relatively high signal in preterm infants on T1-weighted imaging. Repeat imaging will show persistence of this signal beyond term age and then a reversal of the signal intensity. Infants with these MR abnormalities show motor impairment in the form of an athetoid quadriplegia, intellectual and hearing deficits. Kernicterus is relatively rare in the developed world and there are no serial MR studies that describe the evolution of the lesions and their exact association with outcome.

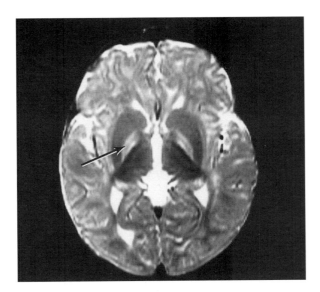

Figure 11.10 Kernicterus. Term-born infant with hyperbilirubin-emia. Neonatal imaging was equivocal with some increased signal intensity within the globus pallidus on T1-weighted imaging but at 11 months of age there are obvious abnormal areas of increased signal intensity on the T2-weighted images (arrow).

11.10.1.9 *Congenital infection*

Lesions in the caudate nuclei are often present in congenital infections such as cytomegalovirus. They form subependymal cysts that protrude into the ventricle. Atrophy of the caudate nucleus may occur with consequent widening of the caudothalamic notch (see Fig. 11.33a). These BG findings may coexist with abnormal signal intensities within the white matter (Fig. 11.33b).

11.10.1.10 *Inherited metabolic disorders*

Bilateral BGT lesions may also be seen in certain metabolic disorders that present in the neonatal period (Fig. 11.11). These infants may be differentiated from those with HIE by the evolution of their clinical signs, but there is often overlap.[22]

> All infants with HIE or those with basal ganglia lesions should have a full metabolic screen and a congenital infection screen.

11.10.2 Unilateral basal ganglia and thalamic lesions

11.10.2.1 *Infarction of the basal ganglia*

A unilateral lesion within the thalamus or basal ganglia may be infarctive and/or hemorrhagic.

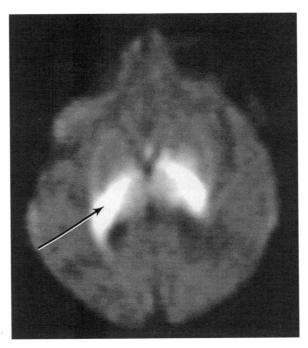

Figure 11.11 Metabolic disease. Term-born infant born to consanguineous parents. He presented with convulsions on day 5. The images were markedly abnormal with increased signal intensity in the corticospinal tracts, the globus pallidus, and cerebellum. The changes were particularly striking on diffusion-weighted imaging which is pathognomonic of maple syrup urine disease. This image shows striking abnormalities within the globus pallidus and posterior limb of the internal capsule (arrow) on diffusion-weighted imaging. The diagnosis was confirmed using proton magnetic resonance spectroscopy which showed an abnormal peak from the accumulation of branched chain amino acids.

Small lesions, usually within the caudate nucleus or lateral lentiform nucleus and consistent with striate artery infarction, may be found in preterm infants.[23] Occasionally they may be bilateral. Small unilateral cysts consistent with antenatal infarction may also be found incidentally in term infants, thus implying an antenatal etiology. Occasionally they may be found as an additional lesion in infants with neonatal stroke (Fig. 11.12). They may then highlight an inherent predisposition to infarction either because of a thrombotic disorder or because of a maternal embolic source. Infants with small unilateral infarction of the BG usually have a normal neurodevelopmental outcome.

Occasionally term neonates may present with a unilateral BG lesion that appears to be a hemorrhagic infarction (Fig. 11.13). It may be accompanied by hemorrhagic lesions elsewhere in the territory of the middle cerebral artery (Fig. 11.14). These infants may have a hemorrhagic or thrombotic tendency. The neurodevelopmental

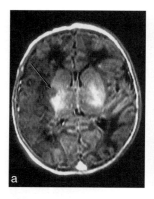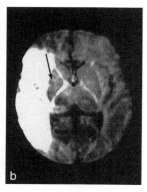

Figure 11.12 Antenatal and perinatal infarction. Infant born at term presenting with neonatal convulsions imaged on day 2. (a) Inversion recovery sequence (IR 3800/30/950). There is a loss of gray/white matter differentiation consistent with perinatally acquired right-sided middle cerebral artery infarction. There is a rounded low signal intensity 'cyst' in the right lateral lentiform nucleus (arrow). (b) Diffusion-weighted imaging shows abnormal high signal intensity within the large infarct consistent with a perinatal onset. The 'cyst' is seen as low signal intensity (arrow). The imaging appearances of the 'cyst' are consistent with it resulting from an antenatal infarction of a striate branch of the middle cerebral artery.

outcome is usually good in isolated unilateral BG lesions.

11.10.2.2 Thalamic hemorrhage

Unilateral hemorrhagic lesions in the thalamus are relatively rare. Very occasionally bilateral thalamic

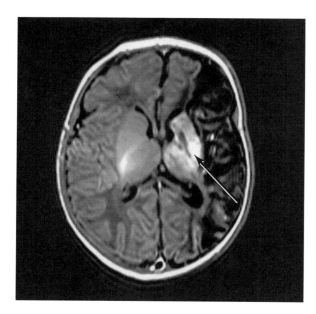

Figure 11.14 Middle cerebral artery infarction. Term-born infant presenting with neonatal convulsions. Inversion recovery sequence (IR 3800/30/850). There is a large left-sided cerebral artery infarction involving the cortex, white matter, the basal ganglia and thalami and the posterior limb of the internal capsule. The basal ganglia lesion s hemorrhagic (arrow). This child now has a mild hemiplegia.

hemorrhage may be seen. The etiology of thalamic hemorrhage is obscure. Neonates with thalamic hemorrhage usually present with convulsions. Imaging may identify associated intraventricular hemorrhage (IVH) (Fig. 11.15) and can help with dating the lesion, although hemorrhage within the thalamus and the ventricle may evolve differently (see Tables 11.2 and 11.3). The IVH may be severe enough to cause ventricular dilatation that requires intervention. The hemorrhage gradually resolves to leave an atrophied thalamus (Fig. 11.15b). These infants may develop a hemiplegia and cognitive problems.

11.11 WHITE MATTER AND CORTEX

Abnormalities in the white matter and cortex may be focal, multifocal, widespread, or in a parasagittal distribution. The assumption that cortical involvement carries a worse prognosis in terms of neurodevelopmental outcome is not founded. The neonatal brain at term is remarkably plastic and appears to compensate well for destruction of large amounts of cortex, particularly if unilateral.

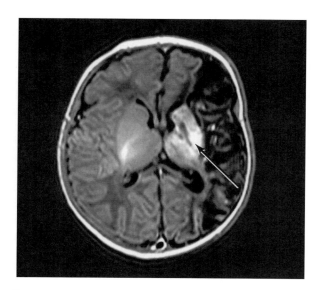

Figure 11.13 Hemorrhagic infarction of the the basal ganglia. Term-born infant who presented with stage I hypoxic-ischemic encephalopathy. Inversion recovery sequence (IR 3800/30/850). There is an abnormal high signal intensity lesion within the head of the left caudate nucleus (arrow) consistent with a hemorrhagic infarct. This child had normal development at 5 years of age.

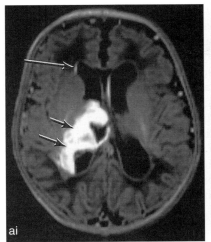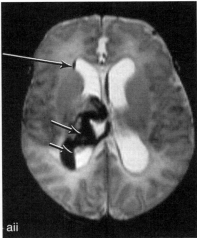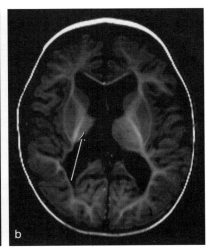

Figure 11.15 Thalamic hemorrhage. Term infant who presented with convulsions. (a) (i) Inversion recovery sequence (IR 3800/30/850). There is unilateral high signal intensity in the thalamus consistent with primary hemorrhage or hemorrhagic infarction (short arrows). There is additional hemorrhage within the right lateral ventricle (long arrow). (ii) T2-weighted spin-echo sequence (SE 2700/120). The hemorrhage is seen as predominantly low signal intensity. (b) Inversion recovery sequence (IR 3600/30/700). At 1 year of age there is marked atrophy of the thalamus (arrow).

Table 11.2   Evolution of signal intensity in parenchymal hemorrhage (personal neonatal data)

Age of hemorrhage	T1-weighted image	T2-weighted image
2 days	nil/high SI rim	low SI
3–10 days	high SI/nil	low SI (with ↑ high SI periphery)
10–21 days	high SI	high SI
3–6 weeks	high SI	high SI (with ↑ low SI periphery)
6 weeks–10 months	nil/min high SI	low SI/nil
10–22 months	nil	min low SI/nil

Table 11.3   Evolution of signal intensity in extracerebral hemorrhage (personal neonatal data)

Age of hemorrhage	T1-weighted image	T2-weighted image
<3 days	high SI	low SI/nil
3 days	high SI	high SI
3–10 days	high SI	low SI (some high SI)[a]
10–21 days	high SI	low SI (some high SI)[a]
3–6 weeks	min high SI/nil	low SI
6 weeks–10 months	nil	low SI/nil

[a]In larger lesions.

11.11.1   Infarction

11.11.1.1   The evolution of white matter infarction on MR imaging

Acute infarction is best detected with DW imaging,[24] then with T2-weighted images and lastly with T1-weighted images (Fig. 11.16). Areas of infarction show restricted diffusion of water molecules, which gives an abnormal high signal intensity on DW imaging. This is probably detectable within hours of the insult and is certainly present at the time the infant comes to imaging. The abnormal high signal intensity on DW imaging gradually decreases over the first 10 days as abnormal SI becomes more obvious on conventional imaging. T2-weighted images will show abnormal high signal intensity and a loss of the normal low SI of cortical markings, presumably due to edema and/or infarction of the cortex. T1-weighted images show loss of gray/white matter differentiation initially. This loss of differentiation returns during the second week and becomes exaggerated, reflecting abnormal low signal intensity within the white matter and abnormal high signal intensity within the cortex. Whilst cranial ultrasound may be unremarkable for the first week, MRI will detect the extent of the lesion and abnormalities in other sites. Infarcts of at least 1 week may show areas of high signal intensity around the periphery on T1-weighted images. This is probably due to capillary proliferation (Fig. 11.17bii). Breakdown and atrophy of the infarcted tissue may become obvious after 2 weeks and generally last about 6 weeks.

This pattern of abnormal SI using the different sequences is similar whatever the extent of infarction. Registration and subtraction of serially acquired images have shown that there is excessive tissue growth in and around areas of white matter infarction (Fig. 11.18).[25] This explains why the area of infarcted tissue appears to shrink over the first few months of life. A large area of perinatal infarction may even look more like an area of schizencephaly within months (Fig. 11.16).

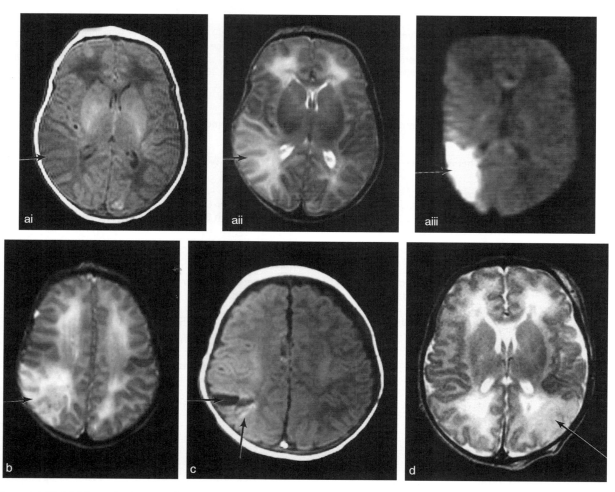

Figure 11.16 Middle cerebral artery infarction. (a) Focal infarction in an infant aged 2 days. Low ventricular level. (i) T1-weighted spin-echo sequence (SE 860/20), (ii) T2-weighted spin-echo (SE 2700/120) sequence, and (iii) diffusion-weighted sequence. The abnormal signal intensity within the parietal lobe (arrow) is seen most clearly on the diffusion-weighted sequences. (b) Centrum semiovale aged 2 days. T2-weighted spin-echo (SE 2700/120) sequence. There is a large area of mainly increased signal intensity with loss of gray/white matter differentiation (arrow). (c) Three months of age, T1-weighted spin-echo sequence (SE 860/20). The infarct (upper arrow) is much smaller than anticipated from the neonatal imaging. There is a residual small area of high signal intensity at the periphery of the infarct (lower arrow) consistent with capillary proliferation. (d) T2-weighted spin-echo sequence (SE 2700/120). Term-born infant recruited as a 'control' for an imaging study unexpectedly found to have a left-sided middle cerebral artery infarct (arrow). The image findings were in keeping with a perinatal onset for the infarction.

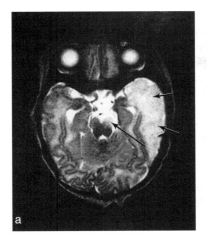 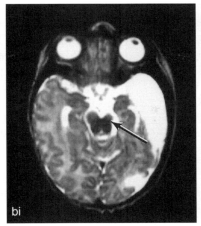 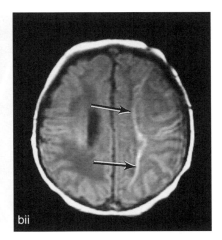

Figure 11.17 Brainstem abnormalities. Infant born at term by elective cesarean section with convulsions on day 1. T1-weighted spin-echo sequence (SE 860/20). (a) Imaged on day 6. There is an extensive left-sided infarct with swelling of the left mesencephalon (long arrow). The infarct is clearly demonstrated (short arrows). (b) Two weeks later. T2-weighted spin-echo sequence (SE 2700/120). (i) The left mesencephalon is now atrophied (arrow). (ii) T1-weighted spin-echo sequence (SE 860/20). There is a linear high signal intensity (arrows) at the borders of the infarct. This also demarcates the territory of the middle cerebral artery.

11.11.1.2   *Focal infarction in the term infant*

Perinatally acquired focal infarction or so-called neonatal stroke is usually left sided and involves the territory supplied by middle cerebral artery. In preterm infants the site of infarction is more often deep, involving the basal ganglia via the striate branches of the middle cerebral artery.[23]

Term-born infants with perinatally acquired infarction may be completely asymptomatic (Fig.

11.16d). More usually neonatal stroke is associated with some specific antenatal factors, e.g. primigravida, history of abdominal pain, fetal distress, or instrumental delivery. The clinical picture is not usually one of 'full blown' HIE and the infants usually go to the postnatal ward following delivery.

It is unusual for focal arterial infarctions in the term infant to be hemorrhagic although there may be hemorrhage in other sites of the brain (Fig. 11.19). A well-recognized combination is the

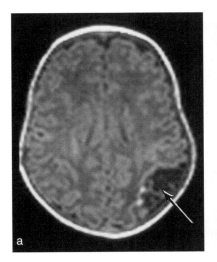 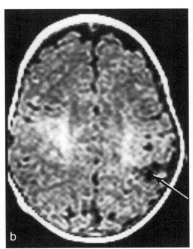 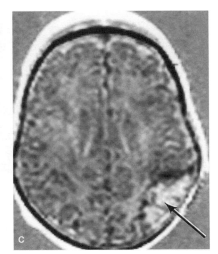

Figure 11.18 (a,b,c) 'Brain regeneration'. T1-weighted volume acquisition sequence at 2 months (a) and 3.5 months (b) in an infant with a perinatally acquired infarction (arrow). The infarct appears much smaller on the later image. The images were registered by computer program and then subtracted from each other. The resulting subtraction image (c) shows high signal intensity (arrow) consistent with excessive tissue growth in the region of the infarct.

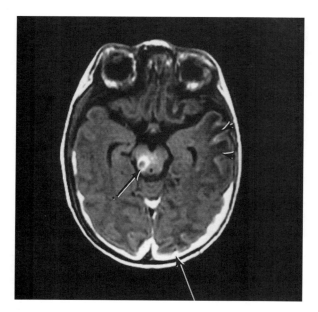

Figure 11.19 Hemorrhagic lesions in association with infarction. Inversion recovery sequence (IR 3800/30/950). Term-born infant with a left-sided middle cerebral artery infarct extending into the anterior temporal lobe (arrowheads). There is extensive subdural hemorrhage (long arrow). This is more marked on the left. There is a hemorrhagic lesion within the right mesencephalon (short arrow).

presence of focal infarction adjacent to an area of subdural hemorrhage (Fig. 11.19).

Outcome following neonatal stroke depends on the sites of involvement, so that those infants that have abnormalities within the hemispheric white matter/cortex, the BGT, and the posterior limb of the internal capsule have a high incidence of later hemiplegia.[26] The development of hemiplegia in children with perinatal stroke has also been associated with the presence of factor V Leiden heterogenicity.[27] More severe hemiplegias that are felt to be 'congenital' in origin may be due to earlier damage including migration defects, other cortical abnormalities, or antenatal infarction.

11.11.1.3   Parasagittal infarction in the term infant

This pattern of white matter injury has been described by Volpe.[28] The areas of infarction involve the deep white matter at border zones of major artery territories (Fig. 11.20). These infants may present with HIE although there may be an abnormal antenatal history. Other infants may have relatively normal Apgar scores but develop seizures during the first 24 hours. Parasagittal lesions may occur in the presence of severe hypoglycaemia (Fig. 11.21).[29,30] Whilst infants with parasagittal infarction usually develop a secondary microcephaly the neurodevelopmental outcome following parasagittal infarction is often surprisingly good, particularly for motor function. This is because there is usually preservation of the BGT. However, underlying pathologies such as severe persistent hypoglycemia are associated with major cognitive problems.

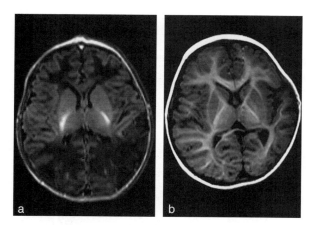

Figure 11.20 Parasagittal infarction. (a) Inversion recovery sequence (IR 3800/30/950) There is loss of gray/white matter differentiation in the parietal, temporal and occipital lobes in an infant with stage II hypoxic-ischemic encephalopathy aged 5 days. There is normal high signal intensity from myelin in the posterior limb of the internal capsule. (b) Inversion recovery (IR 3600/30/70) sequence in the same infant aged 15 months. The areas of tissue atrophy correspond to the abnormalities seen on early images. At aged 5 years this child was microcephalic with a global mild developmental delay and minimal asymmetry of tone.

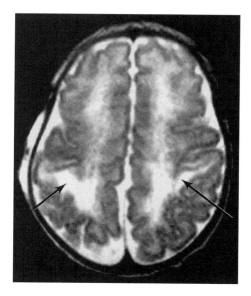

Figure 11.21 Infant with Beckwith Wiederman syndrome complicated by severe, persistent hypoglycemia. T2-weighted image (SE 2700/120) showing abnormal high signal intensity bilaterally (arrows) consistent with ischemia.

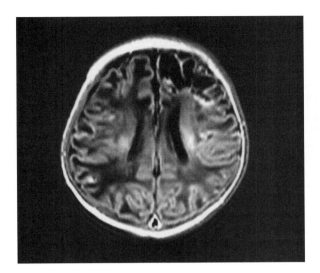

Figure 11.22 Term-born infant with perinatally acquired herpes infection. Inversion recovery sequence (IR 3800/30/950) There are multiple areas of white matter and cortical infarction. These were not confined to the temporal regions.

11.11.1.4 Multifocal infarction

Multifocal areas of infarction that do not appear to be in a parasagittal distribution may be secondary to infection, e.g. herpes (Fig. 11.22), varicella (Fig. 11.23), or listeria (Fig. 11.24). These may be seen at any gestation. Large areas of hemorrhagic white matter infarction may also be seen in infants with signs of HIE. Once again the BGT may be spared. These infants may have more profound metabolic abnormalities such as prolonged conjugated hyperbilirubinemia and recurrent hypoglycemia (Fig. 11.25). They often have marked cognitive impairments and milder motor problems such as mild diplegia. A search for an underlying infection or a metabolic disorder should be carried out but may not be successful.

11.11.2 Destructive white matter abnormalities in the preterm brain

11.11.2.1 Periventricular leukomalacia

The evolution of periventricular leukomalacia (PVL) on ultrasound has been very well documented. There are only a few studies looking at the evolution of PVL with MRI[31] as there are very few units with the ability to safely image preterm infants. Classical cystic lesions in PVL are periventricular (Fig. 11.26) and usually found in the region of the trigone. In severe cases they may be found both anteriorly and posteriorly (Fig. 11.27) and they may also extend out into the subcortical

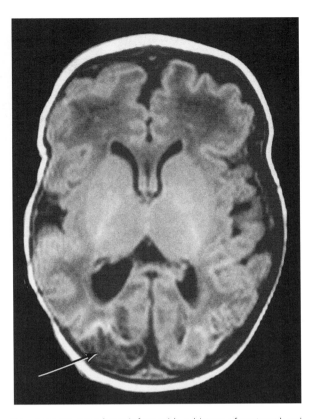

Figure 11.23 Term-born infant with a history of maternal varicella infection at 15 weeks gestation. Inversion recovery sequence (IR 3800/30/950). There were no congenital malformations of the brain. There are areas of infarction within a mature-looking brain (arrow) consistent with infarction within the late third trimester.

white matter. In the precystic stages of PVL, MRI may show the presence of multiple 'hemorrhagic'

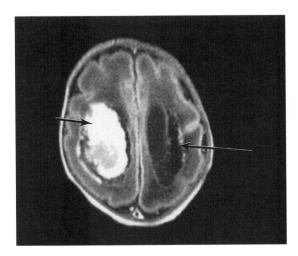

Figure 11.24 Preterm infant at 32 weeks gestation with a history of maternal listeria just prior to delivery. T1-weighted spin-echo sequence (SE 860/20). There are bilateral abnormalities. The lesions on the right are mainly hemorrhagic (short arrow). There is extensive periventricular cyst formation on the left (long arrow).

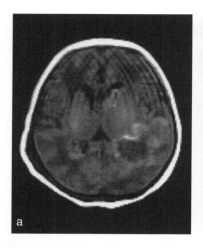 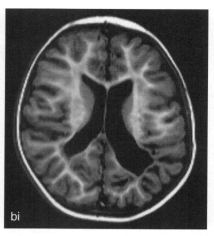 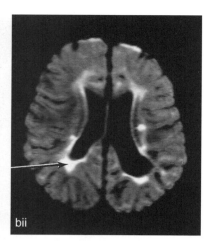

Figure 11.25 Infant with stage II hypoxic-ischemic encephalopathy who also developed persistent hypoglycemia and neonatal hepatitis with prolonged conjugated jaundice. Image taken at 3 days. (a) T1-weighted spin-echo (SE 860/20). There is a large hemorrhagic lesion in the left temporal region. This is slightly low signal intensity with a high signal periphery. The hemorrhage was seen as low signal intensity T2-weighted spin-echo sequence (SE 2700/120). (b) Imaging at 2 years of age. (i) Inversion recovery sequence (IR 3600/30/700). There is bilateral ventricular dilatation with 'squared off' posterior horns and a paucity of myelin posteriorly. (ii) Fluid attenuated inversion recovery (FLAIR) sequence aged 2 years. There is abnormal high signal in the periventricular white matter most marked posteriorly (arrow). This is consistent with glial tissue. These images illustrate how the abnormalities that develop following perinatal white matter injury at term may be reminiscent of those found in more classical periventricular leukomalacia occurring in the preterm infant.

lesions although similar lesions may be seen in infants who do not develop cysts (Fig. 11.28).

PVL was originally thought to always be secondary to ischemia. Many infants with PVL do not have a history of a severe ischemic event and some have a positive history for sepsis. Recent studies confirm that PVL is more likely to be due to a combination of ischemia and inflammation in tissue which is inherently susceptible to damage. Infants with PVL may have had an uneventful clinical course apart, of course, from their prematurity. This has led researchers to try to establish links between the causes of preterm delivery and white matter damage in the preterm infant[32] and the presence of maternal sepsis has been implicated in the etiology of PVL.

By term-equivalent age the majority of cysts in PVL have disappeared. Incorporation into the ventricle results in some ventricular dilatation. The ventricular outline becomes distorted and 'squared off' over the following months. This distortion may be secondary to gliosis that becomes evident on later T2-weighted images (Fig. 11.27b). The late appearance of PVL includes ventricular dilatation, irregular ventricular border, decreased myelination and evidence of gliosis (Fig. 11.27b). These appearances can result from a perinatal injury to the white matter in a term-born infant and cannot be assumed to be secondary to damage to the preterm brain (Fig. 11.25b).

Neurodevelopmental outcome following PVL depends on the site and extent of the cystic lesions.[33] The appearances of the PLIC at term-equivalent age may be valuable in predicting eventual motor outcome. The typical sequelae in infants with PVL are a spastic diplegia with some arm involvement, varying intellectual deficits, and strabismus. The more extensive the lesions the more severe the cerebral palsy with a spastic quadriplegia, more severe intellectual impairment, and cortical blindness.

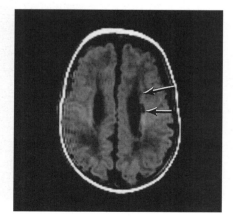

Figure 11.26 Mild periventricular leukomalacia at term-equivalent age. T1-weighted spin-echo sequence (SE 860/20) showing asymmetrical periventricular cyst formation which was more prominent on the left (arrows).

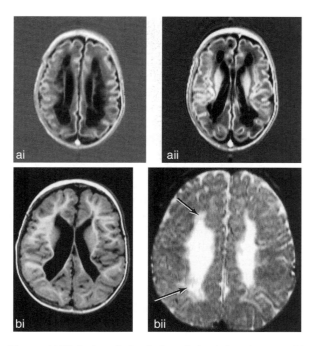

Figure 11.27 Periventricular leukomalacia. Infant born at 32 weeks gestation with evidence of cyst formation on cranial ultrasound a few days later. (a) Inversion recovery sequence (IR 3800/30/950). (i, ii) There is extensive cyst formation all around both ventricles. (b) (i) Inversion recovery sequence (IR 3600/30/700). At follow-up at 15 months of age there is irregular ventricular dilatation and a paucity of myelination. (ii) There is some increased signal intensity consistent with glial tissue (arrows). This may be difficult to distinguish from CSF unless the fluid attenuated inversion recovery (FLAIR) sequence is used (see Fig. 11.25).

11.11.2.2 Venous infarction

Focal white matter infarction in the preterm infant is usually hemorrhagic and associated with intraventricular hemorrhage (IVH). This venous infarction appears to follow impaired venous drainage throughout the terminal veins because of obstruction from germinal matrix hemorrhage (GMH) (Fig. 11.29). Hemorrhagic venous infarction may occur in the presence of isolated GMH. It is usually unilateral but can be bilateral. It is usually seen extending into the frontal white matter from GMH over the head of the caudate nucleus that extends into the frontal horn of the lateral ventricles. Ultrasound is not able to visualize the germinal matrix that persists at the roof of the temporal horn. This may be an additional site of venous infarction with abnormal signal extending out to the cortex of the anterior temporal lobe (Fig. 11.30). Extensive hemorrhagic lesions, which may look very dramatic on MRI (Fig. 11.29), with visualization of distended draining veins, are probably not

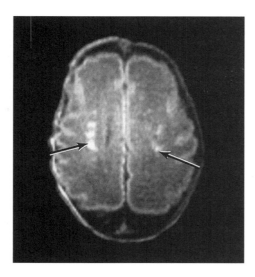

Figure 11.28 Hemorrhagic parenchymal lesions. Preterm infant of 30 weeks gestation imaged at 5 days. T1-weighted fast spin-echo sequence (FSE 3000/208$_{ef}$). There are bilateral high signal intensity lesions in the periventricular white matter (arrows). The enlarged posterior extracerebral space is normal for this gestation. The hemorrhagic lesions had largely cleared by term-equivalent age with no cyst formation or dilatation of the ventricles.

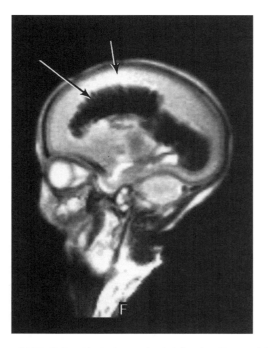

Figure 11.29 Periventricular hemorrhagic infarction. Preterm infant born at 27 weeks gestation and imaged at 3 days. T2-weighted fast spin-echo sequence (FSE 3000/208$_{ef}$). Sagittal plane. There is extensive low signal intensity consistent with intraventricular hemorrhage. There is additional low signal intensity in a fan-shaped distribution in the frontal white matter (long arrow). There is adjacent abnormal increased signal intensity extending out to the cortex (short arrow). This is consistent with edematous or ischemic tissue but was found to show signs of infarction at histology.

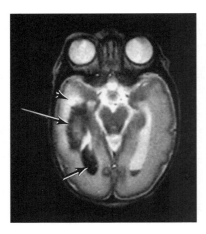

Figure 11.30 Periventricular hemorrhagic infarction. Preterm infant born at 29 weeks gestation. T2-weighted fast spin-echo sequence (FSE 3000/208$_{ef}$). There is bilateral low signal intensity within the ventricles consistent with hemorrhage (short arrow). There is an area of low signal intensity in the periventricular white matter of the right temporal lobe (long arrow). This is surrounded by high signal intensity consistent with edema or infarction (arrowhead).

compatible with survival. Less severe lesions will evolve to form a cyst communicating with the lateral ventricle (porencephalic cyst) or irregular dilatation of the ventricles (Fig. 11.31).

Infants with venous infarction are at risk of developing a later hemiplegia. Involvement of the leg is usually more severe than the arm. De Vries has shown that in preterm infants with focal parenchymal lesions the development of a hemiplegia was related to the appearance of the posterior limb of the internal capsule on MR imaging at term-equivalent age.[34]

11.11.3   Non-infarctive white matter lesions

11.11.3.1   Mild periventricular white matter damage

Infants with HIE with no persistent focal pathology often have some white matter SI changes with slightly long T1 and long T2 in the periventricular white matter (PVWM) on the neonatal scan. This does not behave like infarcted tissue on DW imaging and may just represent an increased water content. These infants may show some excessive high signal intensity on later T2-weighted scans that would be consistent with delayed myelination but could also represent glial tissue. In some infants there may also be some evidence of white matter atrophy which suggests that the original abnormalities have resulted in irreversible damage.

11.11.3.2   Diffuse excessive high signal intensity (DEHSI)

Preterm infants imaged at term-equivalent age may show abnormally long T1 (low signal intensity on T1-weighted images) and abnormally long T2 (high signal intensity on T2-weighted images) in the white matter (Fig. 11.32).[35] This is usually found in the immediate periventricular white matter, more often posteriorly. It may extend out to the subcortical white matter. It has been termed diffuse excessive high signal intensity (DEHSI). The clinical significance of this remains uncertain but it appears to reflect a difference in white matter development in the infant born very preterm. This may be as a result of an ischemic or inflammatory injury or could be secondary to nutritional, hormonal deficiency. This type of damage may correspond to the entity described by pathologists as telencephalic leukoencephalopathy.

11.11.3.3   Congenital infection

Whilst congenital infections can result in destructive white matter lesions, widespread non-infarctive white matter lesions may also be seen in congenital infections such as cytomegalovirus and rubella. These may remain very static and not be associated with atrophy (Fig. 11.33). The appearances of the brain in congenital infections are thought to vary according to the time of the infection in the mother. If there was such a simple relationship then all fetuses with a history of early

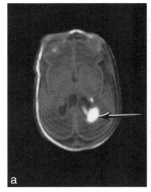
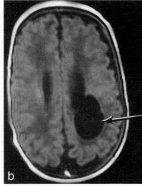

Figure 11.31 Porencephalic cyst formation. T1-weighted spin-echo sequence (SE 860/20). Preterm infant born at 30 weeks gestation. (a) There is abnormal high signal intensity consistent with posterior periventricular hemorrhagic infarction (arrow). (b) At term-equivalent age there is asymmetrical ventricular dilatation with a porencephalic cyst (arrow).

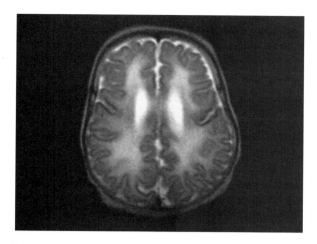

Figure 11.32 Diffuse excessive high signal intensity (DEHSI). Preterm infant born at 26 weeks gestation and imaged at term-equivalent age. T2-weighted fast spin-echo sequence (FSE 3000/208ef). There is excessive high signal intensity throughout the periventricular white matter.

processes and specific immunological and inflammatory responses within the fetal brain.

11.11.3.4 White matter abnormalities in congenital muscular dystrophy

Major white matter changes consistent with a leukoencephalopathy are also associated with muscle diseases, in particular merosin-negative congenital muscular dystrophy (Fig. 11.34).[36] These usually take a few months to become obvious but the white matter may have some subtle abnormalities from birth.

11.12 BRAINSTEM

Lesions in the brainstem may be primary or secondary. Primary lesions include infarction in infants with severe asphyxia (Fig. 11.3) These infarcts tend to involve the dorsal aspects of the brainstem. More diffuse changes can also be detected in infants with severe HIE with generalized short T1, short T2 throughout the mesencephalon (Fig. 11.3). Focal hemorrhagic lesions, often in association with lesions elsewhere in the brain, may occasionally be seen (Fig. 11.19). Acute swelling and signal intensity changes within the brainstem may be detected in neonatal stroke (Fig, 11.17). These abnormalities may be secondary to

first trimester infection would have similar lesions. These would be likely to be major, to interfere with development and mimic congenital malformations, e.g. migration defects. However, this is not always the case as the later brain abnormalities reflect the onset of direct infection or inflammation within the fetal brain not within the mother. The eventual brain abnormalities seen on imaging will result from a combination of these pathological

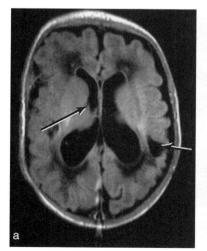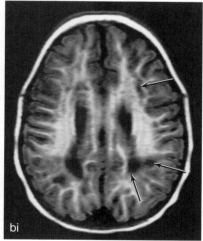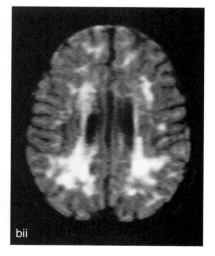

Figure 11.33 Cytomegalovirus infection. (a) Preterm infant with early postnatally acquired cytomegalovirus infection. Imaged at term-equivalent age. Inversion recovery sequence. There is a widened caudothalamic notch (long arrow) consistent with previous subependymal cysts. Subependymal cysts which are clearly visible on ultrasound are easily missed on MR imaging. There is additional abnormal low signal intensity within the white matter (short arrow). (b) Preterm infant born at 35 weeks gestation with a history of maternal cytomegalovirus infection in the first trimester. Imaging at 18 months. (i) Inversion recovery sequence (IR 3600/30/700). There are extensive abnormal signal intensities within the myelinated white matter (arrows). These are most obvious on the fluid attenuated inversion recovery (FLAIR) sequence (ii). This infant has no neurodevelopmental impairments at 6 years of age.

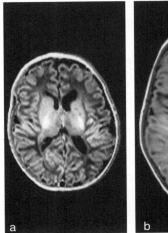
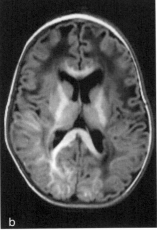

Figure 11.34 Congenital muscular dystrophy. Infant with merosin-negative congenital muscular dystrophy. (a) Inversion recovery sequence (IR 3800/30/950). There are widespread areas of abnormal low signal intensity within the white matter on neonatal imaging. (b) Inversion recovery sequence (IR 3600/30/700). The abnormal signal intensity within the white matter is much more prominent at 1 year of age although there is sparing of the central myelinated white matter.

the phenomenon known as diaschisis where metabolic derangements occur in areas which are remote from, but connected to, an area of ischemia. In neonates with perinatal stroke focal atrophy of the brainstem may occur as a result of secondary atrophy of fibers arising in the damaged area which may follow on from diaschisis (Fig. 11.17). In children with bilateral infarction, bilateral brainstem atrophy may be seen, although this is often more difficult to appreciate because there is no normal side for comparison.

11.13 CEREBELLUM

The cerebellum is apparently sensitive to ischemic damage in the term neonate, particularly the dentate nucleus. However in the presence of global ischemic injury causing atrophy of the entire supratentorial brain, the cerebellum may have an apparently normal appearance on conventional MR images.[37] This may be in part because of the separate circulation through the posterior cerebral arteries. Cerebellar involvement in a term baby is suggestive of a metabolic disease. Cerebellar infarction may occasionally be seen as part of posterior cerebral artery syndrome (Fig. 11.9) and possibly secondary to extensive subdural hemorrhage.

Cerebellar hemorrhage in the term neonate may be devastating and require life-saving surgery to decompress the posterior fossa. In others it may present as an increasing head circumference due to progressive ventricular dilatation (Fig. 11.35).

Small cerebellar hemorrhage may be detected using MRI in very preterm infants. These are usually seen in association with hemorrhagic lesions elsewhere in the brain. Infants with minor bilateral lesions within the cerebellar hemispheres or with a major unilateral infarction may escape without motor impairment (Figs 11.35 and 11.36). An association of the cerebellum with cognitive function has become increasingly well recognized and these children may be at risk of developing later cognitive deficits.

11.14 VENTRICLES

Intraventricular hemorrhage (IVH) is typically a disorder of the preterm infant with an increasing incidence with decreasing gestation. The incidence of IVH appears to be decreasing and this has been attributed to the routine use of surfactant and the subsequent decrease in severe respiratory distress syndrome. In the preterm infant IVH originates from the germinal matrix (Fig. 11.37). In the term infant IVH usually originates in the choroid as the

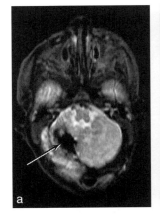
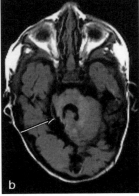

Figure 11.35 Cerebellar hemorrhage. Infant with unremarkable delivery at term who presented with a rapidly enlarging head over the first week of life. (a) T2-weighted spin-echo sequence (SE 2700/120). There is a large low signal intensity hemorrhagic lesion in the right cerebellar hemsiphere (arrow). (b) T1-weighted spin-echo sequence (SE 860/20). At follow-up at 1 year of age there is destruction and atrophy of most of the right cerebellar hemisphere (arrow). Motor development was normal at 2 years of age.

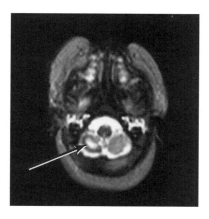

Figure 11.36 Cerebellar infarction. T2-weighted fast spin-echo sequence (FSE 3000/208$_{ef}$). Preterm infant who had intraventricular hemorrhage and some hemorrhagic lesions in the cerebral parenchyma. There is an area of abnormal increased signal intensity within the right cerebellar hemisphere consistent with infarction (arrow).

germinal matrix has largely involuted. Preterm MR imaging allows one to see the full extent of the hemorrhage and to establish whether or not there is parenchymal involvement.

Isolated GMH/IVH is associated with a good neurodevelopmental outcome although the interference of glial cell production and migration from the germinal matrix could be responsible for subtle alterations in cortical and white matter development.

IVH that results in ventricular dilatation that requires intervention is associated with neurodevelopmental impairments.

11.15 EXTRACEREBRAL SPACE

The appearances of the extracerebral space vary with gestational age of the neonate. In the fetus and very preterm neonate it is relatively wide, particularly over the posterior parietal lobe. The space has usually decreased by 32–34 weeks gestation. In preterm infants at term-equivalent age the frontal extracerebral space may be wide (Fig. 11.38). This may be associated with dilatation of the frontal horns of the lateral ventricles and is assumed to be secondary to atrophy but may be due to local CSF dynamics. A similar so-called benign enlargement of the extracerebral space can be seen in infants presenting with macrocephaly. It seems to reduce to normal by about 1 year of age.

Hemorrhage within the extracerebral space may be seen at all gestational ages. Subarachnoid and subdural hemorrhage may be seen in infants with HIE or with a history of a traumatic or instrumental delivery (Fig. 11.39). Subdural hemorrhage may occasionally be found in the preterm infant and may occur apparently spontaneously *in utero*, when a history of trauma should be sought. Large hemorrhages may be seen in fetuses with congenital or acquired clotting abnormalities such as alloimmune thrombocytopenia. Small amounts of

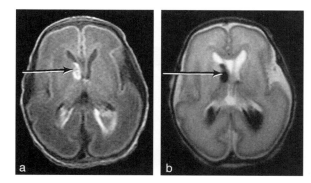

Figure 11.37 Germinal matrix/intraventricular hemorrhage. Preterm infant born at 26 weeks gestation. (a) T1-weighted spin-echo sequence (SE 860/20). There is abnormal high signal intensity in the germinal matrix over the caudate head (arrow). There is additional high signal intensity consistent with hemorrhage within the lateral ventricles. (b) T2-weighted fast spin-echo sequence (FSE 3000/208$_{ef}$). The germinal matrix (arrow) and intraventricular hemorrhage are seen as low signal intensity.

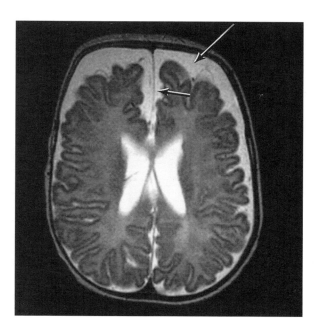

Figure 11.38 Widened extracerebral space. T2-weighted spin-echo sequence (SE 2700/120) of a preterm infant at term-equivalent age. There is widening of the extracerebral space (long arrow) and of the interhemispheric fissure (short arrow) anteriorly. There is dilatation of the lateral ventricles.

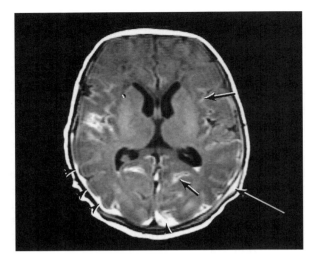

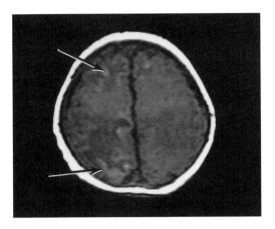

Figure 11.39 Subdural hemorrhage in an infant with stage II hypoxic-ischemic encephalopathy, delivered by vacuum following a failed attempt at forceps. T1-weighted spin-echo sequence (SE 860/20). There is extensive abnormal high signal intensity consistent with hemorrhage in the subdural space over the parietal lobe (arrowheads). There is an additional collection at the site of the vaccuum extraction, consistent with a cephalhematoma (long arrow). There is high signal intensity within the sulcal spaces consistent with subarachnoid hemorrhage (short arrows). There is a small amount of intraventricular hemorrhage in the posterior horns.

Figure 11.41 Sinus thrombosis. A term infant with hypoxic-ischemic encephalopathy who developed abnormal clotting with thrombocytopenia requiring five platelet transfusions. He developed congestive cardiac failure and was grossly edematous at the time of imaging. Liver function was also persistently abnormal. Day 2 imaging was consistent with sagittal sinus thrombosis with some loss of gray/white matter differentiation. T1-weighted (SE 860/20) sequence at 5 days of age. There are multiple areas of abnormal signal intensity in the cortex and subcortical white matter consistent with hemorrhagic infarction (arrows). The sinuses had a normal appearance on the day 5 images (not shown). The evolution of the images in this infant is consistent with a diagnosis of partial sinus thrombosis secondary to congestive cardiac failure, which has resulted in multiple areas of cortical and subcortical infarction.

subarachnoid hemorrhage are difficult to identify on MR imaging but multiplanar MRI is good at detecting small subdural hemorrhages. When subdural hemorrhage is present over the cerebral hemisphere there may be underlying infarction of the brain (Fig. 11.19). In the infant with HIE subdural hemorrhage in the posterior fossa is more frequent. Subdural hemorrhage is best identified using at least two planes, transverse and sagittal or coronal for imaging. In addition the use of

sequences with thin image slices will exclude effects that are secondary to normal blood flow. Posterior fossa subdural hemorrhage usually 'hugs' the cerebellar hemispheres but may be very difficult to differentiate from normal flow in the transverse sinus and with thrombosis in the sinus (Fig. 11.40).

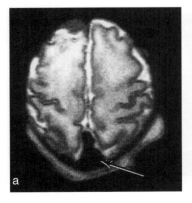 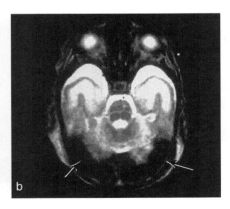 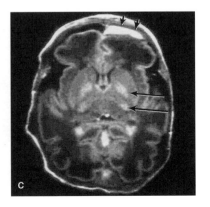

Figure 11.40 Preterm infant with severe sepsis. (a,b,c) T2-weighted spin-echo sequence (SE 2700/120). There was abnormal low signal intensity within the sagittal straight (a) and transverse (b) sinuses (arrows). (c) T1-weighted spin-echo sequence (SE 860/20). There is abnormal high signal intensity within the basal ganglia and thalami (arrows). There is additional abnormal high signal intensity over the left frontal lobe consistent with subdural hemorrhage (arrowheads). This infant subsequently died.

Sinus thrombosis may occur in the infant with polycythemia, in association with sepsis, as a result of trauma or in any condition, congenital or acquired, that increases the viscosity or decreases the flow of blood through the sinuses. Thrombosis of the sagittal sinus will result in infarction of the superficial tissues of the brain (Fig. 11.41). Thrombosis of the straight sinus and transverse sinuses may be associated with infarction of thalamic tissue (Fig. 11.40).

11.16   PARTING COMMENTS

This chapter has only touched on many of the important issues concerning magnetic resonance imaging of brain injury. Readers are referred to excellent, more comprehensive imaging texts listed in the references.

- As with every subject in medicine the more experience you gain the less you feel you understand.
- When imaging the neonate with brain injury never be satisfied with just one explanation but look for predisposing factors.
- Describe appearances and their associations but do not presume a specific pathological process unless histology is available.
- Never say 'never' or 'always' – there are always exceptions.

11.17   REFERENCES

1 Mitchell DG. *MRI principles*. Philadelphia: WB Saunders, 1999.
2 Westbrook C, Kaut C. *MRI in practice*, 2nd edn. Oxford: Blackwell Science, 1998.
3 Barkovich AJ, Latal-Hajnal B, Partridge JC, Sola A, Ferriero DM. MR contrast enhancement of the normal neonatal brain. *AJNR: American Journal of Neuroradiology* 1997; **18**: 1713–17.
4 Noguchi K, Ogawa T, Seto H *et al.* Sub acute and chronic subarachnoid hemorrhage: diagnosis with fluid-attenuated inversion recovery MR imaging. *Radiology* 1997; **203**: 257–62.
5 Bakshi R, Caruthers SD, Janardhan V, Wasay M. Intraventricular CSF pulsation artifact on fast fluid-attenuation inversion recovery MR images: analysis of 100 consecutive normal studies. *AJNR: American Journal of Neuroradiology* 2000; **21**: 503–8.
6 Okuda T, Korogi Y, Ikushima I *et al.* Use of fluid-attenuated inversion recovery (FLAIR) pulse sequences in perinatal hypoxic-ischaemic encephalopathy. *British Journal of Radiology* 1998; **71**: 282–90.
7 Barkovich AJ, Hajnal BL, Vigneron D *et al.* Prediction of neuromotor outcome in perinatal asphyxia: evaluation of MR scoring systems. *AJNR: American Journal of Neuroradiology* 1998a; **19**: 143–9.
8 Barkovich AJ. MR and CT evaluation of profound neonatal and infantile asphyxia. *AJNR: American Journal of Neuroradiology* 1992; **13**: 959–72.
9 Barkovich AJ, Sargent SK. Profound asphyxia in the premature infant: imaging findings. *AJNR: American Journal of Neuroradiology* 1995; **16**: 1837–46.
10 Rutherford MA, Pennock JM, Murdoch-Eaton DM, Cowan FM, Dubowitz LMS. Athetoid cerebral palsy and cysts in the putamen after hypoxic-ischaemic encephalopathy. *Archives of Disease in Childhood* 1992; **67**: 846–50.
11 Rutherford MA, Pennock JM, Dubowitz LMS. Cranial ultrasound and magnetic resonance imaging in hypoxic-ischaemic encephalopathy: a comparison with outcome. *Developmental Medicine and Child Neurology* 1994; **36**: 813–25.
12 Rutherford MA, Pennock JM, Schwieso JE, Cowan FM, Dubowitz LMS. Hypoxic-ischemic encephalopathy: early magnetic resonance imaging findings and their evolution. *Neuropediatrics* 1995; **26**: 183–91.
13 Rutherford MA, Pennock JM, Schwieso JE, Cowan FM, Dubowitz LMS. Hypoxic-ischemic encephalopathy: early and late MRI findings and clinical outcome. *Archives of Disease in Childhood* 1996; **75**: 141–51.
14 Rutherford MA, Pennock J, Counsell S *et al.* Abnormal magnetic resonance signal in the internal capsule predicts poor developmental outcome in infants with hypoxic-ischemic encephalopathy. *Pediatrics* 1998; **102**: 323–8.
15 Rademakers RP, van der Knaap MS, Verbeeten B Jr Barth PG, Valk J. Central cortico-subcortical involvement: a distinct pattern of brain damage caused by perinatal and postnatal asphyxia in term infants. *Journal of Computer Assisted Tomography* 1995; **19**: 252–63.
16 Pasternak JF, Predey TA, Mikhael MA. Neonatal asphyxia: vulnerability of basal ganglia, thalamus and brainstem. *Pediatric Neurology* 1991; **7**: 147–9.
17 Maalouf E, Battin M, Counsell S, Rutherford M, Mansur A. Arthrogryposis multiplex congenita and bilateral midbrain infarction following maternal overdose of coproxamol. *European Journal of Paediatric Neurology* 1997; **5/6**: 1–4.
18 Sarnat HB, Sarnat MS. Neonatal encephalopathy following fetal distress: a clinical and electrophysiological study. *Archives of Neurology* 1976; **33**: 696–705.
19 Chugani HT, Phelps ME. Maturational changes in cerebral function in infants determined by 18 FDG positron emission tomography. *Science* 1986; **231**: 840–3.

20 Malamud N. Status marmoratus: a form of cerebral palsy following birth injury or inflammation of the central nervous system. *Journal of Pediatrics* 1950; **37**: 610

21 Okumura A, Hayakawa F, Kato T, Itomi K, Mimura S, Watanabe K. Preterm infants with athetoid cerebral palsy: kernicterus? *Archives of Disease in Childhood Fetal and Neonatal Edition* 2001; **84**: F136–7.

22 Willis TA, Davidson J, Gray R, Poulton K, Ramani P, Whitehouse W. Cytochrome oxidase deficiency presenting as birth asphyxia. *Developmental Medicine and Child Neurology* 2000; **42**: 414–17.

23 De Vries L, Groenendaal F, Eken P, Haastert IC, Rademaker K, Meiners L. Infarcts in the vascular distribution of the middle cerebral artery in preterm and fullterm infants. *Neuropediatrics* 1997; **27**: 88–96.

24 Cowan FM, Pennock JM, Hanrahan JD, Manji KP, Edwards AD. Early detection of cerebral infarction and hypoxic ischemic encephalopathy in neonates using diffusion weighted magnetic resonance imaging. *Neuropediatrics* 1994; **25**: 172–5.

25 Rutherford MA, Pennock JM, Dubowitz LMS, Cowan FM, Bydder GM. Does the brain regenerate after perinatal infarction? *European Journal of Paediatric Neurology* 1997; **1**: 13–18.

26 Mercuri E, Rutherford M, Cowan F *et al*. Early prognostic indicators of outcome in infants with neonatal cerebral infarction: a clinical, electroencephalogram, and magnetic resonance imaging study. *Pediatrics* 1999; **103**: 39–46.

27 Mercuri I, Cowan F, Gupte G *et al*. Prothrombotic disorders and abnormal neurodevelopmental outcome in infants with neonatal cerebral infarction. *Pediatrics* 2001; **107**: 1400-4.

28 Volpe JJ, Herscovitch P, Perlman JM, Kreusser KL, Raichle ME. Positron emission tomography in the asphyxiated term newborn: parasagittal impairment of cerebral blood flow. *Annals of Neurology* 1985; **17**: 287–96.

29 Barkovich AJ, Ali FA, Rowley HA, Bass N. Imaging patterns of neonatal hypoglycemia. *AJNR: American Journal of Neuroradiology* 1998b; **19**: 523–8.

30 Traill Z, Squier M, Anslow P. Brain imaging in neonatal hypoglycemia. *Archives of Disease in Childhood Fetal and Neonatal Edition* 1998; **79**: F145–7.

31 Sie LT, van der Knapp MS, van Wezel-Meijler G, Taets van Amerongen AH, Lafeber HN, Valk J. Early MR features of hypoxic-ischemic brain injury in neonates with periventricular densities on sonograms. *AJNR: American Journal of Neuroradiology* 2000; **21**: 852–61.

32 Dammann O, Leviton A. Maternal intrauterine infection, cytokines, and brain damage in the preterm newborn. *Pediatric Research* 1997; **42**: 1–8.

33 Van den Hout BM, Eken P, Van der Linden D *et al*. Visual, cognitive, and neurodevelopmental outcome at 5¹/₂ years in children with perinatal haemorrhagic-ischaemic brain lesions. *Developmental Medicine and Child Neurology* 1998; **40**: 820–8.

34 De Vries LS, Groenendaal F, van Haastert IC, Eken P, Rademaker KJ, Meiners LC. Asymmetrical myelination of the posterior limb of the internal capsule in infants with periventricular haemorrhagic infarction: an early predictor of hemiplegia. *Neuropediatrics* 1999; **30**: 314–19.

35 Maalouf E, Duggan PJ, Rutherford MA *et al*. Magnetic resonance imaging of the brain in a cohort of extremely preterm infants. *Journal of Pediatrics* 1999; **135**: 351–7.

36 Mercuri E, Gruter-Andrew J, Philpot J *et al*. Cognitive abilities in children with congenital muscular dystrophy: correlation with brain MRI and merosin status. *Neuromuscular Disorders* 1999; **9**: 383–7.

37 Jouvet P, Cowan FM, Cox P *et al*. Reproducibility and accuracy of MR imaging of the brain after severe birth asphyxia. *AJNR: American Journal of Neuroradiology* 1999; **20**: 1343–8.

12 Radiological assessment of the child with cerebral palsy and its medicolegal implications

Philip Anslow

The purpose of this chapter is to discuss the role of medical imaging in the child with cerebral palsy. Such imaging may be undertaken as part of a clinical investigation into the cause of a neurological disability in an infant or child, or as part of the medicolegal process of causation. This chapter is not intended to cover the acute cerebral imaging of the sick neonate (see Chapters 10 and 11) which is usually undertaken using cranial ultrasound. Cross-sectional imaging using computerized tomography (CT) and magnetic resonance imaging (MRI) is generally reserved for neonatal cases where the diagnosis is in doubt, where a neurosurgical intervention is contemplated, or where there is a research interest.

In clinical practice, the neurological disability associated with cerebral palsy can take many forms. Some neurological disorders are obvious, some are very subtle and only detected during expert neurological assessment. One important feature to stress is that the neurological consequences of non-progressive destructive brain lesions appear from the outside to *change* over time as the nervous system of the child matures in the early years of life. As an example, consider the newborn child who has no purposeful movement of limbs and the normal toddler of 2 years old who is walking, talking, and feeding him or herself. A destructive brain lesion affecting the motor system may well be difficult to detect in the newborn but be obvious to all in the loss of motor function or facility in the toddler. For this reason, the definitive diagnosis of cerebral palsy is usually deferred until the age of 5 when normal motor and intellectual functions are expected to be well established.

Cerebral palsy is frequently defined as a disorder of the *motor* system of a child, but other neurological functions are frequently also impaired. The reasons why motor involvement predominates in discussions surrounding cerebral palsy are complex:

- Motor lesions are more easily detected and quantified than, say, visual or intellectual impairment.
- Motor abnormalities are more easily perceived as 'handicaps'.
- Damage to the motor cortex of the brain results in specific functional loss, while damage to

other less eloquent areas of brain may be more difficult to identify.

- Due to anatomical and physiological factors, the motor areas of the brain are particularly sensitive to hypoxic-ischemic damage.

12.1 THE CLINICAL DIAGNOSTIC PROCESS

The classical diagnostic process consists of clinical history taking and examination followed by special investigations to confirm the initial diagnosis or to refine a differential diagnosis. Of the special investigations available in neurology, cranial CT and MRI scanning are of supreme importance.

The two major forms of cross-sectional imaging have various strengths and weaknesses (Table 12.1). In the context of cerebral palsy, the disadvantages and difficulties of MRI are far outweighed by its supreme tissue contrast, spatial resolution, and ability to demonstrate pathology.

Once neurological disability is detected by carers it will generally be assessed by a pediatrician. This may well be the neonatal pediatrician who cared for the child after a difficult birth, or it may be a 'general' pediatrician referred to by a general practitioner. Given the clinical history of the child (a difficult birth perhaps), the cause of the neuro-

logical disability may be deemed 'obvious' and it is a bald fact that in the year 2000, after clinical history taking and examination almost none of these children will be actively investigated. A recent review of all the children on the Oxford cerebral palsy register found that only 10 percent had ever had a CT or MR brain scan and that almost none of these investigations had been requested by a neonatal or general pediatrician. A majority of the requests for examination had come from pediatric neurologists.

Given the huge emotional and financial burdens of cerebral palsy to a family and to the state, it is perhaps surprising that the rate of investigation is so low. The following reasons are frequently quoted:

- The financial cost of investigation
- The necessity for general anesthetic
- The lack of an effective medical treatment for the disorder.

12.1.1 The cost of investigation

In a cash-limited health service, costs are always important. The marginal cost of a CT or MRI scan is, however, relatively small and is absolutely trivial when compared with the cost of life-time care. There is another cost – the cost of *not* performing an investigation. Without an MRI scan:

Table 12.1 Strengths and weaknesses of the two major forms of cross-sectional imaging

	Advantages	Disadvantages
Computerized tomography (CT)	• Widely available • Images are produced a slice at a time (this means that patient movement may only degrade part of a study) • Quick: most of the current machines will produce a good-quality image slice in a few seconds; newer machines are capable of producing high-quality images in less than 1 second • Hemorrhage is easily detected and characterized	• Involves the use of ionizing radiation • Relatively poor brain (gray matter/white matter) contrast • Imaging effectively limited to axial scan plane • Limited range of scan techniques in brain imaging
Magnetic resonance imaging	• Excellent brain contrast • Multiple pulse sequences and scan planes available	• Slow in comparison to CT • Patient movement during the course of a scan degrades all the images • Limited access to patient during scan • Claustrophobia is a real problem • High capital cost of equipment • Limited availability (in UK)

- An incorrect clinical diagnosis may go unrecognized
- The diagnosis (of cerebral palsy) may be correct, but no clues as to the cause of the disability can be confirmed or offered
- The severity of the damage cannot be accurately assessed
- A prognosis cannot be refined
- Research into the disorder is profoundly hampered by the lack of correct diagnosis.

The parents of a child with cerebral palsy are often assailed by guilt and deeply in need of explanation. Investigation of this diagnosis helps parents come to terms with the disability their child suffers from. Seeing the scan and having it explained may have a profoundly beneficial effect on this process.

12.1.2 The necessity for general anesthetic

Very small babies can usually be scanned after a feed when they are relaxed and sleepy. Children from the age of 5 years can frequently be scanned with explanation and (parental) reassurance. Bribery is commonly very helpful! Children in the age range 6 months to 5 or more years will need some help – either sedation or anesthesia. Older children with a movement disorder or an abnormality of understanding will always need either sedation or anesthesia if the scan is to be successful.

Both sedation and anesthesia have risks (Table 12.2). Both techniques need understanding and close cooperation of the parent, nursing, and medical staff. Rigid protocols need to be established if the techniques are to be successful with minimum disruption to the lives of the parents and child.

12.1.3 The lack of an effective medical treatment for the disorder

This is a real problem when the decision to request a scan is being made. It is reasonable to ask, 'Why put the child at risk, however small, when in the absence of an effective treatment, there will be no improvement in management?'

In clinical practice, a very real balance needs to be struck. It is clear that in the majority of cases of cerebral palsy the balance is such that, in the clinician's mind, no investigation is merited.

In medicolegal practice, however, the decision is much clearer. In order for a case to be successful, causation will have to be established and accurate diagnosis of the cause of the cerebral palsy is essential. It may be possible to make the causation link on

Table 12.2 Advantages and disadvantages of anesthesia and sedation

	Advantages	Disadvantages
Anesthesia	• If protocols are adhered to (e.g. periods of fasting) the procedure is always successful • A high-quality and comprehensive scan will always be obtained • The effect of the anesthetic agents is very brief and there is minimal 'hang-over' • All age groups can be scanned	• Every anesthetic carries with it the risk of death; in the hands of a consultant pediatric anesthetist, the risk is tiny (less than 1:10 000 is usually quoted) • An admission to hospital is mandatory
Sedation	• Sedation is usually given orally; the dose is calculated by the weight of the patient	• It is sometimes unsuccessful: various series have reported a 10–20% failure rate • Even when successful, the scan may have to be modified or curtailed because of patent movement or imminent 'wake-up' • There is a morbidity and mortality to the procedure, but problems are poorly reported and the real risks are not known • Only the age range 6 months to 18–24 months can be routinely sedated successfully • There is a long period of 'hang-over' after the scan and the child's stay in hospital may be protracted

history and examination alone without special investigation, but in the British adversarial system a case is much strengthened by a scan showing damage and an indication of the likely cause of that damage.

12.2 RADIOLOGY IN THE INVESTIGATION OF A CHILD WITH CEREBRAL PALSY

The brain is clearly a hugely complicated structure. The process of its formation and how that process of formation might go wrong were discussed in Chapter 7. Other chapters have dealt with the various insults that may disrupt the development of the brain. Radiological imaging is the demonstration of pathology in life. The role of radiology is to determine 'what sort' of injury has been sustained and, from a knowledge of topographical brain function, 'how might' this damage affect function and disability.

After a diagnosis of cerebral palsy is established on clinical grounds, radiology suggests the likely mechanism for the associated brain damage. Once the mechanism is known, more detailed investigation of the clinical history or special biochemical tests and genetic tests can be set in motion. Radio-

logy can be considered a sophisticated sorting process between the various diagnostic possibilities.

Radiology is not infallible. The adage, 'The easy cases are easy and the hard hard' is frequently demonstrated. Problems in interpreting scans include the fact that they vary in technical quality: they are performed on machines of different quality, age, and resolution. Further, they are performed on children of different ages, and structural lesions must be interpreted against a background of a brain which is constantly changing in the normal process of growth and development.

Scans are interpreted by radiologists, only some of whom have the necessary knowledge and expertise. The routine radiological report from a general radiologist in a district general hospital often cannot be relied upon. As an absolute minimum, the scans must be interpreted by a specialist neuroradiologist and preferably a neuroradiologist with a special interest in pediatrics.

Given that MRI is able to demonstrate pathology in life, it may demonstrate one or other of the following pathologies:

- Congenital brain malformations, failures of brain development
- Hypoglycemic damage

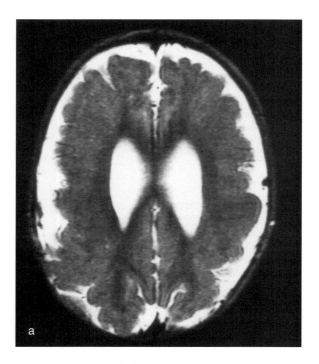
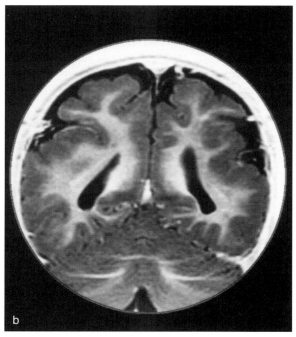

Figure 12.1 Lissencephaly. (a) Axial T2 shows a very abnormal cortical pattern with few gyral markings and a smooth, thickened, malformed cortex. The brain has failed to grow properly and there are large ventricles and extra-axial fluid spaces. (b) Coronal T2 (video-inverted) shows the abnormal cortex to better advantage. Note again the thickened, poorly gyrated cortex.

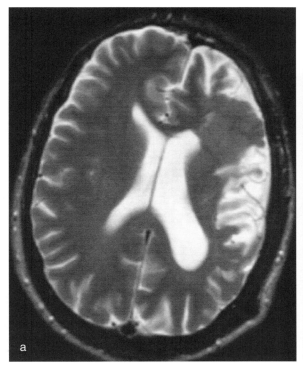
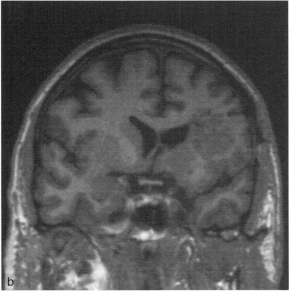

Figure 12.2 Cortical malformations. (a) Axial T2-weighted scan. Whilst the bulk of the brain is well formed, the left frontal region is obviously abnormal. There is a mass of chaotic and disorganized cortex and white matter in this region. (b) Coronal T1-weighted scan from a high-resolution SPGR (General Electric Medical Systems) sequence. Note the very thin superficial cortex and the mass of chaotic gray matter beneath it. It almost appears that the heterotopic mass is 'trying' to form cortical gyrae.

- White matter damage
- Periventricular leukomalacia (PVL)
- Multicystic leukoencephalomalacia (MCLE)
- Leukodystrophy
- Delayed myelination
- Germinal matrix hemorrhages
- Strokes
- Hypoxic-ischemic damage

12.2.1 Congenital brain malformations and failures of brain development

Chapter 7 has illustrated the process whereby the brain is formed. It is a hugely complex process which requires cells to divide, differentiate, migrate, and a proportion to die by a predetermined program to reveal the final structure of the brain. This process is genetically programmed and its events happen in a precisely controlled and specific order. Errors in the process will result in brain malformations. The subject is simply too large to illustrate comprehensively in this chapter, but the following have all been seen in cases labeled as cerebral palsy.

- Lissencephaly (smooth brain) (Fig. 12.1)
- Cortical malformations (Fig. 12.2)
- Migrational disorders such as nodular and laminar heterotopia (Fig. 12.3)
- Agenesis of certain structures, e.g. corpus callosum, inferior vermis of cerebellum (Fig. 12.4).

12.2.2 Hypoglycemic damage

Hypoglycemia is relatively common in the neonatal period, but it is rarely symptomatic. Features include jitteriness, which may progress to proper seizures. Even in symptomatic infants, it is uncommon for brain damage to occur. There are therefore few cases of brain damage following hypoglycemia in the literature.

The pathological literature indicates that the parietal and occipital cortex is the region of the brain most at risk from a hypoglycemic insult. Damage to the cortex will result in secondary atrophy of the associated white matter so that by the time the child is imaged the appearances are of focal cortical and subcortical white matter loss in the parieto-occipital region of the brain (Fig. 12.5).

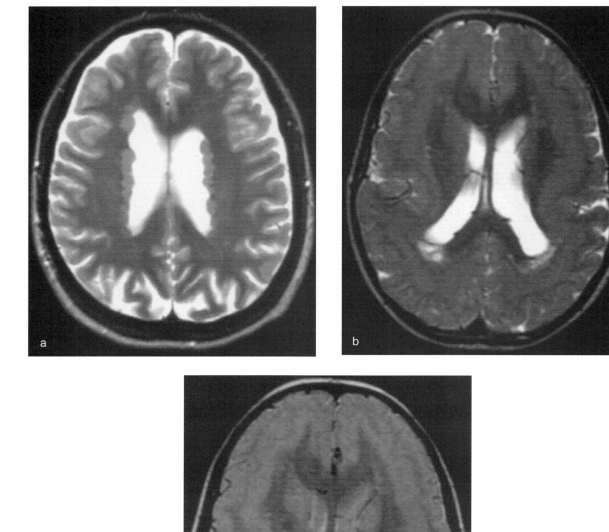

Figure 12.3 Migrational disorders (nodular and laminar heterotopia). (a) Nodular heterotopia. Axial T2-weighted scan shows small nodules of gray matter in the walls of the lateral ventricles. (b,c) Laminar heterotopia. Axial T2 and proton density scans. Note the thin superficial cortex and the much thicker layer of cortex deep to it. (Images courtesy of Dr Khalifa, Royal Berkshire Hospital.)

Very little is known about the effect of uncontrolled maternal diabetes on the brain of a baby. The author has several such cases which appear to be associated with PVL in the newborn child.

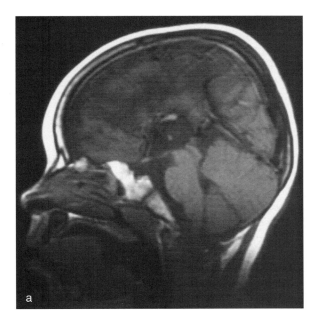
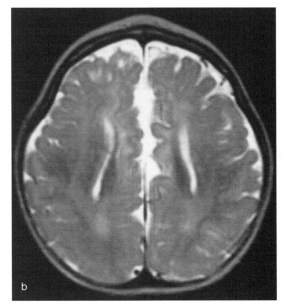
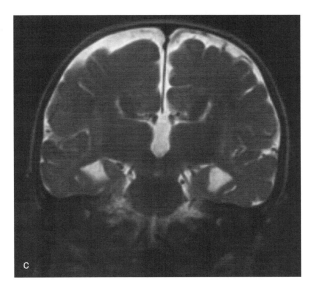

Figure 12.4 Agenesis of corpus callosum. (a) Midline sagittal T1-weighted scan reveals no corpus callosum in the midline. Note the prominent forniceal commissure. (b) Axial T2-weighted scan at the level of the lateral ventricles. Normally the ventricles meet in the midline, but instead they run parallel. Note the white matter tracts parallel to the ventricles (bundles of Probst). (c) Coronal proton density image shows the characteristic 'handlebar' shape of the lateral ventricles. Note the bundles of Probst once more, medial to the upturned lateral ventricles.

12.2.3   White matter damage

In this section, the following need to be considered:

- Periventricular leukomalacia
- Multicystic leukomalacia
- Leukodystrophy
- Delayed myelination.

12.2.3.1   *Periventricular leukomalacia (PVL)*

In the weeks surrounding the 32nd week of gestation, the periventricular white matter is undergoing active myelination and is metabolically highly active and therefore susceptible to injury whenever the supply of oxygen (brain perfusion)

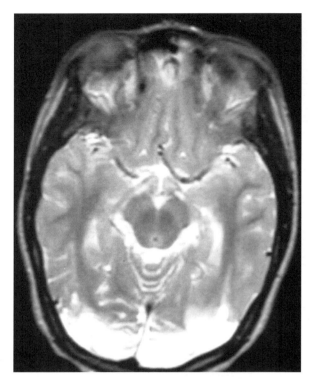

Figure 12.5 Hypoglycemic brain damage. Axial T2-weighted scan in a child who became severely hypoglycemic in the days after delivery. Note the damage to the occipital cortex and secondarily to the subcortical white matter.

is compromised. The causes of such compromise are discussed in Chapters 4 and 8.

Such an injury will result in characteristic changes on MRI scans, including white matter volume loss and abnormal high signal on T2-weighted scans.

The changes range from subtle to gross. The peritrigonal periventricular white matter is particularly susceptible and the fibers of the corticospinal tract are then frequently compromised. This explains the common clinical association of four-limb spasticity (spastic diplegia – legs affected more than arms) with PVL. In injuries inflicted before the 32nd week of gestation, volume loss predominates. After the 32nd week, white matter signal change is more obvious. This may be explained by the increasing reactivity of astrocytes in the infant brain in this critical period, with later injuries thought to be more prone to elicit an astrocytic response and leave a glial scar (Fig. 12.6).

12.2.3.2 Multicystic leukoencephalomalacia (MCLE)

This is a descriptive term for a condition where large areas of the brain are destroyed to leave numerous cystic cavities separated from one another by glial membranes.

MCLE is typically seen in the distribution of the carotid arteries and there is sparing of the posterior cerebral territory – the occipital cortex and inferior temporal lobe (Fig. 12.7).

12.2.3.3 Leukodystrophy

Dysmyelination refers to a process by which enzymatic deficiency or absence causes abnormal formation or increased breakdown of myelin. The pattern of abnormal myelination depends on the exact genetic defect involved. The subject is extremely complex and as biochemical understanding, genetics, and MR imaging develop, more and more disorders are being identified and properly studied.

12.2.3.4 Delayed myelination

It is helpful to think of myelination as the process by which the 'wiring' of the different regions of the brain is insulated to enable nerve impulses to pass rapidly and efficiently. Put a different way, without myelination, electrical impulses cannot be transmitted and the brain cannot function properly.

A newborn term infant can suck and cry, but do very little else. Myelin is seen in the brainstem and has started to appear in the white matter regions involved in motor function. By 2 years of life the toddler is walking, talking, feeding, and becoming increasingly determined. Myelination is virtually complete. The physical and mental development of the child in these first 2 years is almost exactly mirrored by the process of myelination in the brain.

Myelination delay is relatively common, but may be completely recoverable. If the white matter is damaged myelination may never occur, with consequent disability.

12.2.4 Germinal matrix hemorrhage

The walls of the ventricles are pivotal in the process of brain development. All the neurons which go to form the cortex are derived from this structure by a complex process of division and cell migration. In early brain development (8–20 weeks) it is hugely active and millions of cells are involved in cell division. This requires a large blood supply.

Germinal matrix hemorrhage is typically seen in premature infants while a large volume of germinal matrix persists. Diagnosis is usually made by

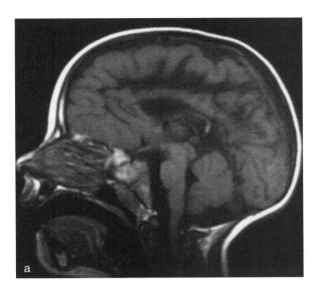

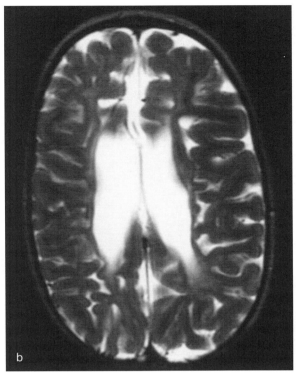

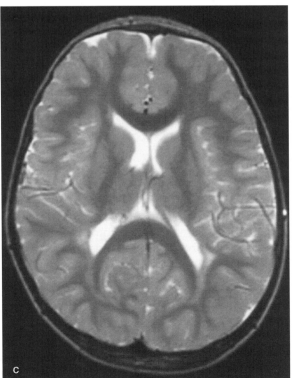

Figure 12.6 Periventricular leukomalacia. (a) Sagittal T1 shows a profoundly atrophic corpus callosum. (b) Axial T2 shows virtually no white matter with dilatation of the ventricles so that in places the undamaged cortex appears to indent the ventricular wall. (c) Axial T2 of a different case where the white matter loss is minimal, but there is more gliosis in the periventricular white matter. It is the author's view that lesions inflicted before the 32nd week tend to have little gliosis and more white matter loss, whereas later lesions have more gliosis and less white matter loss.

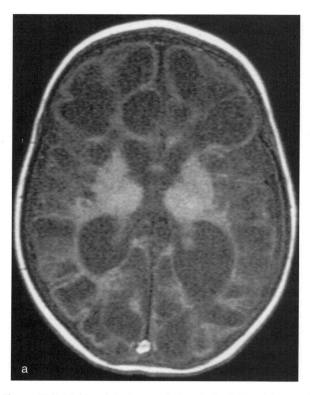 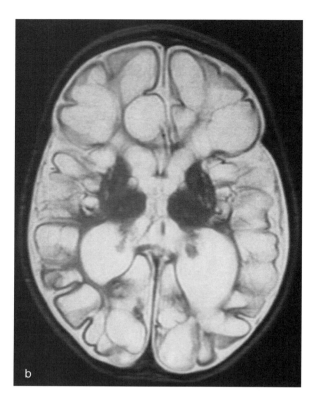

Figure 12.7 Multicystic leukoencephalomalacia. (a,b) Axial T1 and T2-weighted images. The whole of the brain has been replaced by countless cysts of varying size. Only the basal ganglia remain. The outline of the enlarged ventricles can just be appreciated.

ultrasound scans in the neonatal period. It can be graded from small hemorrhages confined to the ventricular wall to massive hemorrhages which rupture into the ventricular system.

Small hemorrhages can disappear without trace and prognosis is very good. Larger lesions associated with significant parenchymal damage have a much worse prognosis (Fig. 12.8).

12.2.5 Stroke

As in adults, children can sustain brain damage when a fragment of solid material (embolus) passes into the cerebral circulation and occludes a vessel. This results in death of the tissue supplied by the occluded vessel unless there is the rapid development of a collateral circulation.

The vessel most commonly involved in the fetus or neonate is the middle cerebral artery and the resulting infarct will involve variable amounts of the frontal, parietal, and temporal lobes. Very little is known about the source or nature of the embolic material. In adults the source is usually blood clot or fragments of atheroma from vascular degeneration. In fetuses, placental fragments may be a potential cause.

There is no doubt that infarcts may be spontaneous events occurring while the fetus is still in the uterus. More frequently strokes seem to occur at or about the time of placental separation. Fragments of tissue may pass into the umbilical vein to the heart, by-pass the lungs through the normal fetal intracardiac shunting and embolize to the brain.

Initially, such infarcts may be completely silent or they may give rise to transient focal seizure activity. Such seizures invariably involve the limb destined to become weak after the acute phase has passed. It is common for the motor consequences of such infarcts to gradually become more obvious with time as the motor system of the child develops and becomes more sophisticated (Fig. 12.9).

12.2.6 Hypoxic-ischemic injury

When a fetus is subjected to an hypoxic-ischemic event, three broad radiological patterns of damage emerge: PVL, basal ganglion damage, and watershed cortical infarction.

Chapters 4 and 8 detail different age-dependent patterns of damage and describe some of the mechanisms thought responsible for them. These mechanisms include:

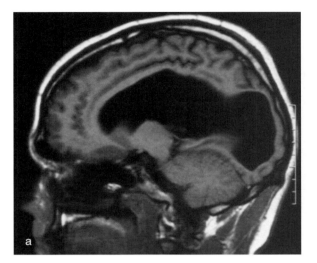
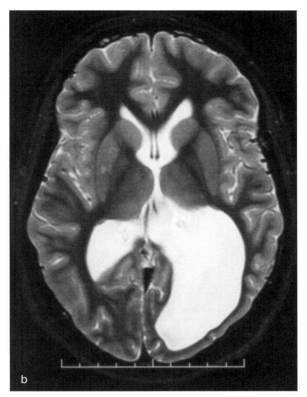
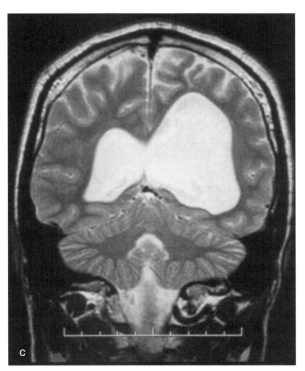

Figure 12.8 Germinal matrix hemorrhage. (a) Parasagittal T1 fluid attenuated inversion recovery (FLAIR) sequence shows hugely dilated left ventricle as the end-stage of changes following a germinal matrix hemorrhage in a premature infant. (b) Axial T2 STIR shows the dilated left ventricle, secondary to severe focal periventricular cerebral volume loss. It also shows some dilatation of the right ventricle. The patient has a coexistent mild degree of periventricular leukomalacia. (c) Coronal T2 demonstrating that the bulk of the cerebral volume loss is at the expense of the white matter.

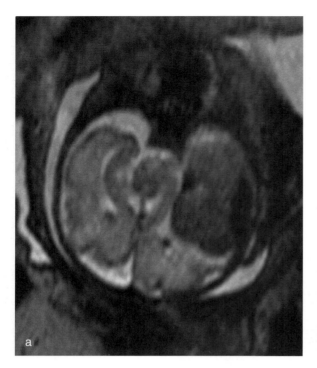 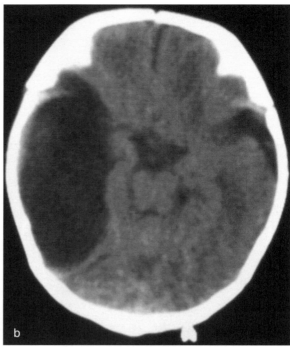

Figure 12.9 Stroke. (a) Axial T2-weighted scan of a fetus still in the uterus. An abnormality detected on ultrasound was shown to be of very low signal on T2, consistent with a subacute hematoma. After delivery, the child was subsequently shown to have a clotting disorder (alloimmune thrombocytopenia). (b) CT scan after birth shows a classical 'middle cerebral' pattern of infarction.

- The maturity of the fetus. An injury at 32 weeks is likely to result in PVL. At later stages of gestation, gray matter damage is more commonly seen.
- The oxygen demand of different tissues. Myelination is very energy dependent and those tissues actively myelinating at the time of insult are more susceptible to damage.
- The anatomy of cerebral perfusion. When perfusion starts to fail, the proximal fields of supply of vessels may contain sufficient blood to sustain brain tissue. More distal branches of the system may contain blood flowing below the critical rate to maintain tissue viability. This may lead to watershed infarction where areas of brain between the territories of supply of the main cerebral vessels are predominantly damaged.
- Neurotransmitter activity. Neurotransmitters are extremely potent chemicals which have an energy-dependent uptake system. When this uptake system is inactivated, unopposed activity can be lethal to cells.
- The nature of the hypoxic-ischemic insult. A short period of severe hypoxemia has a different effect on brain than a prolonged period of less severe hypoxemia.

PVL has been discussed earlier in this chapter. The radiographic findings of term hypoxemia fall into two groups which appear to be related to the nature of the insult:

1 Acute, severe hypoxic-ischemic injury
2 Chronic partial hypoxic-ischemic injury.

12.2.6.1   Acute, severe hypoxic-ischemic injury

In a classical case, an identifiable abrupt and catastrophic event occurs to disrupt the feto-maternal circulation. Examples include placental abruption, cord prolapse, and maternal circulatory collapse.

The fetus, immediately prior to the event, is well oxygenated and perfused. After the insult, carbon dioxide will accumulate within the tissues (hypercapnia). The fetus becomes hypoxic, hypercapnic, and acidotic. Despite this, no immediate cerebral damage will occur. However, at some point, the heart, which obviously has an oxygen demand of its own, starts to fail and at this point damage will start to occur due to the superimposed effect of hypotension and perfusion failure on hypoxia.

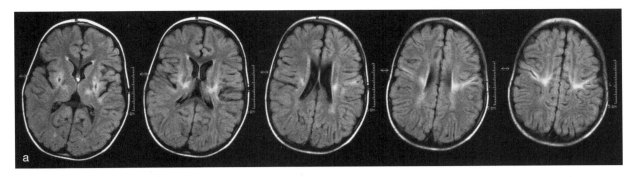

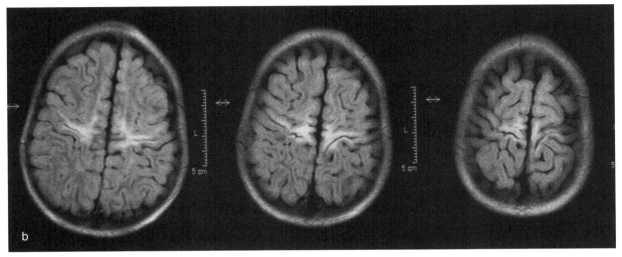

Figure 12.10 Basal ganglion damage. (a) FLAIR images are heavily T2-weighted, but CSF is dark. Lesions therefore stand out against a dark background. In acute severe cases of hypoxic-ischemic damage, the posterior putamen and the dorsal thalamus undergo (often hemorrhagic) infarction which years later is seen as a focal high signal lesion on T2-weighted scans. This is most marked in the left picture; the other images show the associated damage in the peri-Rolandic cortex and underlying white matter. (b) FLAIR scan of the same case through the upper part of the brain shows characteristic high signal change, probably gliosis, in the white matter of the posterior frontal lobe – the corticospinal tract.

Damage first falls to the basal ganglia – the posterior putamen and dorsal thalamus. Shortly after this, damage falls to the motor cortex, which is situated at the watershed of the middle and posterior cerebral vessels (Fig. 12.10).

Infants who survive damage to the basal ganglia may develop athetoid or dystonic cerebral palsy. If this is the only injury, intelligence may be preserved. If the cortex is involved, spasticity is dominant, but intellectual damage may also occur.

12.2.6.2 Chronic partial hypoxic-ischemic injury

In a classical case, there is an intermittent or incomplete disturbance of placental function. The same metabolic changes occur as in acute severe hypoxemia, but gradually over a much longer period. The cause of this sort of hypox-

emia is never as well defined. Intermittent cord compromise is frequently invoked, but rarely proven.

Hypoxia, hypercapnia, and acidosis develop over time, but the heart continues to pump and for a considerable period there is no over-arching perfusion failure. Re-distribution of blood occurs in favor of the posterior circulation, sparing the brainstem and cerebellum. The hallmarks of a chronic partial hypoxic-ischemic insult are:

- Damage to the motor cortex at the watershed between anterior, middle and posterior circulations.
- Ulegyria. In this condition, the crests of the gyrae are relatively preserved, the depths of the sulci are destroyed. This is frequently most easily visible at the edge of a region of more complete damage.

- White matter damage. White matter underneath or adjacent to the damaged cortex is involved in the destructive process.
- Diffuse brain damage. These children frequently develop microcephaly.

As a consequence of focal damage to the motor cortex, spasticity dominates. Such children are frequently also developmentally delayed and microcephalic (Fig. 12.11).

It is very important to stress that the above account refers to two highly stylized forms of hypoxic-ischemic damage. In a typical case, the events are rarely as clear-cut as those described. The infant may start the whole process with a dysfunctional placenta, be growth retarded and acidolic. In such a compromised fetus even minor adverse events during labor and delivery may precipitate damage. The only fetal parameter monitored more or less continuously in labor is the heart rate and this measures the heart rate and nothing else. Remarkably little is known about the compensatory and adaptive processes of the fetus to stress and distress during labor.

12.3   RADIOLOGICAL IMAGING AND THE MEDICOLEGAL PROCESS

How should MRI fit into the medicolegal investigation of a patient? The process of clinical diagnosis – history taking, examination, and special investigation – was set out at the start of this chapter. The medicolegal diagnostic process is similar but there are important differences. For successful preparation of a case, the following are required:

- An accurate statement of the disability of the child (see Statement of disability)
- An MRI scan to identify the lesions responsible for that condition (see Identification of the brain lesion)
- Examination of the clinical record to try to identify the events responsible for the MRI changes.

Note that this process produces a shift in the chain of evidence from 'clinical circumstances of the case causing clinical disability' to clinical circumstances of the case causing changes on the MRI scan which in turn are responsible for clinical disability.

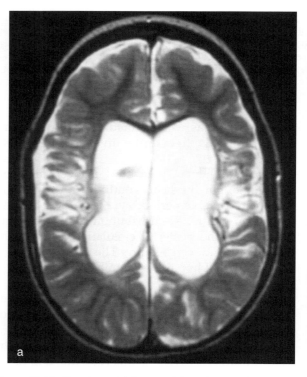 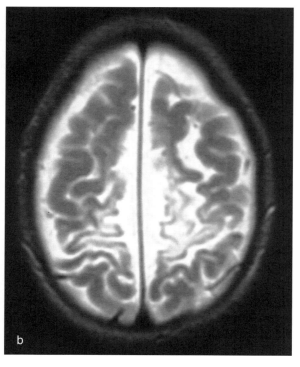

Figure 12.11 Chronic partial damage. (a) Axial T2-weighted scan in a chronic partial type of hypoxic-ischemic injury. Note the small skull and the small brain within it. Note also the extensive cortical damage, most marked in the insular cortex bilaterally. (b) Axial T2 at a higher level shows specific damage in the posterior frontal cortex and diffuse effect on the rest of the brain, which has failed to grow properly.

Inserting MRI evidence into this chain adds an important link. It demonstrates the anatomical substrate of the disability and confirms the timing and causation of the circumstances leading to disability.

12.3.1 Statement of disability

The court is asked to decide whether an individual child should receive damages for the disability suffered. The key word is disability and huge effort goes into assessing disability so that damages (assuming the case is successful) of an appropriate level can be awarded. The assessment of disability is ideally made by a specialist in pediatrics or pediatric neurology with experience in caring for children with handicaps. The assessment is described in detail in Chapter 1. Since the level of disability governs the quality of life achieved by the child and the level of damages awarded, it is proper to start radiological consideration of a medicolegal case by having a clear understanding of exactly what is wrong with the child. This should include:

* Motor function
* Intellectual performance
* Vision and hearing
* Organizational problems (dyspraxia)
* Epilepsy

These data are available in a 'condition and prognosis' report which is always obtained in a cerebral palsy case. Note that this report does not attempt to say 'why' a child is damaged or disabled. The report is simply to say in what way the child is unable to pursue normal activities and achieve normal skills.

12.3.2 Identification of the brain lesion – where, what, and when

The next step is to ask the questions, 'Where in the central nervous system is there a lesion responsible for these disabilities, what might that lesion be, and when did it occur?' From an understanding of anatomy and normal topographical brain function, a competent pediatric neurologist can frequently answer the 'where' question. If the child is blind, then clearly the lesion responsible for that blindness must lie within the visual pathway. Clinical and electrophysiological tests may determine where the lesion must lie with a great degree of precision.

The 'what' question is answered by detailed clinical history taking and radiological imaging. Most of the time there is concordance between these two options. A history is obtained of a difficult birth and of an hypoxic-ischemic encephalopathy. The scan shows evidence of hypoxic-ischemic damage in the brain. Occasionally, there is discordance and the quality of the two sorts of data has to be assessed. The huge value of imaging is that the location of the damage is strongly correlated to the disability from which the child suffers, whilst the morphology of the different destructive processes gives a very strong clue as to the cause of the underlying damage. In a complex case in a child with a very stormy neonatal course, it may allow separation of the actual cause of brain damage from a mass of potential causes (e.g. hypoglycemia, sepsis, renal failure, liver failure, etc.).

An MRI scan will identify the lesion responsible for disability in a majority of cases. Some disabilities will almost always have visible lesions on an MRI scan and others are very poorly correlated with imaging findings. In general it is those areas of brain function where there is a close topographical correlation with function which are easier to identify responsible lesions (Table 12.3).

In a medicolegal case, the issue of when the lesion occurred is of paramount importance. Radiology can be extremely helpful in timing brain injuries. Malformations due to early damage may be identified, and in some cases precise time periods for an injury specified. These are described in Chapter 7. In the second half of pregnancy timing is less precise but patterns of brain damage, characteristic of a particular developmental stage, may be recognized. These are not precise and show some overlap but the information gained from recognizing such patterns on scan can be extremely useful in conjunction with careful examination of the clinical record.

12.3.3 Examination of the clinical record

In a typical medicolegal case, the disability is known and set out in the condition and prognosis report. Further points of issue are the cause of that disability and, most importantly, the issue of when the damage responsible for that disability was sustained. MRI imaging is crucial to determining the site and often the cause of the damage.

In the life of a child from conception to present time, there is a 'window of liability' opened up by expert examination of the clinical record. For

Table 12.3 Correlation of disability with structural brain lesion

Disabilities strongly correlated with structural brain lesions	Motor problems – especially some specific subsets of cerebral palsy Spastic quadriplegia Spastic diplegia Hemiplegia Athetoid or dystonic cerebral palsy Defects in vision Focal epilepsy
Disabilities poorly correlated with structural brain lesions	Ataxic cerebral palsy Developmental delay and learning disability Behavior problems Generalized epilepsy

example, an obstetric expert may say that at a certain time in the labor, the standard of care offered by the midwifery and obstetric staff fell below an acceptable level – the window opens. At a later time, their behavior comes back to standard and the window closes. For a case to be successful, the damage to the brain must fall into the window of liability or, at the very least, a chain of events must be initiated within that period of time which results in unavoidable damage at a later stage.

The nature of the injury as demonstrated on scan is clearly of prime importance. If the damage seen on the scan is characteristic of an hypoxic-ischemic injury, then the clinical notes need to be examined to identify when an hypoxic-ischemic injury could have been inflicted. Similarly if the lesion on the scan is some sort of brain malformation which must have occurred in early gestational life, the clinical record needs to be examined for some injury to the mother and fetus at the appropriate gestational age. Examples may include an amniocentesis needlestick injury to the fetus or a maternal trauma such as a road traffic injury.

The radiology is rarely able to give an answer to the 'when' question with the required degree of precision in a medicolegal case. In the three classical patterns of hypoxic-ischemic damage, for example, the event responsible for the development of PVL can never be identified by examination of the scan. In 'chronic partial' hypoxic-ischemic injury, the radiology can say that the lesion occurred over a period of time – but it cannot say over what period and when in relation to the birth the injury occurred. In 'acute severe', the radiology may allow a very small window to be opened, but it is still the close examination of the clinical record which will allow precise delineation of the moment of injury. It follows that a radiological finding must be closely coupled to the clinical narrative if it is to be useful in a clinical negligence case.

12.4 CONCLUSION

This chapter has set out the role of radiology in cerebral palsy. MRI scans can be of assistance in both the clinical and the medicolegal understanding of a case. Such scans:

- Will identify the lesion responsible for disability in a majority of cases
- Will give specific clues as to the pathological cause of a lesion
- Will allow research into the epidemiology and causes of cerebral palsy
- May allow detection of inherited disorders and initiate counseling of parents.

It is a scandal that children with cerebral palsy are not properly investigated in the same way that children with other neurological disabilities are investigated.

13 Causation – legal proof

Michael J Powers

In cerebral palsy clinical negligence actions, proof of causation is usually more difficult than proof of breach of duty. Legal proof of causation has often presented difficulty and practical proof often has to over-ride philosophical argument. Issues of causation will continue to pervade litigation despite an effort to treat the whole issue as one of common sense.

13.1 FACT AND HYPOTHESIS

Whether or not an event happened in the past may or may not be capable of being decided. There is a process for this. Evidence is called before a Judge and, on the balance of probabilities – that is the prevailing weight of the evidence – the Judge will reach a conclusion as to whether or not that event happened. Once that decision has been made, it is treated in law as having been resolved. Effectively the doubt about whether or not the event happened thereafter becomes a matter of certainty. It did not happen or it did happen. For legal purposes, it becomes a matter of historical fact.

So too with such issues as to where and when that event occurred. These are determinable in the same way so as to become matters of certainty. Even when it comes to what caused the event to occur, sometimes this can be determined simply by a finding of fact as to what happened. Answering the question 'Whose elbow pushed the glass off the bar?', determines who caused the glass to break. This may be the only relevant issue (subject to any argument about state of mind) in such an example as the effect of gravity, the fragility of the glass, and the hardness of the floor are beyond question.

However, causation in medical cases is often very complex. The event may have been going to happen anyway. Indeed, it may, unknown to the prospective tortfeasor, already have happened. The insult giving rise to the cerebral palsy may have occurred in the antenatal period and have nothing to do with how well or poorly the labor was managed. The act or omission of a treating doctor may or may not have caused or contributed to the injury about which complaint is made. In order to reach a conclusion about the causation of injury it may be necessary to test the evidence with hypotheses. For example, in an attempt to determine whether or not the negligent failure to deliver the baby within, say, 15 minutes of a grossly abnormal cardiotocograph (CTG) , it may be helpful to answer the question what *would* have happened if the baby had been delivered within 15 minutes. As what *would* have happened cannot, *ex hypothesi*, be determined with certainty, this kind of 'fact' may be called *hypothetical fact*.

It is the proof of hypothetical fact that presents the philosophical and legal problems. Certainty in respect of any future event is beyond even the ingenuity of lawyers.

> When the question is whether a certain thing is or is not true – whether a certain event did or did not happen – then the court must decide one way or the other. There is no question of chance or probability. Either it did or it did not happen. But the standard of civil proof is a balance of probabilities. If the evidence shows a balance in favour of it having happened then it is proved that it did in fact happen. But here we are not and could not be seeking a decision either that the wife would or that she would not have returned to her husband. You can prove that a past event happened, but you cannot prove that a future event will happen and I do not think that the law is so foolish as to suppose that you can. All that you can do is to evaluate the chance.
> Per Lord Reid in *Davies* v. *Taylor* [1974] A.C. 207, 212–13

The absurdity of the balance of probability test in respect of the likelihood of some future event occurring is made clear in the argument of Lord Reid. By the time an action is brought for clinical negligence there has to be evidence of some injury having occurred. The timing of this injury may be difficult if not impossible. Nevertheless whatever its cause, it is clearly a past event. If the timing is relevant, as it is something which *has* happened, this has to be determined on the evidence on the balance of probabilities. On occasion this can lead to unfairness. However, causation in law is not closely tied to philosophical argument; on the contrary it is often more a matter of common sense and the issue of causation is often linked to the issue of responsibility:

> The courts have repeatedly said that the notion of 'causing' is one of common sense. So in Alphacell Ltd v Woodward [1972] 2 All ER 475 at 490, [1972] AC 824 at 847 Lord Salmon said:

> '…what or who has caused a certain event to occur is essentially a practical question of fact which can best be answered by ordinary common sense rather than by abstract metaphysical theory.'

> …More guidance is, I think, necessary. The first point to emphasise is that commonsense answers to questions of causation will differ according to the purpose for which the question is asked. Questions of causation often arise for the purpose of attributing responsibility to someone, for example, so as to blame him for something which has happened or to make him guilty of an offence or liable in damages. In such cases, the answer will depend upon the rule by which responsibility is being attributed.
> Per Lord Hoffmann, *Empress Car Co (Abertillery) Ltd* v. *National Rivers Authority* [1998] 1 All ER 481 at 486 (HL)

13.2   WHEN WAS THE DIE CAST?

Take as an example the case of a man who, not wearing protective eye goggles, gets a foreign body in his eye whilst hitting the metal head of a chisel with a steel hammer. In fact he has sustained a penetrating eye injury with a metal fragment. No proper examination is conducted when he attends the casualty department. There is no assessment of visual acuity and no X-ray. He is sent home with palliative treatment. The condition of his eye deteriorates. He is reviewed. The correct diagnosis is made and proper emergency treatment instituted. The sight in the eye is nevertheless lost. There are those who would say that had he been properly treated from the outset the sight in the eye would (probably) have been saved. However, other experts would say there are patients who would loose the sight in such an injured eye *even if* they had been properly treated throughout. How is the law to resolve this problem: undeniably there has been a breach of duty – but did it *cause* the loss of vision?

If the evidence adduced is sufficient to persuade the court that the die was cast at the moment the metal fragment entered the eye in the sense that the odds were more likely than not that the sight would be lost in that eye whatever the treatment, then the case falls into the *Hotson* v. *East Berkshire Area Health Authority* [1987] 3 WLR 232 category. To use this approach is not to depart from the principle that past events are determined conclusively on the balance of probabilities. The issue is: had some biological event happened (or had it happened to such an extent) before the breach of duty? Even if the answer can only be determined using epidemiological evidence, the answer has to be found – and on the balance of probabilities. If the odds were in favor of the sight being retained in the eye, given proper medical treatment, the patient/claimant will recover 100 percent for the loss of the eye and the hapless health authority has to compensate fully for a loss which might have occurred in any event. In such a situation the claimant stands to benefit (in financial terms) from the breach of duty. If the man sustained the injury at work, he might have an action against his employer for negligence or breach of statutory duty but the value of the claim would be reduced by any contributory negligence for, say, failure to wear the goggles which the employer had provided for the purpose. Against his employer he might only recover 50 percent of the value of the claim, whereas against the health authority he could win 100 percent.

This unfairness works in the opposite direction once the die is cast against any patient. If, *on the balance of probabilities*, the child would have had cerebral palsy in any event, it seems that no degree of seriousness of breach of duty on the part of the obstetrician will enable any claim against him or her to succeed in law.

In summary therefore, the first question to be asked is: 'Was the die cast *before* the alleged breach of duty?' If the answer on the basis of all the evidence is yes, that is an end to the matter. If the answer is no, then it is open to the claimant to prove that the alleged breach of duty *caused or materially contributed to* the injury and the claimant is in the position to recover 100 percent.

A solution to the apparent unfairness may lie in the re-emergence of the loss of a chance argument in a recent medical negligence case of Smith (see below). It may apply where the negligence is of omission. The reasoning was based upon the judgment of Stuart-Smith LJ in the Court of Appeal in a well-known solicitors' negligence case *Allied Maples* v. *Simmons & Simmons* [1995] 1 WLR 1602. At page 1610 he said:

(2) If the defendant's negligence consists of an omission, for example to provide proper equipment, given proper instructions or advice, causation depends, not upon a question of historical fact, but on the answer to the hypothetical question, what would the plaintiff have done if the equipment had been provided or the instruction or advice given? This can only be a matter of inference to be determined from all the circumstances. The plaintiff's own evidence that he would have acted to obtain the benefit or avoid

the risk, while important, may not be believed by the judge, especially if there is compelling evidence that he would not. In the ordinary way, where the action required of the plaintiff is clearly for his benefit, the court has little difficulty in concluding that he would have taken it .... Although the question is a hypothetical one, it is well established that the plaintiff must prove on balance of probability that he would have taken action to obtain the benefit or avoid the risk. But again, if he does establish that, there is no discount because the balance is only just tipped in his favour.

And at 1611 Stuart-Smith LJ continued:

(3) In many cases the plaintiff's loss depends on the hypothetical action of a third party, either in addition to action by the plaintiff, as in this case, or independently of it. In such a case, does the plaintiff have to prove on balance of probability, as Mr. Jackson submits, that the third party would have acted so as to confer the benefit or avoid the risk to the plaintiff, or can the plaintiff succeed provided he shows that he had a substantial chance rather than a speculative one, the evaluation of the substantial chance being a question of quantification of damages?

Although there is not a great deal of authority, and none in the Court of Appeal, relating to solicitors failing to give advice which is directly in point, I have no doubt that Mr. Jackson's submission is wrong and the second alternative is correct.

So it was that Andrew Smith J in *Smith* v. *NHS Litigation Authority* [2001] Lloyds Law Reports Medical 90 adopted this reasoning in a medical negligence action where it was alleged the claimant's injuries were caused by a failure to undertake a diagnostic test for congenital dysplasia of the hip (CDH) when she was 6 weeks old. The judge said:

The distinction between ascertaining actual facts on the balance of probability and consideration of 'a hypothetical state of facts' is illustrated by Judge v Huntingdon HA (1995) 6 Med LR 223. The Defendant failed to diagnose a cancerous lump in the Claimant's breast, and when it was later diagnosed she had a reduced expectation of life. The judge found that there had been negligence. The Claimant alleged that, had it been diagnosed promptly, earlier treatment would have meant that she had a better expectation of life. Accordingly, questions arose as to how far in fact the cancer had developed by the time that it should have been diagnosed, and what, in view of that, would have been the chances of her condition being amenable to treatment. The first question was one of actual fact and Mr R. Titheridge QC (sitting as a Deputy High Court Judge) determined on the balance of probabilities what the state of the cancer was when it should have been treated. The second question involved an assessment of what would have happened in an hypothetical situation and the judge assessed the chance of effective treatment. (at 101)

The Defendants submitted that the analysis in *Allied Maples* had no application in cases of clinical negligence, and that I should not apply its reasoning in this case. I do not accept that submission. I read the judgment of Stuart-Smith LJ as laying down principles of general application, and I can see no reason to adopt a difference approach because this case concerns a different category of professional negligence. (at 101)

In considering how the Defendant would have acted in the hypothetical situation, it is assumed that he would have acted in accordance with his obligations to the Claimant, but it is also assumed that he will not have gone beyond his duty.... Accordingly, it seems to me that if the six-week examination had not been done, the proper approach to the question what damage resulted therefrom would be to assume a properly competent, but not an unusually thorough or able, examination and then to assess the chance that this would have resulted in the Claimant not suffering the damage which, in the event, she has suffered. (at 102)

In most cerebral palsy cases the allegation is that the staff failed to act expeditiously – in other words negligence by omission. It is likely that this will lead to a development of the law in the area of a loss of a chance of a better outcome had there been no negligent delay. Proof of loss will be easier for a claimant although damages will be less.

13.3   PROOF OF HYPOTHETICAL FACT

In *Bolitho* v. *City and Hackney Health Authority* [1997] 3 WLR 381 a 2-year-old child suffered a car-

diac arrest, brain damage, and eventual death as a consequence of respiratory obstruction which would have been avoided by tracheal intubation. A doctor was negligent in not attending the child before the arrest. The question arose as to whether the negligence was causative of any damage as the doctor maintained that had she attended she would not have intubated the child in anticipation of total respiratory obstruction. So, it was said, any negligence in failing to attend would have made no difference to the care which the child received. In order to have succeeded, the claimant would have had to have shown that 'but for' the negligence the cardiac arrest would not have occurred. To do that it would have been necessary to prove that attendance would have led to intubation. In other words the claimant would have had to have proved that *if* the doctor had attended either she *would have* or *should have* intubated. Proof of *'would'* is factual but proof of *'should'* requires the Bolam principle to be satisfied. In other words, proof of *'should'* would require proof that for a doctor not to have intubated in those circumstances would itself have been negligent.

Where, as in the present case, a breach of a duty of care is proved or admitted, the burden still lies on the plaintiff to prove that such breach caused the injury suffered: <u>Bonnington Castings Ltd. v. Wardlaw [1956] A.C. 613; Wilsher v. Essex Area Health Authority [1988] A.C. 1074.</u> In all cases the primary question is one of fact: did the wrongful act cause the injury? But in cases where the breach of duty consists of an omission to do an act which ought to be done (e.g. the failure by a doctor to attend) that factual inquiry is, by definition, in the realms of hypothesis. The question is what would have happened if an event which by definition did not occur had occurred. In a case of non-attendance by a doctor, there may be cases in which there is a doubt as to which doctor would have attended if the duty had been fulfilled.... I adopt the analysis of Hobhouse LJ in <u>Joyce v. Merton, Sutton and Wandsworth Health Authority [1996] 7 Med. L.R. 1.</u> In commenting on the decision of the Court of Appeal in the present case, he said, at p. 20:

'Thus a plaintiff can discharge the burden of proof on causation by satisfying the court either that the relevant person would in fact have taken the requisite action (although she would not have been at fault if she had not) or that the proper discharge of the relevant person's duty towards the plaintiff required that she take that action. The former alternative calls for no explanation since it is simply the factual proof of the causative effect of the original fault. The latter is slightly more sophisticated: it involves the factual situation that the original fault did not itself cause the injury but that this was because there would have been some further fault on the part of the defendants; the plaintiff proves his case by proving that his injuries would have been avoided if proper care had continued to be taken.'

Per Lord Browne-Wilkinson at 1157–8

Let us look at a mother in labor whose CTG is evidencing signs of significant fetal distress. It is alleged that the medical staff should have both seen and acted on the trace by delivering the baby by emergency cesarean section. The defense is that it was not negligent for a doctor not to have seen the CTG at the time alleged and, even were that to be found to have been negligent, the doctor would not have acted on the trace at that time in any event. To succeed in a claim for cerebral palsy the claimant would have to prove:

1 the failure (of omission) of the doctor to attend and see the CTG trace at the relevant time was negligent;[1] and
2 had the doctor attended he or she either would (proof of usual practice – difficult) or should (Bolam/Bolitho) have interpreted the CTG as requiring immediate delivery of the baby; and
3 an immediate cesarean section would (or should) have been arranged; and
4 had the cesarean section been undertaken the delivery of the baby at such earlier time would have avoided the cerebral palsy.

13.4 THE 'BUT FOR' TEST AND MATERIAL CONTRIBUTION

The 'but for' test of causation is well established, usually easy to apply and, on occasion, hard on claimants. With single event injuries such as a fracture, an air embolism or a drug overdose, the issue of causation is fairly easily resolved by application of the test. But for the force applied would the bone have fractured? But for the volume of air adminis-

tered would the patient have died? But for the overdose would the patient's hair have fallen out?

However, in situations (such as pneumoconiosis, dermatitis, and intrauterine hypoxia/ischemia) where an accumulation of insults is necessary to produce the damage, some of which are innocent and some of which are culpable, it may be impossible to say that 'but for' the negligence the injury would not have occurred. Where it is impossible to separate out the injury caused by the negligent factors from the non-negligent, proof of material contribution to the injury is sufficient (*Bonnington Castings Ltd*. v. *Wardlaw* [1956] AC 613). Focus was placed on the issue of burden of proof where an employee contracted pneumoconiosis from two sources of silica dust, only one of which was 'guilty'. In resolving firmly that the responsibility lay with the claimant to prove his condition was caused by the 'guilty' dust, their Lordships lightened the burden by saying that proof of a material contribution was sufficient. Remarkably, the issue of apportionment was neither argued before the House of Lords nor considered in the speeches.

In many cases thereafter the apportionment issue was not given birth probably because of the difficulties of proof of the proportion. Where the negligent harm *could* be divided from the non-negligent harm, the defendant was only held responsible for negligent harm. In consequence, Defendant Health Authorities have been held responsible for the entire costs of supporting a child born with cerebral palsy where negligent management only *contributed* to the overall damage.

Recently there has been a significant shift in the legal position. In *Holtby* v. *Brigham & Cowan (Hull) Ltd* [2000] 3 All ER 421 (an asbestosis case where the claimant was negligently exposed to asbestos working with the defendants but only for 50 percent of his total exposure) the Court of Appeal upheld the trial Judge's conclusion that there should be an apportionment of the damages. The claimant's argument that proof of a material contribution was sufficient for him to recover 100 percent against the defendant was rejected and the trial Judge discounted the damages by 25 percent whilst recognizing the inability of using the mathematical approach.

In my judgment…the onus of proving causation is on the claimant; it does not shift to the defendant. He will be entitled to succeed if he can prove that the defendants' tortious conduct made a material contribution to his disability. But strictly speaking the defendant is liable only to the extent of that contribution. However if the point is never raised or argued by the defendant, the claimant will succeed in full as in *Bonnington* and *McGhee*. I agree with Judge Altman that strictly speaking the defendant does not need to plead that others were responsible in part. But at the same time I certainly think it is desirable and preferable that this should be done. Certainly the matter must be raised and dealt with in evidence, otherwise the defendant is at risk that he will be held liable for everything.... The question should be whether at the end of the day and on consideration of all the evidence, the claimant has proved that the defendant is responsible for the whole or a quantifiable part of his disability. The question of quantification may be difficult and the court only has to do the best it can using its common sense.

> Per Stuart-Smith LJ in *Holtby* v. *Brigham &
> Cowan (Hull) Ltd*

Where a defendant raises the defense that it is not responsible for the whole damage, the claimant can probably still overcome the risk of the judge making an apportionment if it can be successfully argued that the material contribution of the defendant was to the whole and cannot be divided. This, of course, is to be distinguished from the cases where there is a difficulty in the quantification of the division. Dissenting in *Holtby* v. *Brigham &
Cowan (Hull) Ltd*, Clark LJ said:

It is I think at least arguable on the basis of those decisions that in a case of this kind, where the claimant proves that two employers have made a material contribution to his condition, he is entitled to judgment in full against each, leaving them to contest issues of contribution between them. That would certainly be the case where the injury was truly indivisible, so that each made a material contribution to the same damage, as in a case of damage caused by, say, a collision. However, in this class of case, as Longmore J observed, the injury or disease is not truly indivisible, but is contributed to by sequential exposure to asbestos which aggravates the condition. In these circumstances, as Mustill J said in similar circumstances (albeit with regard to deafness) in *Thompson v Smiths Shiprepairers (North Shields) Ltd [1984] QB 405* (at page 443D), in the first passage quoted by Stuart-Smith LJ:

'The defendants as well as the plaintiffs are entitled to a just result. If we know – and we do know, for by the end of the case it was no longer seriously in dispute – that a substantial part of the impairment took place before the defendants were in breach, why in fairness should they be made to pay for it? The fact that precise quantification is not impossible should not alter the position.'

In my opinion that approach applies to this class of case.

All this makes the claimant's task more difficult. When the claimant has proven both that the standard of obstetric care fell below the acceptable minimum and further that that failure made a material contribution to the asphyxia and hypoxic ischemia suffered by the baby *in utero* and the child's subsequent development of cerebral palsy, why in fairness should the burden still be on the claimant to prove the *size* of the proportion of that damage simply because the Health Authority shouts 'But not all!'? This was recognized by Clarke LJ a little later in his judgment:

It seems to me that Longmore J's view is the more consistent with the approach in the cases. If the position were that the claimant cannot, as a matter of law, recover anything more than the contribution which the defendant has tortiously made to his disease, it does seem to me to be surprising that none of their Lordships mentioned the point in either *Bonningtons* or *Nicholson*. That seems to me to be so even though (as appears to have been the case) the point was not raised by counsel. Moreover, Mustill J's approach in *Thompson* also seems to me to be consistent with the conclusion that the burden of proof in this regard (whether classified as the legal burden or the evidential burden) is on the defendant. In the passage quoted above, he spoke in terms of what was known at the end of the trial and he said (at page 443H-444A), in the last part of the passage quoted by Stuart-Smith LJ:

'What justice does demand, to my mind, is that the court should make the best estimate which it can, in the light of the evidence, making the fullest allowances in favour of the plaintiffs for the uncertainties known to be involved in the apportionment. In the end, notwithstanding all the care lavished on it by the scientists and by counsel I believe that this has to be regarded as a jury question, and I propose to approach it as such.'

It seems to me that it would not be appropriate to make 'the fullest allowances in favour of the plaintiffs' if the burden of establishing the apportionment were on them and not on the defendants.

I do not share the view that justice demands that the burden on this question should be on the claimant. It seems to me that once the claimant has shown that the defendants' breach of duty has made a material contribution to his disease, justice requires that he should be entitled to recover in full from those defendants unless they show the extent to which some other factor, whether it be 'innocent' dust or tortious dust caused by others, also contributed. It follows that I regard the part of the judgment of the Fifth Circuit of the United States Court of Appeals in *Borel v Fibreboard Paper Products Corp (1973) 493 F2d 1076* at 1095 as expressing a just result and not an unjust result.

Just as the burden is on a negligent defendant to prove contributory negligence, so the burden should be on a negligent defendant who has contributed to the claimant's disease to show that others have also contributed and to what extent. I do not think that it matters in this regard whether such a burden is classified as a legal burden of proof or an evidential burden, the result will be the same and, in either event, in my opinion defendants must plead the point if they wish to rely upon it.

The case of *Allen & Others* v. *British Rail Engineering Ltd & Anr (CA)* 23rd February 2001 involved a claim for damages for vibration white finger (VWF). It was accepted that even if his employer had not been negligent the claimant would have carried on doing the work but he would have done less of it and been less damaged. The trial judge reduced the total award by 50 percent to take account of this. VWF is a progressive and dose-related condition. Nevertheless a similar argument was raised on behalf of the claimant to that in *Holtby* v. *Brigham & Cowan (Hull) Ltd*, namely that a material contribution from the defendant's breach is sufficient for the claimant to recover 100 percent. However, reliance was placed by the Court of Appeal upon what Mustill J had said in

Thompson v. *Smiths Ship Repairers (North Shields) Ltd* [1984] Q.B. 405 at 443:

The defendants as well as the plaintiffs are entitled to a just result. If we know…that a substantial part of the impairment took place before the defendants were in breach, why in fairness should they be made to pay for it? The fact that precise quantification is impossible should not alter the position…. Thus, whatever the position might be if the Court were to find itself unable to make any findings at all on the issue of causation and was accordingly being faced with a choice between awarding for the defendants in full, or for the plaintiff in full, or on some wholly arbitrary basis such as an award of 50%, I see no reason why the present impossibility of making a precise apportionment of impairment and disability in terms of time, should in justice lead to the result that the defendants are adjudged liable to pay in full, when it is known that only part of the damage was their fault. What justice does demand, to my mind, is that the Court should make the best estimate which it can, in the light of the evidence, making the fullest allowance in favour of the plaintiffs for the uncertainties known to be involved in any apportionment. In the end, notwithstanding all the care lavished on it by the scientists and by counsel I believe that it has to be regarded as a jury question, and I propose to approach it as such.

Shiemann LJ, delivering the judgment of the court in *Allen & Others* v. *British Rail Engineering Ltd & Anr (CA)*, drew five propositions from the present law on this point, the first concerned with liability and the others with quantifying the damages:

(i) The employee will establish liability if he can prove that the employer's tortious conduct made a material contribution to the employee's disability.

(ii) There can be cases where the state of the evidence is such that it is just to recognise each of two separate tortfeasors as having caused the whole of the damage of which the claimant complains; for instance where a passenger is killed as the result of a head on collision between two cars each of which was negligently driven and in one of which he was sitting.

(iii) However in principle the amount of the employer's liability will be limited to the extent of the contribution which his tortious conduct made to the employee's disability.

(iv) The court must do the best it can on the evidence to make the apportionment and should not be astute to deny the claimant relief on the basis that he cannot establish with demonstrable accuracy precisely what proportion of his injury is attributable to the defendant's tortious conduct.

(v) The amount of evidence which should be called to enable a judge to make a just apportionment must be proportionate to the amount at stake and the uncertainties which are inherent in making any award of damages for personal injury.

Whilst to date there has been no reported cerebral palsy case where the apportionment (along the lines of *Holtby* v. *Brigham & Cowan (Hull) Ltd* and *Allen & Others* v. *British Rail Engineering Ltd & Anr (CA))* approach has been used, this will doubtlessly be seen in future. A number of cases have failed because claimant's have not satisfied the court that a negligent period of just a few minutes made a material difference. This may be because of the perceived unfairness on a defendant where it is obliged under the *Bonnington Castings Ltd.* v. *Wardlaw* principle to pick up the whole tab for a significant injury which may have happened in any event. Now, a court may be less reluctant to find a material contribution if a substantial discount from the full value of the claim can be made.

13.5   EXPERTS

No matter how refined and esoteric the legal arguments, without the input of expert evidence from specialists who are willing to devote some of their time to the complexities of causation issues, the claims could not be fought or defended. So much turns upon the experts' careful attention to the facts and their knowledge of the literature. They have to be prepared to discuss and justify in great detail the views they express. Many experts are for one reason or another not prepared to suffer close scrutiny of their views. This is one of the principal reasons for cases going all the way to trial and then

failing. Being an expert requires training in the legal approach and relevant legal principles but it is the one course which should not lead to a career.

13.6   THE SCIENTIFIC APPROACH

Studies of the causes of cerebral palsy (largely, we lawyers suspect, spurred on by claims for compensation in every case on the simplistic approach cerebral palsy = birth asphyxia = obstetric negligence) show only a small proportion in the region of 8–15 percent to be associated with perinatal events. Assuming these figures to be correct, one might be tempted to say *in each case* that on the balance of probabilities the cerebral palsy was caused by an antenatal event – usually unknown. This would be an unacceptable approach as in no cerebral palsy case could any claimant succeed.

13.7   EPIDEMIOLOGY AND THE LAW

Epidemiological evidence seeks to show a causal relationship between birth asphyxia and cerebral palsy but this type of evidence does not of itself identify in which individual cases there is a causal relationship. Nevertheless at the generic level, especially in the large pharmaceutical cases where it is alleged drugs have caused injuries which are recognized as having other known and unknown causes, epidemiological evidence is of enormous importance.

Without educated and informed scrutiny, lawyers as well as doctors are apt to fall into the fallacy of *post hoc ergo propter hoc*. As Dr Johnson put it, 'It is incident to physicians...to mistake subsequence for consequence'.[2] In *Shrinking history (on Freud and the failure of pyschohistory)*, David E. Stannard[3] illustrated an extension of the absurdity of drawing conclusions on causation from simple associations:

Not only do Freud, Erikson, and others of much lesser eminence and talent violate basic rules of evidence by inventing numerous facts crucial to their arguments, but in their most common method of doing so they breach one of the most fundamental principles of logic. *Post hoc, ergo propter hoc* describes the error built on the assumption that if event B followed event A, then B must have happened because of A. This is a common enough mistake in all historical writing, but since Freud it has been given a dizzying new twist: it is now apparently no longer necessary to historically establish the existence of A. So long as B is found to exist, it is assumed that A must have happened since B is a psychoanalytically posited consequence of A. Once having ascertained, then (by means of conjecture), the alleged existence of A, the cause of B's existence is made clear: it exists because of A – even though there may be not a shred of real evidence that A ever existed.

The purpose of the statistical approach to causation is to introduce scientific logic and analysis into the evaluation of whether an association (which is often temporal) is in fact causal. First the element of chance has to be removed by the mathematic analysis of the incidence of the effect. Mathematic confidence is expressed in terms as to the likelihood of an association being caused by chance. Sir Ronald Fisher FRS proposed the 0.05 (5 percent) level as an arbitrary divide. If it could be said that it was less than 5 percent likely that the association occurred by chance, the association was deemed to be 'statistically significant'. This is not the same as saying the association is real. Explanations other than chance have to be considered, such as bias in the selection of cases and confounding unidentified further variables. If chance, bias and confounding could be excluded, the association would be causal but this level of perfection can never be achieved.

Having done the best with analysis of the data, support for a causal link is to be gained by satisfying other tests. Usually nine criteria of Sir Austin Bradford Hill[4] or the five of the US Surgeon General:[5] the consistency, the strength, the specificity, the temporal relationship, and the coherence of the association.

There is a risk that a primip with a full-term normal vertex delivery will result in a child with cerebral palsy (absolute risk). In a vaginal twin delivery the after-coming twin faces a higher absolute risk of suffering from cerebral palsy. Comparison of these two risks produces the relative risk (RR) of cerebral palsy for the two children. In this instance the RR would be >1. In what circumstances could a court find that cerebral palsy in the after-coming twin was caused by being in that situation as opposed to what might have happened even if the child had been a singleton cephalic presentation?

In an oral contraceptive case (*Vadera* v. *Shaw* 22 November 1996, unreported), Alliot J relied upon the ratio of relative risks to make a finding on the balance of probabilities that there was no causation:

> …the odds ratio or relative risk…does not in any event exceed the figure of 2, the figure beyond which it would have to go before it could be said that there is more chance than not that an individual picked from the sample had suffered a stroke by reason of the oral contraceptive taken. Having considered the evidence…on the balance of probabilities I am not able to find that the plaintiff sustained her stroke by reason of the oral contraceptive prescribed for her.

Although lawyers are keen to get science into causation, save for the developments I have referred to above, the burden of proof remains with the claimant and it is discharged on the balance of probability. Undoubtedly there will be further development of this link between scientific proof and legal proof in the area of generic causation.

13.8   NOTES AND REFERENCES

1 On the Bolam principle as modified by the second limb of *Bolitho* v. *City and Hackney Health Authority* (namely that it is not sufficient to show that a responsible body of medical practitioners would have acted as the defendant did where such action/inaction cannot withstand reasoned analysis).
2 Dr Johnson. *Review of Dr Lucas's essays on Waters*. 1734.
3 Stannard DE. *Shrinking history (on Freud and the failure of pyschohistory)*. Oxford: Oxford University Press, 1980.
4 Hill AB. The environment and disease: association or causation? *Proceedings of the Royal Society of Medicine* 1965; **58**: 295–300.
5 US Surgeon General Report 1982.

Index

Notes: Figures in the text are denoted by page numbers in italics, those in the colour plate section are denoted as Plate.